AF385716

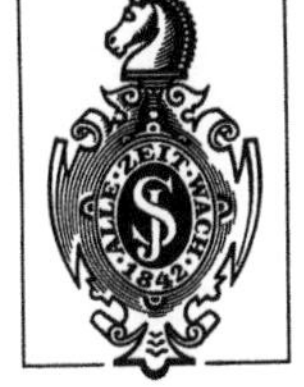

Takeo Nagayo

Histogenesis and Precursors of
Human Gastric Cancer

Research and Practice

With 188 Figures and 45 Tables

Springer-Verlag
Berlin Heidelberg New York Tokyo

Takeo Nagayo

Aichi Cancer Center
Research Institute
81–1159 Kanokoden, Tashiro-Cho
Chikusa-Ku, Nagoya 464
Japan

Library of Congress Cataloging in Publication Data.
Nagayo, Takeo, Histogenesis and precursors of human gastric cancer.
Includes index. 1. Stomach--Cancer. 2. Precancerous conditions. 3. Histology, Pathological.
I. Title. [DNLM: 1. Precancerous Conditions. 2. Stomach Neoplasms--pathology. WI 320 N1 52h]
RC280.S8N34 1986   616.99'433071   85-27792
ISBN-13: 978-3-642-70363-8   e-ISBN:13 978-3-642-70361-4
DOI:10.1007/978-3-642-70361-4

Typesetting, printing and bookbinding: Appl, Wemding
2123/3145-543210

Preface

In the summer of 1952, Dr. Fukuzo Ohshima, Professor of Pathology at the School of Medicine of Nagoya University, advised me to
perform histological examinations of stomachs surgically resected at
Yokoyama Hospital for Gastrointestinal Disease. The main purpose
of these examinations was to establish the pathological and histological nature of human peptic ulcers as against that of the experimental
gastric ulcers we were then trying to induce in rabbits by ligation of
all the gastric arteries.

During the histological examination of individual resected stomachs – almost all of which were affected by peptic ulcer or gastric
cancer – some cases with unusual concomitant mucosal changes
apart from the main lesions were encountered. The atypical epithelial
features of the lesions were quite suggestive of adenocarcinoma, but
owing to lack of knowledge and experience, I asked several col-
leagues to help me with diagnosis of the histological specimens; un-
fortunately no satisfactory answers were achieved.

In the library, I had examined several papers on the histopathology
of early gastric cancer, but to my great regret I was not acquainted at
that time with the brilliant articles already published by Konjetzny,
Gutmann, Bertrand, and Stout et al. One day I chanced upon a case
report entitled "So-called Mucosal Cancer of the Stomach" [Ayabe M
(1949) Rinshō to Kenkyu (Clinic and Research) 26: 514–526].

The close similarity of the macroscopical and histological changes
in the case in this report with those I myself had observerd led me to
make a definitive diagnosis of intramucosal cancer of the stomach,
and the article also led into further literatures on this subject. After
this, my major interest was devoted to the search for superficial cancerous change in the resected stomachs, and all the changes recognizable by naked-eye examination were examined histologically with
great care; records were kept of all the histological findings, including schematic drawings of the lesions.

Arount 1955, most early cancerous changes were found unexpectedly in the mucosa around chronic gastric ulcers diagnosed as such
after X-ray examination and, after resection of the stomach also
macroscopically as nonmalignant chronic peptic ulcers. These observations led me to the opinion that in most cases early gastric cancers
were preceded by chronic gastric ulcer.

V

Thereafter, however, the frequency with which malignant change was detected around ulcers declined over time, in keeping with the remarkable decrease in the number of chronic or callotic peptic ulcers in resected stomachs. Conversely, with the introduction of new diagnostic methods – double-contrast X-ray and fibergastroscopy – into clinical practice in the 1960s, cases with superficial cancerous erosion accompanied by secondary peptic ulceration within the eroded lesion gradually increased in frequency.

These observations and studies were followed by severe criticism of reports on early gastric cancer in which histological evidence of the ulcer-cancer sequence was claimed. I myself also had to reexamine these cases from the viewpoint of possible secondary ulceration of cancerous erosion. These reexaminations confirmed beyond all doubt that, unlike the healthy stomach, gastric mucosa affected by cancerous erosion is quite prone to ulceration as a result of the action of acidic gastric juice: In some cases the diagnosis of ulcer cancer had to be revised since there was after all no concrete evidence of the ulcer-cancer sequence, while others still did fulfill the macroscopical and histological criteria for this sequence. From our present standpoint it can be said that the relative frequency of early gastric cancers preceded by or followed by peptic ulcer is due mainly to the social and medical environments during the period under scrutiny.

The intimate correlation between histological features of gastric cancer and grade of intestinal metaplasia of the cancer-bearing gastric mucosa, which had also long been a subject of vigorous discussion, became clearer following histological studies on intramucosal cancer, especially of microscopic in size. Borderline lesions intermediate between benign and malignant were found during the examinations. The findings in the presence of precancerous change of the stomach and the ways in which it was different from the incipient state of gastric cancer became more recognizable when atypical, dysplastic lesions were examined for comparison. The transition in macroscopical appearance from early to advanced gastric cancer has also been clarified by studies of intermediate-stage cancers.

In the past 30 years gastric cancer has been diagnosed in over 5000 of the resected stomachs subjected to histological examination at this hospital. In recent years I have reached the stage in my life's work as a pathologist of summarizing my studies of gastric cancer, especially of its morphogenesis, and trying to put this knowledge into perspective and apply it as a basis of guidance and criticism for use by a wide range of investigators, not only pathologists, but also radiologists, endoscopists, surgeons, and physicians practicing in this field.

Publication of this monograph could not have been realized without long-term collaboration with Dr. HIDEKICHI YOKOYAMA and several members of the staff in his hospital. It is also certain that this book could not have been published without a great deal of support from the doctors, technicians, and secretaries at Nagoya City Uni-

VI

versity, Department of Pathology and at Aichi Cancer Center Research Institute and Hospital.

I would like to express my sincere thanks to those who have given me so much support, in particular: H. YOKOYAMA, Y. YOKOYAMA, I. YOKOYAMA, T. KOMAGOE, K. KUBOTA, K. YAMASHIRO, K. HANAWA, K. KONDO, H. SUZUKI, E. YAMADA, T. KASUGAI, T. SUCHI, T. KITO, S. KOBAYASHI, and T. SATO (doctors); H. TANASE, Y. KOBAYASHI, J. KIYONO, Y. MIGITAKA, H. MINAMIKAWA, H. KITO, and N. TERASHIMA (technicians); and K. SHINNOBU, K. SUGIYAMA, Y. NAKAMURA, and K. HORI, Y. HAYASHI (secretaries).

My sincere thanks are also due to Dr. A. JOHANSEN (Bispebjerg Hospital, Copenhagen), whose monograph was a great help to me, and to Dr. T. READ (Repatriation General Hospital, Australia), who corrected my manuscript.

Chikusa-Ku Nagoya, March 1986   Takeo Nagayo

Table of Contents

1. History of Pathological Studies

The history of pathological and histological studies on human gastric cancer has to be traced back to about 150 years ago, when the idea of "cellular pathology" proposed later by R. Virchow was not yet established. The studies performed by the pioneers in this field were of various kinds, and the conclusions they yielded concerning the pathogenesis of gastric cancer were immature, uncertain, and sometimes erroneous from our present viewpoint. Nevertheless, we should bear in mind that without such pioneering studies our present knowledge of the histology and histogenesis of gastric cancer could not have been obtained. In this chapter, I will attempt a brief chronological review of the classic work on pathology carried out by the pioneers (Table 1).

In 1829, CRUVEILHIER [9] cited observations of gastric cancer preceded by chronic peptic ulcer, which were later a recurrent topic of discussion among clinicians and pathologists for more than 100 years.

BRINTON [5] in 1859 reported a specific type of gastric cancer having the following three characteristics;

a) small stomach;
b) diffuse thickening of the gastric wall;
c) narrowing of the gastric cavity.

He named this change "linitis plastica," as he thought it resulted from inflammation.

After several animal experiments, in 1881 BILLROTH and his coworkers succeeded for the first time in performing surgical resection of pyloric cancer in a 43-year-old female patient. Even though successful results did not become very frequent until the end of the nineteenth century, BILLROTH's original methods are still useful in present-day surgery, and they greatly enhanced the knowledge of surgical pathology in this field. He himself did not publish any original papers, but his procedure was reported in detail by his coworker WÖLFLER [42].

In the same year, KUPFFER [26] mentioned intestinal epithelium in gastric mucosa. He described goblet cells and was of the opinion that any epithelial cells in the gastric mucosa might become goblet cells.

In 1883, HAUSER [19] reported on the development of gastric cancer from the mucosa around chronic peptic ulcer and proposed histological criteria for "ulcer cancer." He also stressed this possibility on subsequent occasions [16–18].

BIZZOZERO [3] studied the histology of gastric mucosa and named it "elementi labili" in 1888. The name indicated that the mucosa maintained a state of dynamic equilibrium. His study attracted no great attention at that time, but was certain-

Table 1. Summarized history of pathological studies on gastric carcinoma

1829	J. Cruveilher	Pointed out the presence of *Ulcus-carcinoma*
1859	W. Brinton	Described "Linitis plastica"
1881	A. Wölfler	Reported first success of surgical resection of gastric cancer by Billroth's method
1883	G. Hauser	Described histological criteria of *Ulcuskrebs*
1888	G. Bizzozero	Cited *elementi labili* of gastric mucosa
1894	G. Hauser	Described *Histogenese des Magenkrebses*
1896	A. Schmidt	Described intestinal metaplasia of gastric mucosa
1903	M. Versé	Described *Schleimhautkarzinom*
1905	K. Yamagiwa	Cited development of carcinoma from edge of gastric ulcer
1909	L. Aschoff	Supported the theory of *Ulcuskrebs*
1909	M. Versé	Cited the possibility of secondary ulceration of gastric cancer
1912	F. Stromyer	Same as above
1913	F. Saltzman	Cited gastric cancer not preceded by ulcer or polyp
1913	G. E. Konjetzny	Pointed out the importance of chronic gastritis as a precursor of gastric cancer
1926	M. J. Stewart	Described severe criteria for "ulcer-cancer"
1926	R. Borrmann	Proposed criteria for macroscopical classification of gastric cancer
1931	H. Hamperl	Stressed the importance of *Umbau* in development of gastric cancer
1933	R. A. Gutmann	Reported on 15 cases of early gastric cancer including eroded type
1936	J. Ewing	Stressed the importance of "superficial carcinoma"
1940	T. B. Mallory	Same as above
1942	A. P. Stout	Reported on 15 cases of "superficial spreading type" of gastric cancer

ly a real forerunner in cell kinetics of the gastric mucosa from the aspect of the present study.

After the first report by KUPFFER, SCHMIDT [32] in 1896 described intestinal epithelial cells in gastric mucosa and came to the conclusion that these epithelial cells resulted from a metaplastic process following the degeneration of normal gastric mucosa.

In 1903, VERSÉ [40] reported seven cases of mucosal or submucosal gastric cancer from his large autopsy material. He was of the opinion that secondary ulceration of cancerous lesions could not be denied even in that state. He also referred to the development of gastric cancer from polyposis ventriculi [38, 39].

In 1905, YAMAGIWA [43] published a monograph entitled Theory on the Development of Gastric Carcinoma, in which he came to the conclusion that the development of gastric cancer resulted from the birth of "new altered cells" (HAUSER) or of "anaplastic cells" (HANSEMAN) and that these cells grow slowly in gastric mucosa. He also mentioned that the origin of gastric cancer is not necessarily unifocal. The book was written only in Japanese and did not became so widely known as his brilliant animal experiments later did.

In 1909, Aschoff [1] published the second edition of his textbook, and in this book he described the histogenesis of gastric cancer: "Malignant transformation of gastric mucosae can occur from chronic round ulcer, ulcer scar or glandular polyp, even though the etiology of this disease is not known."

Stromeyer [37] reported in 1912, on the basis of his extensive work, that ulcerated cancers were more common than ulcer cancer. Like Versé's, his opinion called Hauser's theory into question.

Konjetzny [24] reported in 1913 that there were some types of gastric cancer which were not related morphologically to gastric ulcer or gastric polyp. The same conclusion was also reached by Saltzman [31] in the same year. Later on, Konjetzny described and illustrated this type of gastric cancer in great detail in Henke-Lubarsch's textbook [24] and in his monograph [23]. He stressed in this book and in other publications [23–25] that this type of cancer might result from or be preceded by chronic gastritis.

A macroscopical classification of advanced gastric cancer was proposed in 1926 by Borrmann [4]. On the basis of gross appearance, he classified the cancer into four main types. His original classification has since been used by many investigators, with or without modification.

In 1926, Stewart [33], who had strict criteria for ulcer cancer, calculated its frequency in cases of preexisting chronic gastric ulcer as 9.5%. Similar results (6%–14%) were also reported by Orator [29] and Büchner [6]. Later on, Büchner [7] stressed that repeated destruction and regeneration of the glandular epithelia not only at the margin of chronic peptic ulcer but also in chronic *Umbaugastritis* leading to faulty regeneration, might be the cause of gastric cancer.

Hamperl [15], in 1931, stressed the significance of the histological changes in gastric mucosa called *Umbau* (modified structure) for the development of gastric cancer. From his description, it seemed that *Umbau* of the gastric mucosa resulted from faulty cellular differentiation following damage to the mucosa or from the process of physiological cell renewal.

Among 154 cases of simple chronic gastric ulcer, Newcomb [28] in 1932 found six cases fulfilling his criteria for ulcer cancer. He also observed "quite atypical and proliferated epithelia suspicious of malignancy" in the margin of the ulcer.

From 1933 to 1939 Gutmann [14], Bertrand [2], Gutmann and Bertrand [13], and Gutmann et al. [12] reported 15 cases of early gastric cancer (le cancer de l'éstomac au début). Together with ulcer cancer and ulcerating cancer, the cases reported included "le cancer gastrique érosif à marche lente" (slow-growing erosive cancer), which seems to have been almost indentical with the type later named "superficial spreading carcinoma" by Stout. Gutmann was a radiologist and pioneered the detection of early gastric cancer by X-ray examination.

Influenced by a case presented by Cabot [8] at a routine conference on clinical pathology, Ewing [10] in 1936 and Mallory [27] in 1940 stressed the importance of a particular type of gastric cancer, "superficial carcinoma." Ewing [10] stated that in the case of this lesion malignant changes were only visible in the upper layer of the mucosa, leaving the surface uninvolved, and that they might result from atypical chronic hyperplastic gastritis. Mallory used the term "carcinoma in situ" for these lesions, and he pointed out that secondary ulceration of such lesions was

3

not uncommon. In 1940, KONJETZNY [22] also reported similar cases, referring to the condition as *"oberflächlicher Schleimhautkrebs."*

In 1942, STOUT [36] reported 15 cases of large and superficial cancerous lesions, in which the surface was relatively flat and growth of the cancer cells did not extend beyond the layer of the submucosa. Almost all lesions were accompanied by erosion or ulceration. He named this type of gastric cancer the "superficial spreading type" and suggested the importance of atrophy and cyst formation of the gastric glands for the development of gastric cancer [34, 35].

In 1943, GUISS and STEWART [11] expressed their opinion that in chronic atrophic gastritis no histological evidence supporting a precancerous nature had been found but it was often caused or intensified by the presence of gastric cancer. Conversely, WARREN and MEISSNER [41] presented the conclusion in 1944 that some cases of gastric carcinoma arose on a background of chronic gastritis with epithelial changes. On the grounds of analysis of a case of protruded and unifocal gastric cancer with its growth confined entirely to the mucosa, RÖSSLE [30] stated in 1944 that hypertrophic gastritis could be a precursor of this lesion.

As described briefly above and summarized in Table 1, the histopathological relationship between ulcer or polyp of the stomach and the development of gastric cancer were the main topics in this field of study until the late 1920s, except in Konjetzny's work. Since most gastric cancer specimens obtained at that time by autopsy or by surgery were from advanced cancers, it is not surprising that they did not allow an adequate approach to the study of the histogenesis of gastric cancer. Later on, gastric cancers related macroscopically to neither ulcers nor polyps were found mostly by chance in resected stomachs, and this type of cancer became another main subject of study. The gradual increase in the number of resected stomachs since then and the progress in diagnosis and in surgical pathology, especially of the earlier stages of cancer, have greatly advanced the study of its histogenesis.

Since the middle of this century great progress has been made in the early detection of gastric cancer, the main avenues being the development of double-contrast radiography and of endoscopic fibergastroscopy. These new methods, together with the histological examination of biopsied specimens taken from doubtful lesions under direct vision by the endoscope, have greatly enhanced the reliability of early detection and early diagnosis of gastric cancer, and with this progress in diagnosis studies on the histogenesis of gastric cancer have made great advances in recent years.

Thus, the studies on the histogenesis of gastric cancer are derived from and dependent upon the pioneering work of several investigators, as described above. In particular, the work done by Georg Ernst KONJETZNY (photo), who was the first to describe *oberflächlicher Schleimhautkrebs* and did so in great detail, is certainly of immortal merit [26 a].

References

1. Aschoff L (1909) Das Karcinom des Magens. In: Pathologische Anatomie, vol 2/1. Fischer, Jena, pp 330–337
2. Bertrand I (1937) Diagnostic histologique précoxe du cancer de léstomac. 2nd International Congress of Gastroenterology, Paris
3. Bizzozero G (1888) Über die Regeneration der Elemente der schlauchförmigen Drüsen und des Epithels des Magendarmkanals. Anat Anz 3: 781–784
4. Borrmann R (1926) Geschwülste des Magens. In: Henke F, Lubarsch O (eds) Handbuch der speziellen pathologischen Anatomie und Histologie, vol 4/1. Springer, Berlin, pp 864–871
5. Brinton W (1859) The diseases of the stomach. London
6. Büchner F (1927) Kriegs-Konst. Pathologie. Jena
7. Büchner F (1956) Die Pathogenese des Magenkarzinomas. In: Spezielle Pathologie. Urban & Schwarzenberg, Munich, pp 231–248
8. Cabot RC (1935) Ante mortem and post mortem records as used in weekly clinical-pathologic exercises. N Engl J Med 212: 481–485
9. Cruveilhier J (1829) Anatomie pathologique du corps humain. Baillère, Paris
10. Ewing J (1936) The beginnings of gastric cancer. Am J Surg 31: 204–205
11. Guiss LW, Stewart FW (1943) Chronic atrophic gastritis and cancer of the stomach. Arch Surg 46: 823–843
12. Gutmann RA, et al. (1939) Le cancer de léstomac au début. Etude clinique radiologique et anatomopathologique. Doin, Paris
13. Gutmann RA, Bertrand I (1938) Le cancer gastrique érosif á marche lente. Presse Med 46: 814–817
14. Gutmann RA (1933) De quelques signes radiologiques aux cancer gastrique au début. Bull Soc Radiol Med Fr 21: 347–351
15. Hamperl H (1931) Über Umbauvorgänge in der Magenschleimhaut. Verh Dtsch Pathol Ges 26: 392–395
16. Hauser G (1926) Die krebsige Entartung des chronischen Magen- und Duodenalgeschwürs. In: Henke F, Lubarsch O (eds) Handbuch der speziellen pathologischen Anatomie und Histologie, vol 4/1. Springer, Berlin, pp 497–518
17. Hauser G (1910) Zur Frage von krebsiger Entartung des chronischen Magengeschwüres. MMW 57: 1209–1213
18. Hauser G (1894) Zur Histogenese des Krebses. Virchow's Arch Pathol Anat 138: 482–499
19. Hauser G (1883) Das chronische Magengeschwür und dessen Beziehungen zur Entwicklung des Magencarcinoms. Hirschfeld, Leipzig
20. Konjetzny GE (1953) The superficial cancer of the gastric mucosa. Am J Dig Dis 20: 91–96
21. Konjetzny GE (1943) Die Beziehungen zwischen Gastritis und Magenkrebsentwicklung. Langenbeck's Arch Klin Chir 204: 4–63
22. Konjetzny GE (1940) Der oberflächliche Schleimhautkrebs des Magens. Chirurg 12: 192–202
23. Konjetzny GE (1938) Der Magenkrebs. Enke, Stuttgart
24. Konjetzny GE (1928) Die Entzündung des Magens. In: Henke F, Lubarsch O (eds) Handbuch der speziellen pathologischen Anatomie und Histologie, vol 4/2. Springer, Berlin, pp 768–1175
25. Konjetzny GE (1913) Über die Beziehung der chronischen Gastritis mit ihren Folgeerscheinungen und des chronischen Magenulkus zur Entwicklung des Magenkrebses. Brun's Beitr Klin Chir 85: 455–519
26. Kupffer C (1883) Epithel und Drüsen des menschlichen Magens. In: Festschrift dem Ärztlichen Verein München, zur Feier seines fünfzigjährigen Jubiläums
26a. Lindenschmidt TO (1980) Meister der deutschen Chirurgie – Georg Ernst Konjetzny. Zu seinem hundertsten Geburtstage. Dtsch Ges Chir Mitt 2: 42–47
27. Mallory TB (1940) Carcinoma in situ of the stomach and its bearing on the histogenesis of malignant ulcers. Arch Pathol 30: 348–362
28. Newcomb WD (1932) The relationship between peptic ulceration and gastric carcinoma. Br J Surg 20: 279–308
29. Orator V (1925) Beiträge zur Magenpathologie. II. Zur Pathologie und Genese des Carcinomas und Ulcuscarcinoms des Magens. Virchow's Arch Pathol Anat 256: 202–229

30. Rössle R (1944) Über einen frühen Oberflächenkrebs der Magenschleimhaut. Zentralbl Allg Pathol Pathol Anat 82: 165–170
31. Saltzman F (1913) Studien über Magenkrebs. Arb Pathol Inst Helsingfors [Neue Folge] 1: 335–440
32. Schmidt A (1896) Untersuchungen über das menschliche Magenepithel unter normalen und pathologischen Verhältnissen. Virchow's Arch Pathol Anat 143: 477–508
33. Stewart MJ (1926) The histological criteria of ulcer cancer of the stomach. J Pathol Bacteriol 29: 321–324
34. Stout AP (1945) Gastric mucosal atrophy and carcinoma of the stomach. NY State J Med 45: 973–977
35. Stout AP (1943) Pathology of carcinoma of the stomach. Arch Surg 46: 807–822
36. Stout AP (1942) Superficial spreading type of carcinoma of the stomach. Arch Surg 44: 651–657
37. Stromeyer F (1912) Die Pathogenese des Ulcus ventriculi zugleich ein Beitrag zur Frage nach den Beziehungen zwischen Ulcus und Carcinoma. Beitr Pathol Anat 54: 1–67
38. Versé M (1909) Über die Entstehung von Karzinomen aus altem Ulcus ventriculi und bei Polyposis ventriculi. Verh Dtsch Pathol Ges 13: 374–379
39. Versé M (1908) Über die Histogenese der Schleimhautkarzinome. Verh Dtsch Pathol Ges 12: 95–99
40. Versé M (1903) Die Histogenese der Schleimhautcarcinome. Leipzig
41. Warren S, Meissner WA (1944) Chronic gastritis and carcinoma of the stomach. Gastroenterology 3: 251–258
42. Wölfler A (1881) Über einem neuen Fall von gelungener Resektion des carzinomatösen Pylorus. Wien Med Wochenschr 51
43. Yamagiwa K (1981) Theory on development of gastric carcinoma (in Japanese). Keiseisha, Tokyo

2. Statistics, Epidemiology, and Etiology

Carcinoma of the stomach is one of the commonest malignant neoplasms throughout the world, even though the frequency varies widely in different countries, areas, and races. According to the most recent published data from Segi's Institute [63], the age-adjusted death rate per 100000 population from this disease in 1977 was highest in Japan (m: 52.3, f: 26.8), followed by Costa Rica (m: 48.7, f: 17.2), and Chile (m: 46.4, f: 21.3), and lowest in Thailand (m: 1.5, f: 0,8) and Egypt (m: 1.2, f: 0,8). The rate is relatively high in Hungary (m: 34.5, f: 16.3), Poland (m: 33.9, f: 12.9), Czechoslovakia (m: 33.7, f: 16.3 in 1979), Romania (m: 27.9, f: 12.9), Bulgaria (m: 27.8, f: 15.6), and Iceland (m: 27.6, f: 12.9), and fairly low in New Zealand (m: 12.9, f: 5.7), Canada (m: 12.9, f: 5.9 in 1979), Australia (m: 10.8, f: 5.8), and the United States of America (m: 6.6, f: 3.1). It

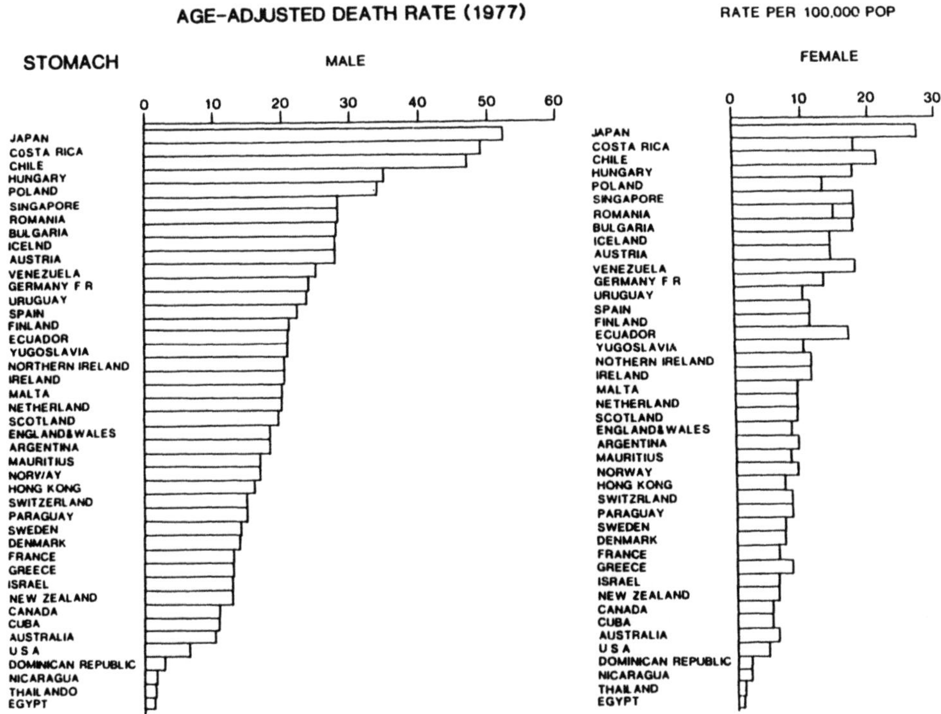

Fig. 1. Age-adjusted mortality rates for gastric cancer in different countries in 1977 (Chap. 2 [63])

should be mentioned at this point that regardless of differences in frequency, the male incidence is about twice the female incidence in almost all countries (Fig. 1).

Several investigators [2, 20, 24, 37, 44, 61, 62, 70, 78, 83, 84, 86] have pointed out that during the last 50 years the mortality rate for gastric cancer has been decreasing in most countries (Fig. 2), and according to HAENSZEL [15], the decrease commenced in U.S. whites in the 1930s. (Fig. 3). The rate has also recently started to decrease in Japan, which used to have the highest rate [28, 48], but the slighter decline in the curve than might be expected in view of the remarkable reduction in frequency in middle-aged people is explained by the prolongation of the average life-span among the Japanese (Fig. 4).

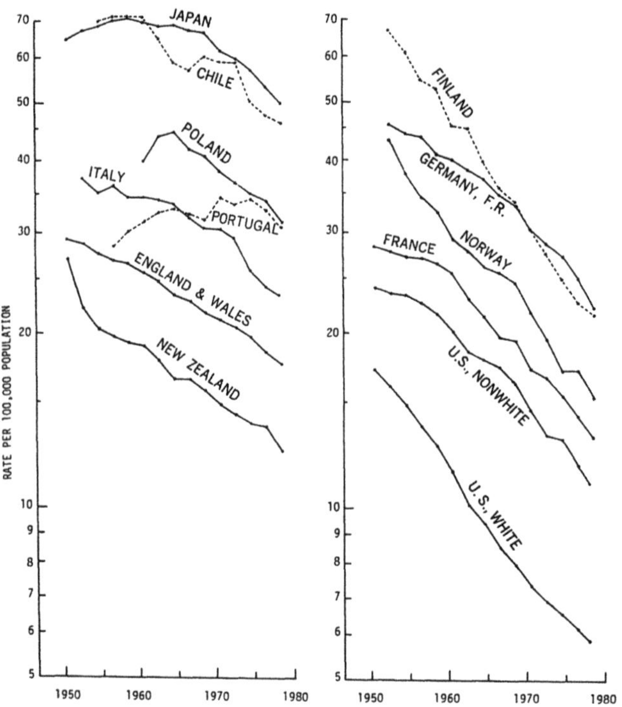

Fig. 2. Trends in age-adjusted male mortality rates for gastric cancer in selected countries (Chap. 2 [2])

As shown in Fig. 4, the age-adjusted death rate for gastric cancer is highest in the age group 80–84 years, followed by the 8th, 7th, 6th, 5th, and 4th decades in declining order. The overall male:female ratio is 1.5:1.0, but as shown in Fig. 4, it is less than 1.0 for people under the age of 40. Similar sex ratios were obtained in 72 756 cases of surgically resected gastric cancer for which the recorded data were registered at the National Cancer Center·WHO-CC in Tokyo during the 10 years 1963–1973 (Fig. 5).

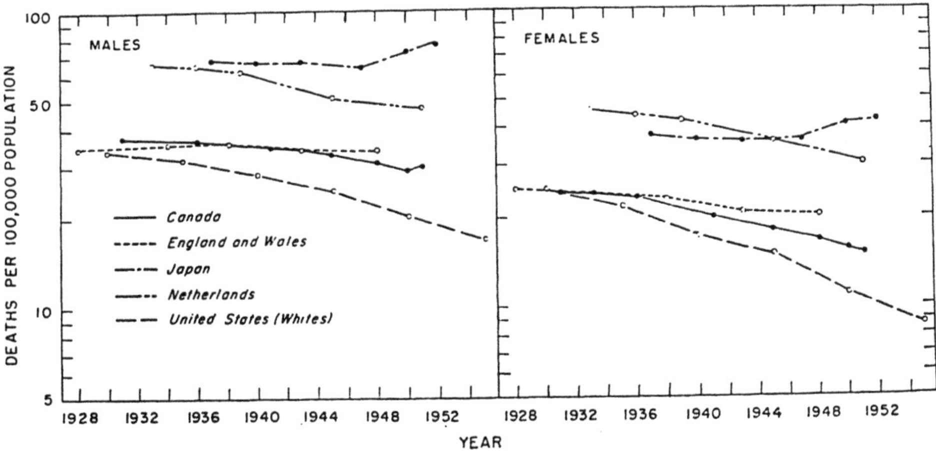

Fig. 3. Trends in age-adjusted mortality rates (per 100 000 population) for gastric cancer by sex for five countries (Chap. 2 [19])

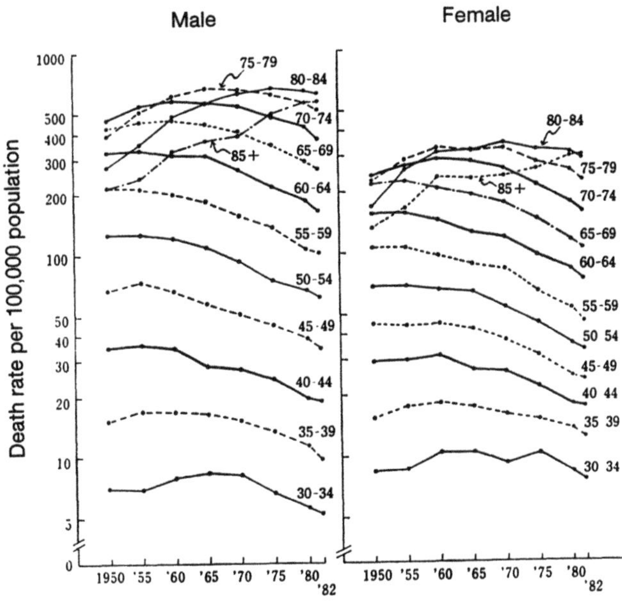

Fig. 4. Trends in age- and sex-specific mortality rate for gastric cancer in Japan from 1950 to 1982 (Data source: Ministry of Health and Welfare, Japan vital statistics series 1950–1982)

Even though the etiology of gastric cancer is not yet fully understood, from epidemiological and experimental studies done in the last 30 years it has become evident that the development of gastric cancer is due mainly to the environment, especially factors concerning diet. This conclusion first emerged from the results of statistical and epidemiological studies on immigrants from high-risk to low-

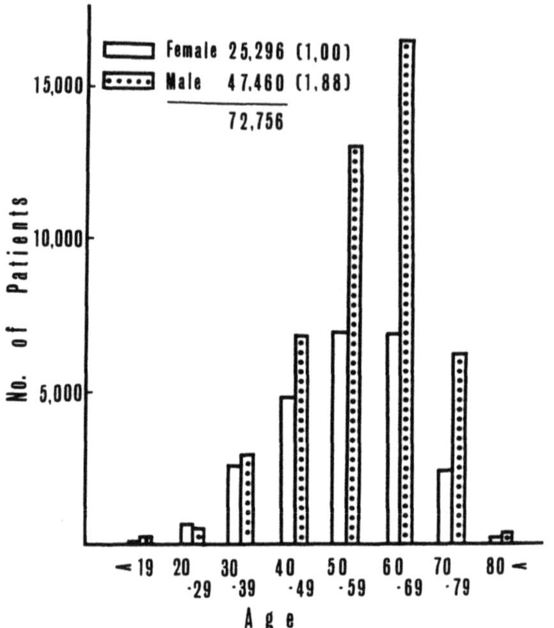

Fig. 5. Distribution of gastric cancer patients ($n = 72756$) by age and sex (Data source: Japanese Society for Gastric Cancer Research and National Cancer Center, Tokyo 1963–1973)

risk coutries [4, 8, 17, 18, 54, 68–72]. For example, Hawaii Japanese born in Hawaii showed a higher mortality rate from gastric cancer than Hawaii Caucasians and U.S. whites, but this mortality rate was still significantly lower than that of the Hawaii Japanese who had been born and brought up in Japan and later moved to Hawaii (Fig. 6).

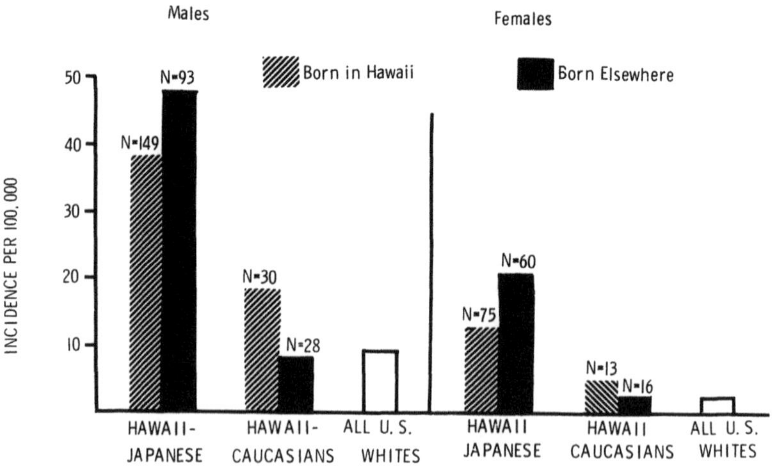

Fig. 6. Age-adjusted incidence of gastric cancer in Hawaii Japanese and Caucasians (1973–1977) by place of birth (Chap. 2 [34])

Following this observation, a cooperative epidemiological study on the development of gastric cancer in the United States of America and Japan was started in 1960 [8, 15–19, 26, 27, 34, 54, 61, 67, 71, 72], and the conclusions reached in the epidemiologic investigations included the identification of salty food, salty dried fish, salty pickles, smoked food, too much broiled or roasted fish and meat, low calorie intake, smoking, alcohol drinking, and irregular meals as risk factors [2, 7, 8, 11, 14, 15, 16, 25, 29, 32, 34, 52, 58, 65, 82, 85]. The risk factors were also analyzed from the standpoint of soil and water [21, 53], social class [5], vitamin C deficiency [11], genetics [22], and high- and low-risk areas within a country [11, 66]. The histological nature not only of gastric cancers but of grades of intestinal metaplasia of the gastric mucosa between high- and low-risk countries was also compared [8, 30, 46, 47].

Comparative statistical and epidemiologic studies carried out at national and international levels also revealed that the death rates of gastric cancer and of colon cancer are inversely proportional and the cause of both diseases is closely associated with diet [18, 67, 86].

The success of animal experiments aimed at inducing cancer of the glandular stomach in rodents and dogs by oral administration of chemical carcinogens [10, 40, 45, 60, 73, 74 a], especially of nitroso compounds [38, 39] such as MNNG or ENNG [74], reinforced this conclusion enormously. With such methods, the induction of gastric cancer in experimental animals became feasible, and some of the cancers induced metastasized not only to the regional lymph nodes but also to remote organs such as liver, lung, and peritoneal cavity, as in human cases. Later it became known that following oral administration of two kinds of noncarcinogenic substances, such as secondary amine or amide and nitrite, carcinogenic nitroso compounds are formed in the stomach under the influence of acidic gastric juice [57]. The analysis of several foodstuffs revealed that these noncarcinogenic but potentially precarcinogenic substances were contained in several naturally occurring and artificial foodstuffs, albeit in small amounts. The presence or absence of carcinogenicity in several substances can now confirmed by Ames' mutagenicity test in vitro (Table 2).

On the other hand, animal experiments aimed at promoting the development of gastric cancer have been tried in several institutions, and surfactants such as al-

Table 2. Summary of experimental studies on induction of gastric cancer

P. N. Magee	(1956)	Development of hepatoma induced by diethyl-nitorosamine. Rat
H. Druckrey	(1961)	Induction of gastric cancer by nitosamide. Rat
H. L. Stewart	(1961)	Induction of gastric cancer by N, N'-2, 7-fluolenylenebisacetamide. Rat
R. Schoental	(1963)	Induction of gastric cancer by N-nitroso-N-alkylurethane. Rat and mouse
K. Mori	(1967)	Induction of gastric cancer by 4-nitroquinoline 1-oxide. Mouse
T. Sugimura	(1967)	Induction of gastric cancer by N-methyl-N'-nitro-N-nitrosoguanidine. Rat
J. Sander	(1969)	Induction of malignant tumor by nitrite and secondary amine
W. Lijinsky	(1970)	Nitrosamine as environmental carcinogen
T. Sugimura	(1971)	Induction of gastric cancer by N-methyl-N'-nitro-N-nitrosoguanidine. Dog

kylbenzene sulfonate or Tween 60 [77], highly concentrated salts [75, 76, 81], and regurgitated bile [9, 33a, 33b, 35] are known to have promoting activities. Animal experiments also suggest that immature regenerative epithelium following erosion or ulceration of the gastric mucosa is more susceptible to orally introduced carcinogens than the steady-state epithelium [64].

Following the progress made in such experimental studies, epidemiologic studies have now entered on a new stage of analysis, with the aim of preventing the development of this disease. The amounts of nitroso compounds or their precursors contained in water, soil, foodstuffs, urine, blood, saliva, or gastric juice are being examined from various aspects [3, 21, 23, 31, 38, 39, 43, 50, 56, 59, 79, 80]. Cohort studies of high-risk patients with long followup periods [12, 13, 51] will give more information on the precancerous changes in the stomach.

Other papers report that gastric cancer is more frequent in coalminers [1, 33, 41] and in the survivors of the atomic bomb [42, 49, 88] than in the general population.

The role of genetic factors in the development of human gastric cancer, which has been underestimated in recent years, is also important. A recent report [49a] stresses that the percentage of cancer patients who have a family history of the same condition is far higher for gastric cancer than for other cancers (Fig. 7). These data strongly suggest family clustering and the involvement of a genetic factor in the development of gastric cancer.

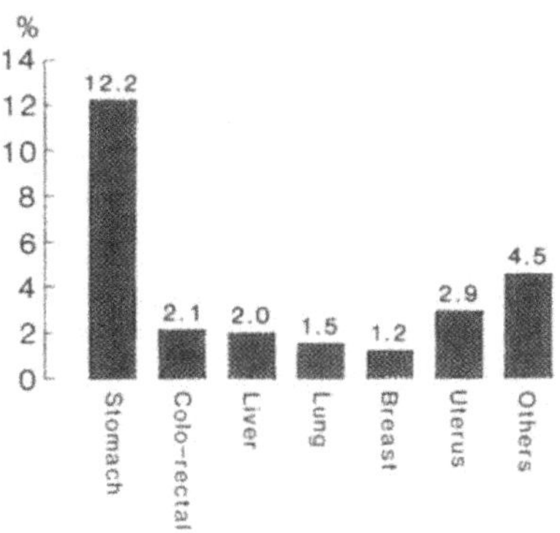

Fig. 7. Percentages of cancer patients with family history of cancer at same specific sites (Chap. 2 [49a])

It is certain that the etiology of human gastric cancer cannot be fully known without the summation and incorporation of results obtained from epidemiologic, physical, analytical, experimental, and biological studies, and as a background to these studies a knowledge of histopathology is indispensable.

From the several studies presently in hand, the cause of human gastric cancer might be assumed to be not unifactorial but rather multifactorial, even though the main causative role is played by chemical substances introduced to the stomach by mouth (Fig. 8).

Recently a new approach has been attempted to determination of the mechanism of development of gastric cancer; this is based on molecular biology and at-

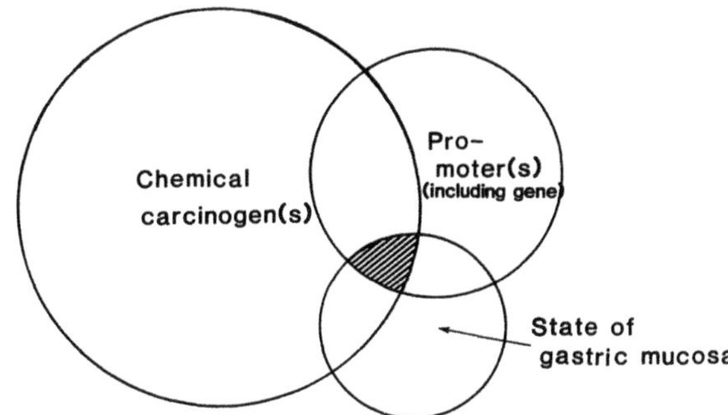

Fig. 8. Hypothesis concerning development of human gastric cancer

tempts by several investigators to obtain specific oncogene from DNA of human gastric cancer cells. The identification of specific oncogene and its product will be an enormous step forward, not only for our basic understanding of the mechanism of development of human gastric cancer but also for the elaboration of procedures useful in the prevention of this disease and detection of it in its earliest stage.

References

1. Ames RG (1983) Gastric cancer and coal mine dust exposure. A Case-control study. Cancer 52: 1346–1350
2. Aoki K, Tominaga S, Kuroishi T (1981) Age-adjusted death rates for cancer by site (ICD. 8th Revision) in 50 countries. Gann Monogr Cancer Res 26: 251–274
3. Bartsch H, Ohshima H, Munōz N, Crespi M, Lu SH (1983) Measurement of endogenous nitrosation in humans. Potential applications of a new method and initial results. In: Harris CC, Antrup HN (eds) Human carcinogenesis. Academic, New York, pp 833–855
4. Buell P, Dunn JE (1965) Cancer mortality among Japanese Issei and Nisei of California. Cancer 18: 656–664
5. Clemmesen J, Nielsen A (1951) The social districution of cancer in Copenhagen, 1943 to 1947. Br J Cancer 5: 159–171
6. Correa P, Cuello C, Fajardo LF et al. (1983) Diet and gastric cancer: Nutrition survey in a high-risk area. J Natl Cancer Inst 70: 673–678
7. Correa P, Cuello C, Montes G (1979) Pathogenesis of gastric carcinoma: The role of the micro-environment. In: Herfath C, Schlag P (eds) Gastric cancer. Springer, Berlin Heidelberg New York, pp 9–12
8. Correa P, Sasano N, Stemmermann G (1973) Pathology of gastric carcinoma in Japanese populations: Comparisons between Miyagi Prefecture, Japan, and Hawaii. J Natl Cancer Inst 51: 1449–1459
9. Dahm K, Werner B (1973) Experimentelles Anastomosencarcinom. Ein Beitrag zur Pathogenese des Magenstumpfcarcinoms. Langenbecks Arch Chir 333: 211–236
10. Druckrey H, Preussmann R (1961) Chemische Konstitution und carcinogene Wirkung bei Nitros-aminen. Naturwissenschaften 48: 134
11. Dungal N, Sigurjonsson J (1967) Gastric cancer and diet. A pilot study on dietery habits in two districts differing markedly in respect to mortality from gastric cancer. Br J Cancer 21: 270–276
12. Fujimoto I, Hanai A (1981) Cancer incidence in Japan 1975. Cancer registry statistics. Gann Monogr Cancer Res 26: 92–120

13. Fujimoto I, Hanai A, Sakagami F et al. (1977) Cancer registries in Japan: Activities and incidence data. Natl Cancer Inst Monogr 47: 7–15
14. Graham S, Schotz W, Martino P (1972) Alimentary factors in the epidemiology of gastric cancer. Cancer 30: 927–938
15. Haenszel W, Kurihara M, Locke FB, Shimizu K, Segi M (1976) Stomach cancer in Japan. J Natl Cancer Inst 56: 265–274
16. Haenszel W, Kurihara M, Segi M, Lee RKC (1972) Stomach cancer among Japanese in Hawaii. J Natl Cancer Inst 49: 969–988
17. Haenszel W, Kurihara M (1968) Studies of Japanese migrants. I. Mortality from cancer and other diseases among Japanese in the United States. J Natl Cancer Inst. 42: 43–68
18. Haenszel W (1961) Cancer mortality among the foreign born in the United States. J Natl Cancer Inst 26: 37–132
19. Haenszel W (1958) Variation in incidence of and mortality from stomach cancer with particular reference to the United States. J Natl Cancer Inst 21: 213–262
20. Hanai A, Fujimoto I (1982) Cancer incidence in Japan in 1975 and changes of epidemiological features for cancer in Osaka. Natl Cancer Inst Monogr 62: 3–7
21. Hawksworth G, Hill MJ, Gordillo G, Cuello C (1974) Possible relationship between nitrates, nitrosamines and gastric cancer in south west Colombia. IARC Sci Publ 9: 229–234
22. Hill MJ (1983) Environmental and genetic factors in gastorointestinal cancer. In: Sherlock P, Morson BC, Barbara L, Veronesi U (eds) Precancerous lesion of the gastrointestinal tract. Raven, New York, pp 1–22
23. Hill MJ, Hawkworth G, Tattersal G (1973) Bacteria, nitrosamines and cancer of the stomach. Br J Cancer 28: 562–567
24. Hirayama T (1975) Epidemiology of cancer of the stomach with special reference to its recent decrease in Japan. Cancer Res 35: 3460–3463
25. Hirayama T (1968) The epidemiology of cancer of the stomach in Japan, with special reference to the role of diet. Gann Monogr 3: 15–27
26. Hirohata T (1982) Age-adjusted death rates of malignant neoplasms of various sites for 33 selected countries in the world. Kurume Med J 29: 1–18
27. Hirohata T, Kolonel L, Nomura A (1977) Epidemiologic cancer research programs of the cancer center of Hawaii. Natl Cancer Inst Monogr 47: 67–70
28. Hisamichi S (1984) Mass screening for gastric cancer by X-ray examination. Jpn J Clin Oncol 14: 211–223
29. Ikeda M, Yoshimoto K, Yoshimura T et al. (1983) A cohort study on the possible association between broiled fish intake and cancer. Gann 74: 640–648
30. Imai T, Kubo T, Watanabe H (1971) Chronic gastritis in Japanese with reference to high incidence of gastric carcinoma. J Natl Cancer Inst 47: 179–195
31. Jones SM, Davis PW, Savage A (1978) Gastric juice nitrate and gastric cancer. Lancet 1: 1355
32. Joossens JV, Geboers J (1983) Epidemiology of gastric cancer: A clue to etiology. In: Sherlock P, Morson BC, Barbara L, Veronesi U (eds) Precancerous lesions of the gastrointestinal tract. Raven, New York, pp 97–114
33. Klauber MR, Lyon JL (1978) Gastric cancer in a coal mining region. Cancer 4: 2355–2358
33a. Kobori O, Shimizu T, Maeda M, Atomi Y, Watanabe J (1984) Enhancing effect of bile and bile acid on stomach tumorigenesis induced by N-methyl-N'nitro-N nitrosoguanidine in Wistar rats. J Natl Cancer Inst 73: 853–861
33b. Kobori O, Watanabe J, Shimizu T, Shoji M, Morioka Y (1984) Enhancing effect of sodium taurocholate on N-methyl-nitro-N-nitroso quanidine-induced stomach tumorigenesis in rats. Gann 75: 651–654
34. Kolonel LN, Nomura AMY, Hirohata T et al. (1981) Association of diet and place of birth with stomach cancer incidence in Hawaii Japanese and Caucasians. Am J Clin Nutr 34: 2478–2485
35. Kondo K, Suzuki H, Nagayo T (1984) The influence of gastrojejunal anastomosis on gastric carcinogenesis in rats. Gann 75: 362–369
36. Kubo T (1971) Histologic appearance of gastric carcinoma in high and low mortality countries: comparison between Kyushu, Japan and Minnesota, USA. Cancer 28: 726–734
37. Kuroishi T, Tominaga S, Hirose K, Aoki K, Segi M (1981) Cancer mortality in Japan. Gann Monograph Cancer Res 26: 1–91

38. Lijinsky W (1977) Nitrosamines and nitrosamides in the etiology of gastrointestinal cancer. Cancer 40: 2446–2449
39. Lijinsky M, Epstein SS (1970) Nitrosamines as environmental carcinogens. Nature 225: 21–23
40. Magee PN, Barnes JM (1956) The production of malignant primary hepatic tumour in the rat by feeding diethylnitrosamine. Br J Cancer 16: 114–122
41. Matolo NM, Klauber MR, Gorishek WM, Dixon JA (1972) High incidence of gastric carcinoma in a coal mining region. Cancer 29: 733–737
42. Matsuura H, Yamamoto T, Sekine L, Ochi Y, Otake M (1984) Pathological and epidemiological study of gastric cancer in atomic bomb survivors, Hiroshima and Nagasaki, 1959–77. J Radiat Res 25: 111–129
43. Mirvish SS (1983) The etiology of gastric cancer. Intragastric nitrosamide formation and other theories. J Natl Cancer Inst 7: 629–647
44. Moore GE (1962) Decrease in incidence of cancer in the stomach. Surg Gynecol Obstet 114: 209–210
45. Mori K (1967) Carcinoma of the glandular stomach of mice by instillation of 4-nitroquinoline 1-oxide. Gann 58: 389–393
46. Muñoz N, Asvall J (1971) Time trends of intestinal and diffuse type of gastric cancer in Norway. Int J Cancer 8: 144–157
47. Muñoz N, Connelly P (1971) Time trends in intestinal and diffuse types of gastric cancer in the United States. Int J Cancer 8: 158–164
48. Nagayo M (1933) Statistical studies on cancer in Japan. Gann [Special Issue]
49. Nakamura K (1977) Stomach cancer in atomic-bomb survivors. Lancet 2: 866–867
49a. Ogawa H, Kato I, Tominaga S (1985) Family history of cancer among cancer patients. Gann 76: 113–118
50. Ohshima H, Bartsch (1981) Quantitative estimation of endogenous nitrosation in humans by monitoring N-nitrosoproline excreted in the urine. Cancer Res 41: 3658–3662
51. Oshima A (1976) Evaluation of a mass screening program for stomach cancer. Natl Cancer Inst Monogr 53: 181–186
52. Palmer S, Bakshi K (1983) Diet, nutrition and cancer: Interim dietary guidelines. J Natl Cancer Inst. 70: 1151–1170
53. Pfeiffer CJ, Foder G (1979) Gastric cancer mortality and watertrace elements: International study of Iceland, Newfoundland and Japan. In: Pfeiffer CJ (ed) Gastric cancer. Etiology and pathogenesis. Witzstock, Baden-Baden, pp 45–59
54. Quisenberry WB (1961) Stomach cancer among Japanese in Hawaii and the United States mainland. Acta Unio Int Contra Cancrum 17: 858–866
55. Reed PI, Smith PL, Haines K, House FR, Walters CL (1981) Gastric juice N-nitrosamine in health and gastroduodenal disease. Lancet 2: 550–552
56. Ruddel WS, Bone ES, Hill MJ, Blendis LM, Walters CL (1976) Gastric juice nitrite. A risk factor for cancer in the hypochlorhydric stomach? Lancet 2: 1037–1039
57. Sander J, Bürkle G (1969) Induktion maligner Tumoren bei Ratten durch gleichzeitige Verfütterung von Nitrit und sekundären Aminen. Z Krebsforsch 73: 54–66
58. Saxen EA, Hakama M (1967) The different incidence of gastric cancer all over the world and possible reasons for this difference. UICC Monogr Ser 10: 49–54
59. Schlag P, Bockler R, Peter M (1982) Nitrite and nitrosamines in gastric juice: Risk factors for gastric cancer? Scand J Gastroenterol 17: 145–150
60. Schoental R (1963) Induction of tumours of the stomach in rats and mice by N-nitroso-N-alkylurethane. Nature 199: 190
61. Segi M, Fujisaku S, Kurihara M (1957) Geographical observation on cancer mortality by selected sites on the basis of standardised death rate. Gann 48: 219–225
62. Segi M, Fukushima I, Fujisaku S et al. (1957) An epidemiological study on cancer in Japan (Report of the Committee for Epidemiological Study on Cancer, sponsored by the Ministry of Welfare and Public Health). Gann 48 (Suppl): 1–62
63. Segi Institute of Cancer Epidemiology (1982) Age-adjusted death rate for cancer for selected sites (A-classification) in 43-countries in 1979
64. Shirai T, et al. (1978) Induction of preneoplastic hyperplasia and carcinoma by N-methyl-N-nitro-N-nitrosoguanidine from regenerated mucosa of ulcer by iodoacetamide in fundus of rat stomach. Gann 69: 361–366

65. Sigurjonsson J (1967) Occupational variation's in mortality from gastric cancer in relation to dietary differences. Br J Cancer 21: 651–656
66. Sigurjonsson J (1966) Geographical variations in mortality from cancer in Iceland, with particular reference to stomach cancer. J Natl Cancer Inst 37: 337–346
67. Smith RL (1956) Recorded and expected mortality among Japanese of the United States and Hawaii with special reference to cancer. J Natl Cancer Inst 17: 459–473
68. Staszewski J (1972) Migrant studies in alimentary tract cancer. Recent Res Cancer Res 39: 85–97
69. Steiner PE (1954) Carcinoma of stomach. In: Cancer. race and geography. Williams and Willkins, Baltimore, pp 60–74
70. Steiner PE (1949) Etiologic implications of the racial incidences of gastric cancer. J Natl Cancer Inst 10: 429–437
71. Stemmermann G (1977) Gastric cancer in the Hawaii Japanese. Gann 68: 525–535
72. Stemmermann G, Haenszel W, Locke F (1977) Epidemiologic pathology of gastric ulcer and gastric carcinoma among Japanese in Hawaii. J Natl Cancer Inst 58: 13–20
73. Stewart HL, Snell KC, Morris HP, Wagner BP, Ray FE (1961) Carcinoma of the glandular stomach of rats ingesting N, N-2, 7-fluorenylenebisacetamide. Natl Cancer Inst Monogr 5: 105–139
74. Sugimura T, Fujimura S (1967) Tumor production of glandular stomach of rats by N-methyl-N-nitro-N-nitrosoguanidine. Nature 216: 943–944
74a. Sugimura T, Tanaka N, Kawachi T et al. (1971) Production of stomach cancer in dogs by N-methyl-N'-nitro-N-nitrosoguanidine. Gann 62: 67–68
75. Suzuki H, Kondo K, Nagayo T (to be published) Sex difference of the enhancing effects of sodium chloride on rat stomach carcinogenesis induced by N-methyl-N'-nitro-N-nitrosoguanidine. Gann
76. Takahashi M, Kokubo T, Furukawa F et al. (1983) Effect of high salt diet on rat gastric carcinogenesis induced by N-methyl-N'-nitro-N-nitrosoguanidine. Gann 74: 28–34
77. Takahashi M (1970) Effect of alkylbenzene sulfonate as a vehicle for 4-nitroquinoline 1-oxide on gastric carcinogenesis in rats. Gann 61: 27–33
78. Tanaka A (1977) Mortality from stomach cancer. In: Hirayama T (ed) Epidemiology of stomach cancer. WHO, Geneva, pp 13–20 (WHO-CC monograph)
79. Tannenbaum SR, Moran D, Rand W, Cuello C, Correa P (1979) Gastric cancer in Colombia. IV. Nitrite and other ions in gastric contents of residents from a high risk region. J Natl Cancer Inst 62: 9–12
80. Tannenbaum SR, Archer MC, Wishnok JS, Bishop WW (1978) Nitrosamine formation in human saliva. J Natl Cancer Inst 60: 251–253
81. Tatematsu M, Takahashi M, Fukushima S, Hananouchi M, Shirai T (1975) Effects sodium chloride on experimental gastric cancer in rats induced by N-methyl-N'-nitro-N-nitrosoguanidine or 4-nitroquinoline 1-oxide. J Natl Cancer Inst 55: 101–106
82. Tominaga S, Ogawa H, Kuroishi T (1982) Usefulness of correlation analyses in the epidemiology of stomach cancer. Natl Cancer Inst Monogr 2: 135–140
83. Tulnius H (1974) Geographical distribution of malignant neoplasms and some other epidemiological features. 6 Geographical distribution of cancer of the stomach. In: Grundmann E (ed) Geschwülste/Tumors I. Springer, Berlin Heidelberg New York, pp 436–438 (Handbuch der allgemeinen Pathologie, vol 4/5)
84. Waterhouse J, Muir C, Correa P, Powell J (eds) (1976) Cancer incidence in five continents. IARC, Lyon (IARC scientific publications, no 15, vol 3)
85. Weisburger JH (1977) Current views on mechanisms concerned with the etiology of cancer in the digestive tract. In: Faber F et al. (eds) Pathophysiology in the digestive organs. University of Tokyo Press, Tokyo, pp 1–20
86. Wynder EL, Hyams L, Shigematsu T (1967) Correlation of international cancer death rates. An epidemiological exercise. Cancer 20: 113–126
87. Wynder EL, Kmet J, Dungal N, Segi M (1963) An epidemiological investigation of gastric cancer. Cancer 16: 1461–1496
88. Yamamoto T, Kato H, Ishida K, Tahara E, McGregor DH (1970) Gastric carcinoma in a fixed population Hiroshima and Nagasaki. Gann 61: 473–483

3. Background Data to the Study of Advanced Gastric Cancer

During the 25 years from 1957 to 1981, a series of 264693 outpatients underwent X-ray examination of the stomach in Yokoyama Hospital, with whom the author have been collaborated. In 9826 of these patients (3.7%) a diagnosis of gastric cancer or suspected gastric cancer was recorded. In 5051 patients (51.4%) gastric resection was performed in the hospital. The proportion of outpatients undergoing stomach X-ray and subsequent surgery was thus 1.9% (Table 3).

Table 3. Background data to the study

Calendar years	No. of patients examined by X-ray (A)	Gastric cancer				
		No. of patients diagnosed as having gastric cancer (B)	$\frac{B}{A}$ %	No. of patients subjected to surgery (C)	$\frac{C}{B}$ %	$\frac{C}{A}$ %
1957–60	23767	1555	6.5	668	43.0	1.9
1961–63	30625	1549	5.1	675	43.6	2.2
1964–66	37785	1633	4.3	806	49.4	2.1
1967–69	38665	1399	3.6	807	57.7	2.1
1970–72	38549	1272	3.3	724	56.9	1.9
1973–75	36000	987	2.7	570	57.8	1.6
1976–78	33512	781	2.3	401	51.3	1.2
1979–81	25790	650	2.5	400	61.5	1.5
Total	264693	9826	3.7	5051	51.4	1.9

The frequency with which gastric cancer was diagnosed or suspected on the basis of X-ray examination was 6.5% for the years 1957–1960, but it subsequently decreased each year, being 2.5% for the years 1979–1981.

During these years, 10221 cases of peptic ulcer (5358 cases of gastric ulcer, 3198 cases of duodenal ulcer, and 1665 cases of combined gastric and duodenal ulcer) and 493 cases of other gastric diseases (252 cases of gastric polyp, including "borderline" elevated lesion, 140 cases of gastritis of several types, and 101 cases of gastric tumors other than cancer, mostly malignant lymphoma and myoma) were surgically treated and their natures were histologically confirmed. The ratio of surgically resected peptic ulcers to gastric cancers was therefore 2.02:1.00 (Table 4).

The gross appearance of gastric cancer varies quite widely, not only with the nature of the cancer but also with the stage of the cancerous growth. For macro-

Table 4. Number and diagnoses of surgically resected stomachs (1957–1981)

Gastric cancer	5051 cases
Peptic ulcer	10 221 cases
Gastric	5358 cases
Duodenal	3198 cases
Gastric and duodenal	1665 cases
Other diseases	493 cases
Polyp	252 cases
Gastritis	140 cases
Tumor	101 cases
Total	15 765 cases

scopical classification, therefore, it is necessary first to separate various features of gastric cancer into early and advanced stages, even though in every type of gastric cancer the growth is transitional from the initial stage to the terminal one. In this chapter, the morphology of advanced gastric cancer and its related subjects will be described.

Gross Appearances

Advanced gastric cancer (AGC) can be classified by its common macroscopical characteristics into the following four main types, as proposed by BORRMANN in 1926 [2] (Fig. 9).

- Polypoid or fungating type (Type I)
- Circumscribed excavating type (Type II)

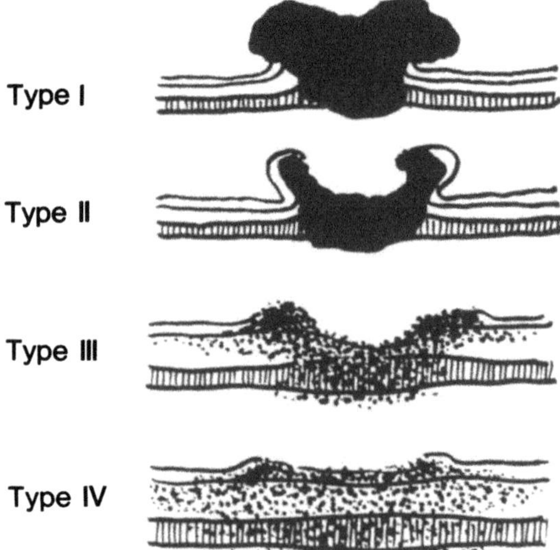

Fig. 9. Macroscopical types of AGC by Borrmann's classification

18

- Ulcerated and infiltrating type (Type III)
- Diffusely thickened type (Type IV)

The classification is based on the presence or absence in the lesions of

a) well-defined boundary,
b) ulceration,
c) convergence of the mucosal folds,
d) thickening of the wall,
e) deformation of the stomach.

The usefulness of the classification not only for clinical purposes but also for statistical and research investigations is also an important factor.

Polypoid or Fungating Type

This type of AGC (type I in Borrmann's classification) is characterized macroscopically by a large polypoid or fungating protrusion of the mucosa toward the lumen of the stomach, with a well-defined boundary. Unlike the early stages of this type, the shape of this large protrusion is irregular, its surface is uneven or bumpy, not infrequently assuming an appearance reminiscent of cauliflower or velvet, and in almost all cases it is sessile with a broad base. Deep ulceration at the surface of the polypoid tumor is scarcely visible, even though erosion, hemorrhage, or necrosis is not uncommon. The protruded mass is usually not hard but rather soft, fragile, and dark red in color owing to venous congestion. In many cases the tumor-bearing mucosa is affected by obvious atrophy (Fig. 10).

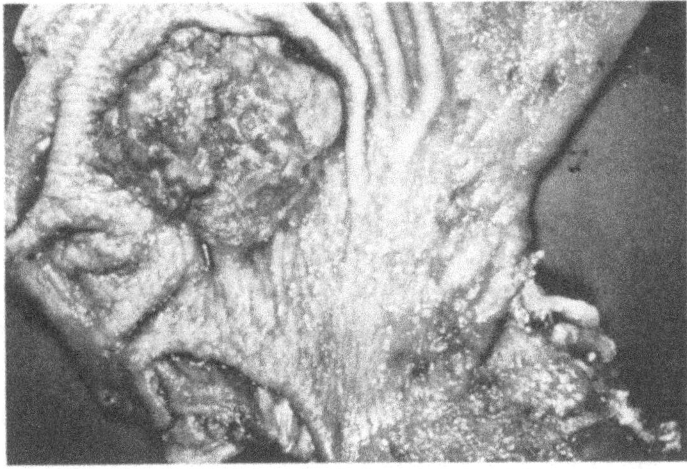

Fig. 10. Large, circumscribed and protruding cancerous lesion (Borrmann type I) in the antrum. The surface of the tumor is partly eroded (Pt no. 6365, 64 years, m)

The site of the lesion is variable, but it is found more often (71.2%) in the antrum or angulus than in the corpus or fundus, and it is mostly more than 3 cm in diameter. In most cases the lesion is unifocal and it affects elderly people (the average age among 81 patients was 59.0 years). Borrmann designated this type of AGC as type I. The frequency of this type among all the cases of AGC treated by resection is around 2.0% in almost every years and the sex ratio (m/f) is 2.4 (Table 5 and Fig. 11).

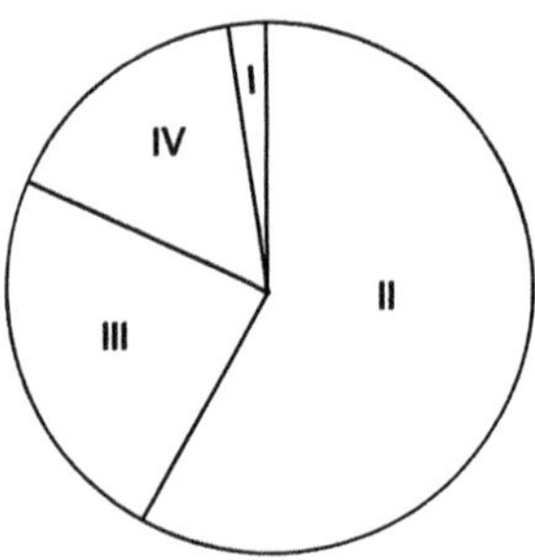

Fig. 11. Relative frequencies of the different macroscopical types of AGC according to Borrmann's classification

Table 5. Frequency of macroscopical types of AGC by site of development (1955–1980)

| Type | Frequency (%) | | | Total no. of cases |
	Antrum	Angulus	Corpus	
Borrmann I	39.7	31.5	28.8	81
Borrmann II	55.3	30.4	14.3	2287
Borrmann III	51.8	32.1	16.1	965
Borrmann IV	37.8	40.6	21.6	612
Total	51.6	32.3	16.1	3945

Circumscribed Excavating Type

Circumscribed excavating AGC (Borrmann's type II) also has a clear boundary from the surrounding mucosa, but its characteristic feature is wide and deep excavation of the central part of the cancerous lesion owing to necrosis of the medullary cancerous tissues, giving a crater-like appearance. The base of the crater is uneven, hemorrhagic, sometimes nodular, and often covered by a grayish-white exudate with a necrotic mass. It is also characteristic of this type that the deep crater is almost always surrounded by elevated mucosa, which forms a prominent rampart-like marginal wall. This type differs from the ulcerated and infiltrating types, which will be described below, in that convergency of mucosal folds toward the center of the excavation is seldom seen (Fig. 12).

This type of lesion is seen most frequently in the mucosa of the antrum (55.3%), especially of elderly persons (average age of the patients was 56.3 years), and is accompanied quite often by widespread severe intestinal metaplasia. This type of AGC was predominant in frequency (58.7%) up to 1978 in Japan, but its

20

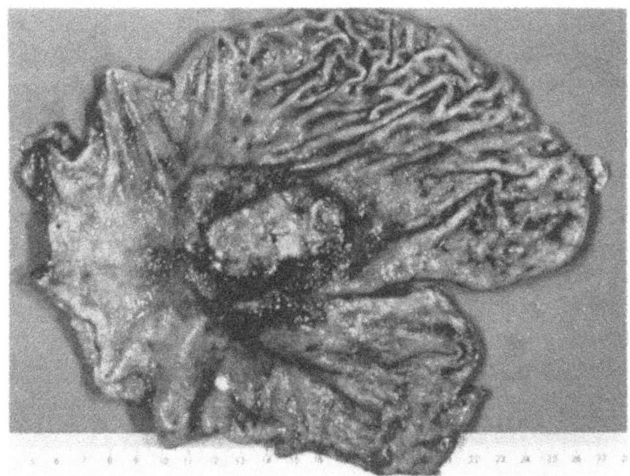

Fig. 12. Large circumscribed and heavily excavated cancer surrounded by elevated mucosa (Borrmann type II) in the angulus (Pt no. 17 684, 69 years, m)

frequency has been declining in recent years, as will be described later (s. Chapt. 7). The characteristic features are more often seen in male than in female patients (sex ratio is 2.6) (Table 5 and Fig. 11).

Ulcerated Infiltrating Type

Unlike the previous two types, the boundary of ulcerated and growing cancerous lesions (Borrmann's type III) is entirely or partly ill defined, while ulceration in the central part of the indurated cancerous lesion is the major change in this type (Fig. 13).

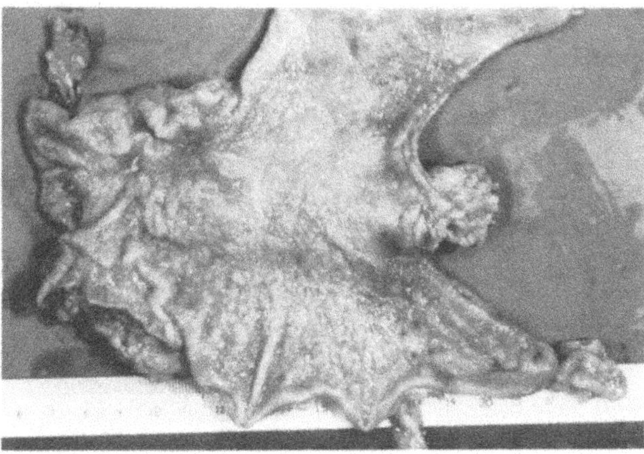

Fig. 13. Ill-defined induration of gastric wall with central shallow ulceration (Borrmann type III) in anterior wall of the antrum (Pt no. 14 487, 46 years, m)

The ulceration, which is easily recognizable by routine X-ray and endoscopic examinations, is irregular in shape, variable in size, but mostly not very deep; it is seen most frequently in or around the area of the angulus. The mucosa around the ulcer is slightly elevated, and its margin with the surrounding mucosa is vague owing to the infiltrative and indurative nature of the cancerous growth. Convergency of the mucosal folds toward the center of the ulcerated lesion, owing to fibrosis and contraction of the ulcerated lesion, is characteristic of this type.

In most respects, this type of AGC is intermediate in nature between the circumscribed excavated type and the diffuse thickened type, and Borrmann classified it as type III. The frequency of this type among all AGCs resected is next to that of the circumscribed excavated type (24.1%), and the average age of the patients is the lowest (51.3 years) for all types of AGC. The sex ratio (m/f) is lower than the previous two types (Table 5 and Fig. 11).

Diffusely Thickened Type

No circumscribed lesion can be recognized at all in the diffusely thickened type (Borrmann's type IV), and the main change in the stomach is diffuse thickening and hardening of the gastric wall with the nature of scirrhous cancer. Even though the surface of the thickened gastric wall is relatively flat, detailed macroscopical examination may reveal shallow ulceration or, widespread erosion, in the central part of the indurated lesions, most of which are located near the angulus or in the corpus.

When these changes occur in the area of the prepylorus or of the antrum, stenosis of the pylorus due to constriction of the thickened gastric wall inevitably occurs in the advanced stage, and dilatation of the proximal part of the stomach may result (Fig. 14).

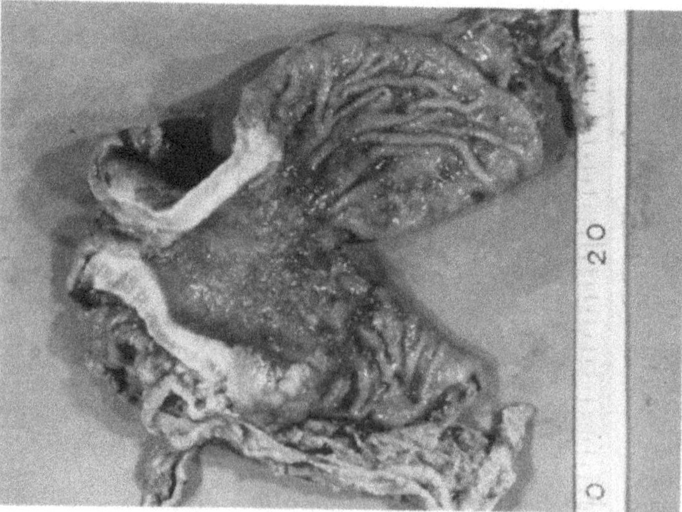

Fig. 14. Diffuse thickening and hardening of the antrum without prominent focal lesion (Borrmann type IV) has resulted in pyloric stenosis (Pt no. 11 201, 57 years, m)

Linitis plastica, which shows diffuse thickening and hardening of almost the entire gastric wall with no noticeable deformity of the stomach, is an extreme example of this type of AGC and is characterized also by concomitant giant hypertrophy of the mucosal folds in the area of the corpus and fundus, which at first glance looks like the giant rugae of Menetrier's disease. It is evident that this specific type of gastric cancer commences as small cancerous erosions in the mucosa of the anterior or posterior wall of the corpus, which is rich in mucosal folds.

This scirrhous type of gastric cancer is relatively frequent in younger age groups and in middle-aged women (average age in our series was 52.7 years), even though the type as a whole belongs to a minor group (15.1%). The sex ratio is nearly 1.0 in this type (Table 5 and Fig. 11).

Owing to the wide variability of the gross appearance, AGC is classified by several investigators in different ways [1, 5, 6, 13, 14, 18, 20, 22–24, 39]. Even though the criteria and the terms of the classification are slightly different, most investigators have grouped the macroscopical features of AGC principally into

a) polypoid,
b) ulcerating, and
c) diffuse types.

It is reasonable to classify the various features of AGC under this minimum three prototypes, but from the viewpoints of surgical pathology and of histogenesis, these macroscopical classifications seem to have some inadequacies. This applies especially in the case of the ulcerating types. As is well known, when intramural growth of the cancer reaches the deeper layers secondary ulceration of the cancerous lesion is quite often observed regardless of the macroscopical type, but the gross appearance of the secondary ulceration differs fairly characteristically between well-demarcated and ill-defined AGC. In the former, the expansive cancerous lesion is heavily and deeply excavated in its central part owing to necrosis of the cancerous tissues, and the boundary of the ulcerated lesion is well demarcated owing to reactive hyperplastic growth of the marginal mucosa, while in the latter the peptic ulceration varies in size, shape and depth and the area adjacent to the ulcer is diffusely indurated and ill defined owing to the infiltrative nature of the cancerous growth.

For study of the clinical pathology and histogenesis of gastric cancer, the inadequacy of the classification seems to be largely overcome by the macroscopical classification proposed by Borrmann. The criteria of the classification proposed by WILLIS [41] are not very different in principle from those of BORRMANN [2].

Morphological classification itself almost always involves some difficulty in cases showing intermediate or complex changes into one or another type, and this is also true in the case of AGC. There are cases in which the appearance seems to be between the excavated and the ulcerated types or between the ulcerated and the diffusely thickened type, while in other cases the macroscopical changes are more complex than in the prototypes described above, owing to fusion of double or multiple cancerous foci with different morphologies or to heterogeneity of the original cancer itself. Thus, it is unavoidable that the same case is sometimes classified into different types by different examiners.

To understand the clinical and biological nature of AGC, it is necessary for the pathologist to use a simple but useful macroscopical classification. With this in mind, MING [22] classified diverse gastric cancers into two main types, expanding and infiltrative. According to his criteria, the types described in this paper as polypoid or fungating and as circumscribed excavated can be included with the expanding type, whereas the ulcerated and infiltrative type and the diffusely thickened type correspond to the infiltrative type.

Histological Features

In contrast to colorectal cancer, in which there is almost always a relatively simple histological picture of highly differentiated tubular or tubulopapillary adenocarcinoma composed of columnar epithelial cells, gastric cancer takes several histological forms even in its early stage, and this variability of the histology increases as the cancerous growth within the stomach progresses.

The wide variety in the histology of AGC is due mainly to the histological structure of normal gastric mucosa itself. For example, the mucosa covering the several parts of the stomach is composed histologically of fairly different glandular components, even though the basic structure of the mucosa is identical. In the fundus and corpus, most layers of the mucosa underlying the surface are composed of densely arranged and perpendicularly running fine tubules of fundic glands made up of mucous neck cells, parietal cells, and chief cells, while in the antrum the thinner layer of the lower half of the mucosa is composed of the acinar structures of pyloric glands; except for a few endocrine cells these contain no specifically differentiated cells and the appearance is the same as that of mucous glands elsewhere in the body. In the intermediate zone between corpus and antrum, which corresponds macroscopically to the mucosa of the angulus, the glands show transitional features from fundic to pyloric glands.

These histological features of normal gastric mucusa, together with the results obtained from the studies on cell kinetics of gastric mucosa with tritiated thymidine autoradiography, suggest that immature stem cells in the generative cell zone (G zone) situated in the neck zone between the foveolae and the gastric glands proper are the only epithelial cells that are capable of synthesizing DNA and undergoing mitosis, and they also have the latent potential for cell differentiation. The biologically different potential nature of the stem cells may be manifested as several histological features when they are transformed into malignant cells.

It has also been noticed that in some cases of AGC the original histological features of gastric cancer are modified not infrequently by secondary changes in the intramural tissue environment, such as circulatory disturbances, ulceration, fibrosis, or scar formation, and that this variability of the histological picture can sometimes be accelerated by intrinsic heterogeneity of the cancer. The multiple

24

development of gastric cancer of different histologies might be involved in this complex phenomenon in some cases.

Owing to this diversity, the histological features of AGC have been classified by different investigators into different types [7, 17, 18, 22–25, 31, 33, 34, 36]. Some investigators take the lesion showing least differentiated changes as their standard, as suggested by BRODERS [3], while others classify the cancer according to the lesions that have the most characteristic features, naming it mucoid, mucinous, mucocellular, diffuse-infiltrating, medullary, or scirrhous adenocarcinoma, etc. A histological classification of gastric cancer into two main types – intestinal and diffuse – was proposed by Laurén and Järvi in 1965 [21] and has been used recently by many investigators, contributing greatly to epidemiologic, geopathological, and chronological studies; but from the viewpoint of the histogenesis of gastric cancer, the classification seems to be in some measure inadequate or oversimple. At the present time, classification criteria are based mainly on grades of the glandular formation of the cancerous tissues showing predominant changes within the lesion. Classifications proposed by the World Health Organization and other organizations base their standards on this principle [11, 16, 37, 38, 40].

In my experience it seems most reasonable and practical to classify histological features of AGC into the following three types on the basis of the grade of glandular formation of the cancerous tissues (Fig. 15):

- Well-differentiated adenocarcinoma
- Moderately differentiated adenocarcinoma
- Poorly differentiated adenocarcinoma

Regardless of histological type, when the connective tissue stroma in the cancerous tissue is extremely sparse or extremely abundant, the above classification can be supplemented by the terms medullary or scirrhous pattern (e. g., well-differentiated medullary or poorly differentiated scirrhous adenocarcinoma).

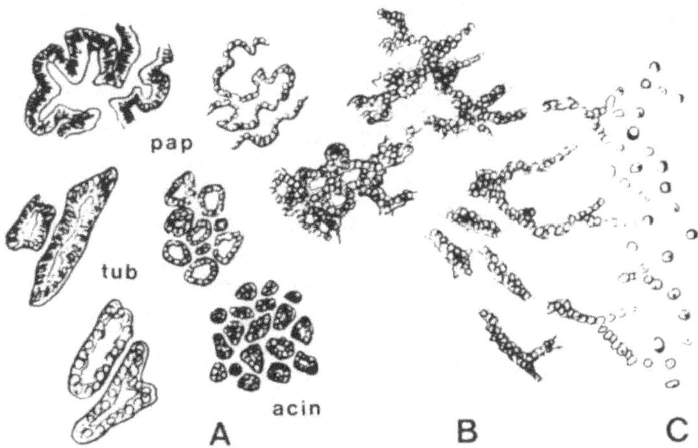

Fig. 15. Histological types of mucosal cancer: **A,** well-differentiated adenocarcinoma: **B,** moderately differentiated adenocarcinoma: **C,** poorly differentiated adenocarcinoma

Well-Differentiated Adenocarcinoma

This type of cancer is characterized histologically by high grades of glandular or tubular formation. For example, the lesion obviously has the structure of tubular, tubulopapillary, or cystopapillary adenocarcinomas when the glandular lumina are sufficiently wide. The adenocarcinomas of this type are composed of tall columnar epithelial cells, with a brush border sometimes containing goblet cells and Paneth's cells, and their elongated or oval nuclei show atypia, ranging from a relatively monotonous shape with regular arrangement to a more or less pleomorphic and piled-up distribution (Fig. 16).

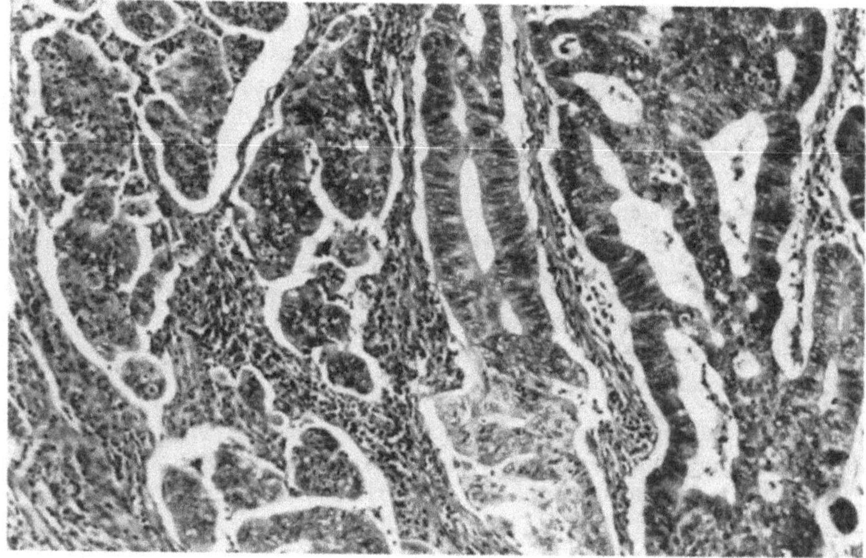

Fig. 16. Well-differentiated tubular and medullary adenocarcinoma composed of tall columnar epithelial cells (gastric cancer of intestinal type). (Pt no. 13 294, × 100)

The stroma of the cancer is generally sparse but rich in capillaries, especially when the cancerous tissues show polypoid protrusion, and focal degeneration or necrosis of cancerous tissue is quite often seen in the central part of the medullary cancer. In most cases, mucus production is entirely lost in the cancerous epithelial cells, but in others it is quite abundant and of the same kind as in mucinous, gelatinous, or mucoid adenocarcinoma.

Adenocarcinomas with this histology tend to grow massively inside and outside the stomach without losing the tight connection of the cancerous epithelial cells, while invasion of the cancer cells into the lymphatics and metastasis to regional lymph nodes are quite frequently seen in its advanced stages. Furthermore, direct invasion of the cancer cells into intra- and extramural venules, causing liver metastasis, is also not uncommon in this type.

Thus the histological and biologic nature of this type of cancer is similar in several respects to that of colorectal cancer, and for these reasons together with

26

the histochemical [10, 11] and electronmicroscopic findings [30], Laurén and Järvi named this type of gastric cancer the "intestinal type."

Moderately Differentiated Adenocarcinoma

Even though the glandular origin of the cancer is obvious from its structure, nests of cancerous tissue are relatively small and the cancerous epithelia forming the glands are mostly cuboidal or sometimes flat and lacking in brush border, goblet cells, and Paneth cells. Thus, unlike the case of the previous type, intestinal metaplasia of the cancerous epithelia is not apparent in this type (Fig. 17).

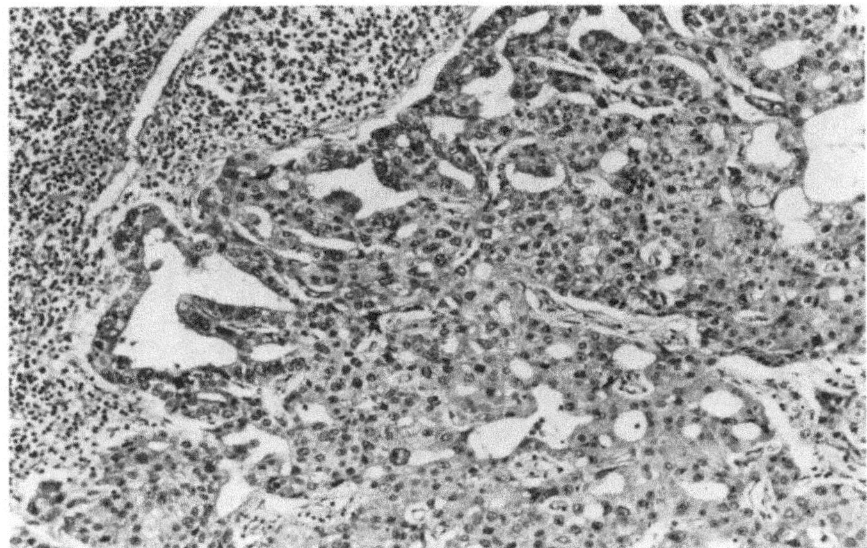

Fig. 17. Moderately differentiated adenocarcinoma of acinar or cribriform structure composed mainly of small cuboidal epithelial cells (gastric cancer of mixed intestinal and diffuse type). (Pt. no. 12955, × 100)

Adenocarcinoma of a purely tubular or tubulopapillary pattern is seldom seen, and most of the lesions show alveolar structures with several glandular patterns (e. g., cribriform, acinar, solid, reticular) similar in nature to those of lobular carcinoma of the breast. It is by no means uncommon to see cancerous tissues composed of this type of cancer intermingled with well-differentiated or poorly differentiated adenocarcinoma in a single focus, and both types quite often show transitional features. The amount of stroma is moderate in most cases, but a scirrhous lesion is not so rare. The border of the cancerous lesion with the surrounding tissue is not expanding and not infiltrating, but ragged or zig-zagged, and these features are well seen in low-power views of the histological specimens.

From the findings described above, it is said that this type corresponds neither to the intestinal type nor to the diffuse type as defined in the Laurén-Järvi classification, but rather has the nature of "gastric type" adenocarcinoma.

Poorly Differentiated Adenocarcinoma

In this type, the glandular formation of the cancerous tissues is very poor, and they often take the form of minute solid clusters, anastomosing or trabecular patterns composed of non-mucin-producing small immature cells, diffuse infiltration, or isolated cancer cells detached from the clusters or trabecules. In fact, the histological diagnosis of adenocarcinoma is often reached only on the basis of glandular arrangements faintly seen in some parts of the lesion (Fig. 18).

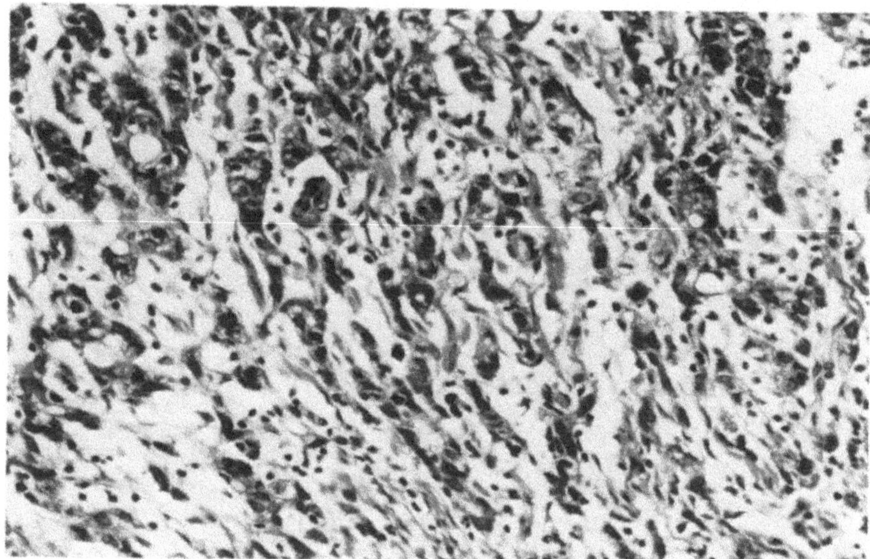

Fig. 18. Poorly differentiated adenocarcinoma showing trabecular and infiltrating growth pattern composed of small loosely connected cancer cells (gastric cancer of diffuse type). (Pt no. 14 860, ×200)

Unlike the cases of well and moderately differentiated adenocarcinoma, mutual cohesion of the cancer cells tends to cease, and the cells thus liberated infiltrate diffusely into the surrounding stroma. When small groups of cancer cells or free cells infiltrate diffusely into the submucosa or deeper layers they almost always provoke fibrous proliferation of the connective tissue by specific epithelial cell-mesenchyma correlation, and this growth pattern results in diffuse and desmoplastic changes of the gastric wall with ill-defined boundaries at advanced stages. Because of these macroscopical and microscopical characteristics, this type of cancer is often known clinically as scirrhous cancer.

Permeation of the cancer cells into the lymphatics, especially in the submucosa, is not uncommon, but invasion of cancer cells directly into venules is hardly ever seen. This type of cancer corresponds entirely to gastric cancer of diffuse type in the Laurén-Järvi classification, but poorly differentiated adenocarcinoma of the medullary type, which is also characterized by intense reactive formation of lymph follicles within the well-defined cancerous tissues cannot be excluded from this category.

Relationship Between Gross Appearances and Histological Features

Histological changes in gastric cancers are closely correlated with their gross appearances, and thus, the gross appearance of a cancer allows us to infer its histological nature.

In general, in any kind of AGC with a well-defined boundary visible on gross examination, such as large polypoid or fungating tumors (BORRMANN I) or large and deep excavations surrounded by elevated mucosa (BORRMANN II), the histological picture of well-differentiated adenocarcinoma is found, while carcinoma with an ill-defined boundary and shallow ulceration (BORRMANN III) or with diffuse thickening of the gastric wall and no prominent focal lesion (BORRMANN IV) is mostly accompanied by a histological picture of diffusely infiltrating and poorly differentiated adenocarcinoma of a scirrhous nature to some degree (Table 6).

Table 6. Relationship between macroscopical types and histological types

Histological type (grade of gld. differentiation) Macroscopical type	Well	Moderate	Poor	No. of cases	
Type I	90.7%	9.3%	0%	54	
Type II	74.4%	20.3%	5.3%	2024	Total
Type III	20.4%	32.9%	46.7%	828	3567
Type IV	5.5%	22.0%	72.5%	473	
Type 0	37.7%	39.4%	22.9%	188	

(Borrmann's classification)

Table 7. Crude correlation between macroscopical and histological types of AGC

Macroscopical	Histological
Borrmann I	Intestinal
Borrmann II	Intestinal
Borrmann III	Diffuse
Borrmann IV	Diffuse

As shown in Table 6, the correlation between macroscopical and histological findings in AGC is highest in the cases of BORRMANN I, followed by BORRMANN II and then BORRMANN IV. In the first two types, gastric cancer with an intestinal type of histology is far more frequent, while in the last type, diffuse histology predominates. In the case of BORRMANN III, no such close correlation is observed, even though the histology is inclined to be diffuse in type.

Characteristics of the above-mentioned correlation of the macroscopical types of AGC with their histological types are summarized (Table 7).

Changes in Frequency of Macro- and Microscopical
Types by Age and Sex of Patients and Year of Surgery

For 3567 cases of AGC surgically resected from 1953 to 1974, classification according to the age and sex of the patients was carried out. Most patients were in the 7th decade, followed by the 6th, 5th, 4th, 8th, and 3rd decades in that order. The sex ratio (m/f) was nearly 1.0 up to the age of 40, but subsequently became higher with advancing age. The overall sex ratio was 1.92 (Fig. 19).

Similar age and sex distributions of the patients were also observed on examination of 31 546 surgically resected stomachs, details of which were submitted to the WHO-CC. National Cancer Center in Tokyo from more than 100 institutions in Japan from 1963 to 1969 (Fig. 20).

It is well known that the gross appearance of AGC varies somewhat with patient age and sex. It became apparent from the statistics that in patients aged more

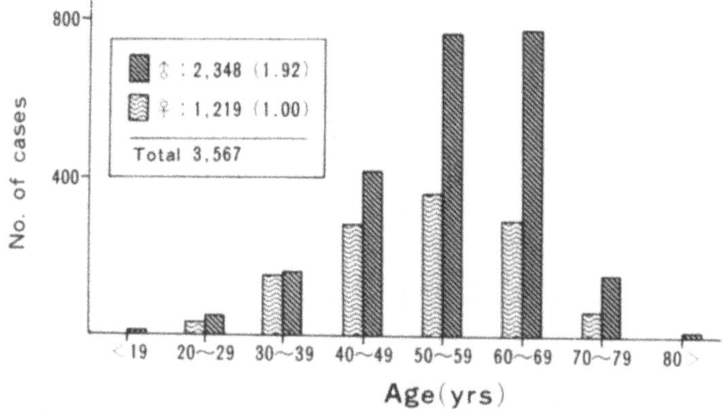

Fig. 19. Distribution of gastric cancer (not including EGC) by age and sex. (Yokoyama Hospital for Gastrointestinal Disease, 1953–1974)

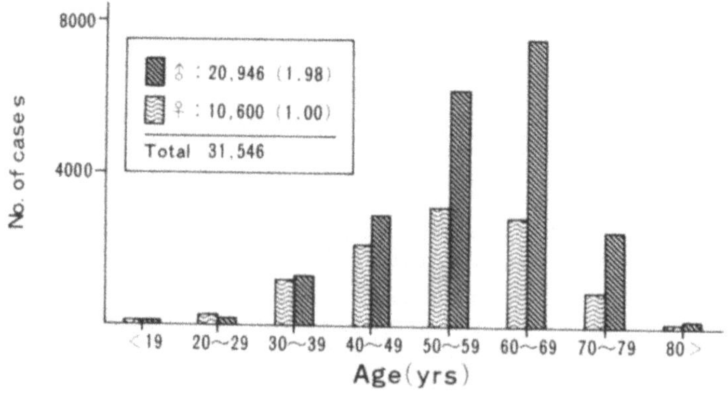

Fig. 20. Distribution of gastric cancer by age and sex. (Cases registered in 1963–1966 and in 1969 with the Japanese Research Society for Gastric Cancer and the National Cancer Center, Tokyo)

30

than 50 years most gastric cancers have the macroscopical appearance of Borrmann's type II in both sexes, while in patients under the age of 35 cancers with an ill-defined boundary, i.e., Borrmann's type III or IV, are relatively frequent. In the middle age group between 35 and 49 year old, especially in women, the pattern is more like that of the younger generation. It is also evident from Fig. 21 that in every decade up to the age of 65 years the frequency of Borrmann II is higher in male than in female patients, while the reverse applies to the frequency of Borrmann III and IV (Fig. 21).

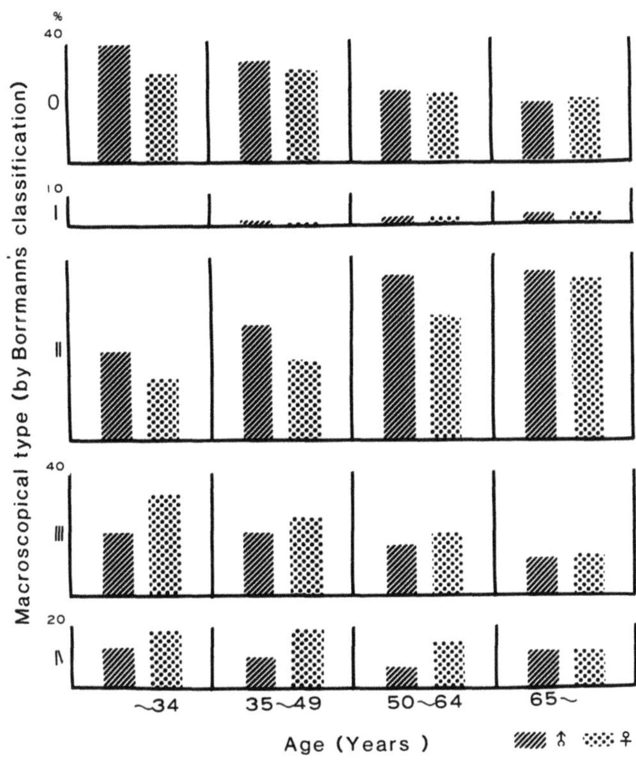

Fig. 21. Frequencies of different macroscopical types of gastric cancer by age and sex of patients

The differing frequency of the macroscopical types in the individual age groups becomes more obvious when compared in patients under 35 and over 65 years of age. In 305 patients under the age 35, Borrmann type 0 was the most frequent (33.8%), which means that macroscopical examination does not allow classification under any rubric in Borrmann's classification, most cases of this type being early or intermediate stages of cancerous growth, followed by types III (26.6%), II (24.9%), and IV (14.7%). Type I was not found at all in this group. In 924 patients over 65, in contrast, type II was extremely frequent (53.9%), followed by types 0 (18.8%), III (12.3%), IV (12.2%), and I (2.7%) (Fig. 22).

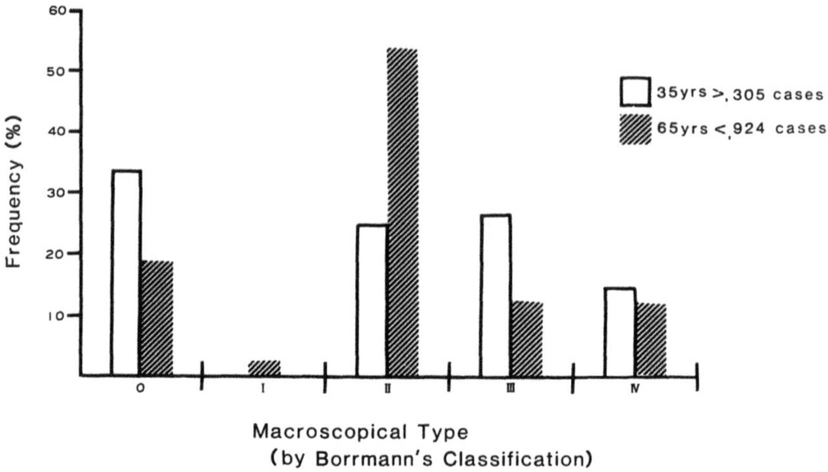

Fig. 22. Differing frequency of macroscopical types of gastric cancer in young and old patients

A comparison of patient age and histological types of cancer reveals that the two factors are closely correlated. For example, in 305 patients under 35 the highest frequency was that of low-grade glandular formation followed by middle-grade and high-grade glandular formation, while the order of frequency was exactly the opposite in 924 patients over 65. These results show that macroscopical and histological types of gastric cancer not only correlate with each other but are a morphological expression varying mainly with patient age (Fig. 23).

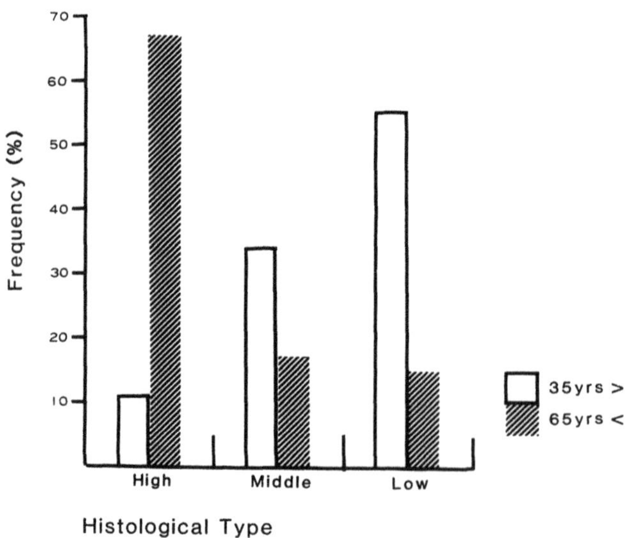

Fig. 23. Differing frequency of histological types of gastric cancer in young and old patients

32

A further statistical analysis of the same material was made from the chronological aspect. From this examination it became apparent that the frequency of BORRMANN's type II, which was more than 60% around 1955 in all AGC, is decreasing each year in both sexes, and has recently become a minor group. In contrast, the frequency of BORRMANN's types III and IV, which constituted a minor group at the beginning of the examination, increased in proportion with the passage of the years. A tendency for Borrmann's type 0 to be more frequent among the surgically resected stomachs at 10-year intervals is also apparent (Figs. 24 and 25).

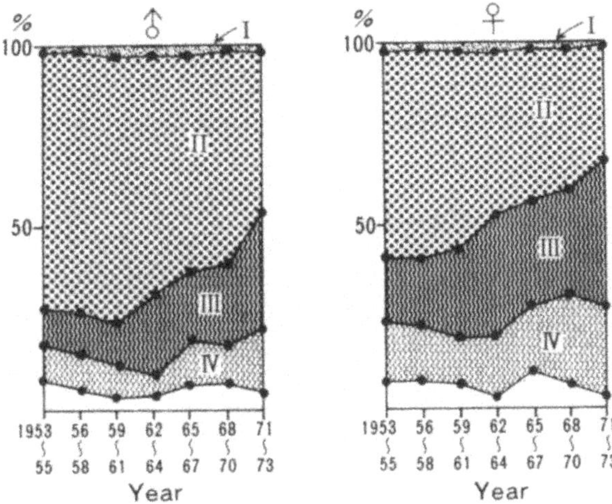

Fig. 24. Changes over time in the relative frequencies of macroscopical types of gastric cancers by Borrmann's classification

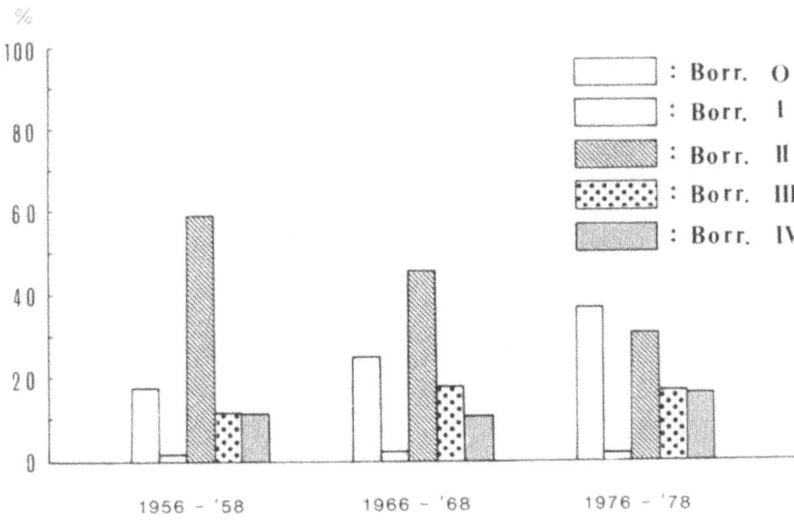

Fig. 25. Changes over time in the relative frequencies of macroscopical types of cancer in stomachs resected for cancer (10 years interval)

It is already known from epidemiologic and geopathological studies that the relative frequency of the intestinal and diffuse types of gastric cancer varies fairly widely among the nations of high- and low-risk countries [4, 8, 18, 27], and even within one country that frequency changes with the passage of time [15, 26, 28, 29]. For example, the frequency of intestinal-type cancer is significantly higher in high-risk countries than in low-risk ones, while in the case of diffuse-type cancer the situation is reversed. Thus, the ratio of the two types is not stable but labile in every country, probably because of changes in the social, nutritional, and medical environment. On the basis of the results described above, it can safely be said that a decreasing frequency of Borrmann's type II indicates a declining tendency of the occurrence of intestinal-type gastric cancer, while an increasing frequency of Borrmann's types III and IV suggests a relative increase in the frequency of diffuse-type gastric cancer. It is concluded from these statistics that the pattern of gastric cancer in Japan is changing from that of a high-risk country to that of a low-risk country, even though the change is still not very prominent.

Site of Development

Gastric cancer can occur in any part of the stomach. In general terms the lower third of the stomach, i.e., antrum and prepylorus, has the highest incidence (51.6%), followed by the middle third – angulus and the adjacent area (32.3%) –

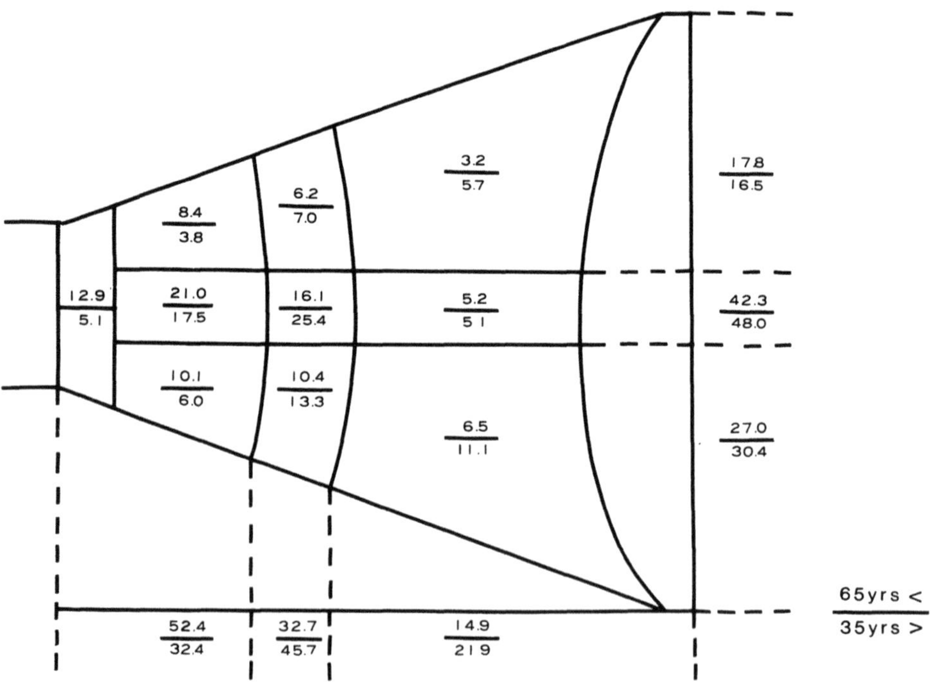

Fig. 26. Differences in relative frequency of sites of development of gastric cancer (%) by patient age

and the upper third, i. e., corpus, fundus, and cardia, has the lowest (16.1%). The macroscopically recognizable types of AGC tend to develop at characteristic sites. In the cases of BORRMANN I no preferential site can be cited, while more than half (55.3%) the cases of Borrmann II cancer occurred in the antrum. Similar results with reference to occurrence were observed with BORRMANN III. In contrast, in cases of BORRMANN IV, the focus of the cancerous lesion was most often (40.6%) located in the angulus and the frequency of cancers in the corpus was higher than average in this group (Table 5).

The relative frequency at different sites of development, however, varied according to the age of the patients. In patients over 65 years the antrum was most often (52.4%) affected by cancer, but in patients under 35 years cancers were most often (45.7%) found in the angulus (Fig. 26).

Several aspects of AGC described above are summarized (Table 8).

Table 8. Data recorded in a sample of 3771 cases of AGC (1955–1978)

Macroscopical type (Borrmann)	No. of cases	Frequency (%)	Av. age (years)	Sex ratio (m/f)	Preferential site
I	79	2.1	59.0	2.4	None
II	2215	58.7	56.3	2.6	Antrum
III	907	24.1	51.3	1.4	Antrum and angulus
IV	570	15.1	52.7	1.1	Angulus and corpus

Terminal Stage

By autonomous, progressive, and invasive growth not only within the stomach but outside of it, AGC advances into the remote organs and sooner or later reaches the terminal stage. There are various growth patterns of AGC outside the stomach:

a) local extension or diffuse infiltration to the surrounding organs;
b) widespread dissemination to the omentum, peritoneum or serosa of the intestine; and
c) metastasis into remote organs by the way of the lymphatics or blood vessels.

The growth characteristics of AGC are by no means random, however, but are subject to certain tendencies according to the macroscopical and histological nature of the cancers. For this reason, we can roughly estimate the prognosis of surgically resected cancers not only from the grade of their intramural growth but also from several of their histological features.

As described previously, AGC can be classified histologically into the three main types:

a) well, b) moderately, and c) poorly differentiated adenocarcinoma, but for the purposes of this discussion dealing with autopsied case of gastric cancer, which were reported in several ways by different pathologists, some modification and summarization of the classification seems to be necessary.

The cases reported as (a) tubular, tubulopapillary, papillary or villous adenocarcinoma and (b) mucinous, mucoid, or gelatinous carcinoma in the autopsy record, can be classed together as well-differentiated adenocarcinoma or gastric cancer of the intestinal type, while the cases reported as carcinoma simplex, adenocarcinoma acinosum, scirrhous cancer, small cell cancer or signet-ring cell carcinoma might be classed jointly as poorly differentiated adenocarcinoma or gastric cancer of diffuse type; but (c) anaplastic carcinoma with medullary stroma which shows no infiltrative growth but has a well-defined boundary, might also be included in this category.

On the basis of the criteria described above, the histological nature of AGC and its mode of growth outside the stomach were reviewed on autopsied cases, which were reported every year by pathological institutions throughout Japan to the Japanese Pathological Society; the summarized data, with the final diagnosis for every case, are published as the Annual Record of Autopsied Cases. In all, 39 021 autopsy cases were reported in the Record in 1981, and these cases were used for the study. Among the cases recorded, malignant neoplasms were 20 499 (52.5%), and a diagnosis of gastric carcinoma was made after the autopsy in 3738 (18.2% of all the malignant neoplasms). Of these 3738 cases, those recorded simply as "adenocarcinoma" and those death occurring shortly after surgical gastrectomy without metastasis were excluded from the statistics and the remaining 1063 cases were classified by the descriptions in the Record into well-differentiated and poorly differentiated adenocarcinoma. The number of cases grouped in the former class was 301 (28.3%) and the number allocated to the latter, 762 (71.7%).

As pointed out previously by several investigators [9, 19, 32, 35, 42], it is also apparent from this examination that the main cause of death in gastric cancer with the histology of well-differentiated adenocarcinoma was liver metastasis (47.9%), but the "peritoneal type," characterized mainly by cancerous infiltration into the peritoneum, was also not infrequent (43.5%). Hematogenous metastasis to other remote organs such as lung, pleura, bone, and ovary was relatively infre-

Table 9. Relationship between macroscopical type and degree of histological differentiation in autopsied cases of gastric cancer from the viewpoint of mode of growth

Macroscopical type / Histological type	Peritoneal		Hepatic		Other		Total no. of cases
	No.	%	No.	%	No.	%	
Well-differentiated adenocarcinoma	131	43.5	144	47.9	26	8.6	301
Poorly differentiated adenocarcinoma	590	77.4	89	11.7	83	10.9	762

Table 10. Relationship between macroscopical and histological types of well-differentiated adenocarcinomas among autopsied cases of gastric cancer

Histological type \ Macroscopical type	Peritoneal %	Hepatic %	Other %	Total no. of cases
Tubular	35.3	53.5	11.4	167
Papillary	37.8	56.1	6.1	82
Mucinous	78.9	17.3	3.8	52
Total	43.5	47.9	8.6	301

quent (8.6%) in this group. However, when the above frequencies were analyzed from the viewpoint of the three histological subtypes, the relative frequency of the "hepatic type" was significantly higher in tubular or papillary adenocarcinoma than in mucinous adenocarcinoma, while in about 80% of the cases diagnosed as mucinous adenocarcinoma peritoneal involvement was the main change (Tables 9 and 10).

On the other hand, more than 75% of AGC cases with the histology of poorly differentiated adenocarcinoma had the growth characteristics of the peritoneal type, and many of them were recorded as "peritonitis carcinomatosa." The frequency of the hepatic type was far lower (11.7%) than that of the peritoneal type, while that of metastasis into remote organs such as lung, pleura, bone, and ovary was a little higher. It was also noted that the hepatic type was significantly more frequent in the anaplastic, medullary type of cancer than in the other two subtypes (Table 11).

Table 11. Relationship between macroscopical and histological types of poorly differentiated adenocarcinomas among autopsied cases of gastric cancer

Histological type \ Macroscopical type	Peritoneal %	Hepatic %	Other %	Total no. of cases
Glandular	77.5	12.7	9.8	560
Mucocellular scirrhous	84.3	1.3	14.4	160
Anaplastic medullary	50.0	38.1	11.9	42
Total	77.4	11.7	10.9	762

From these results, it can be said that the mode of growth of AGC is more varied outside the stomach than in the stomach, but there are trends in the mode of growth according to the histological nature of the cancer that has developed in the stomach. It was confirmed by the examination of these autopsy records that the major site of metastasis in gastric cancer with an intestinal-type histology was the liver and that in the nonintestinal type was the peritoneum.

References

1. Aschoff L (1936) Das Karzinom des Magens. In: Pathologische Anatomie, Spezieller Teil. Fischer, Jena, pp 330–337
2. Borrmann R (1926) Makroskopische Formen des vorgeschritteten Magenkrebses. In: Henke F, Lubarsch O (eds) Handbuch der speziellen pathologischen Anatomie und Histologie, vol 4/1. Springer, Berlin
3. Broders AC (1941) The microscopic grading of cancer. Surg Clin North Am 21: 947–962
4. Correa P, Sasano N, Stemmermann GN, Haenszel W (1973) Pathology of gastric carcinoma in Japanese populations: Comparison between Miyagi Prefecture, Japan and Hawaii. J Natl Cancer Inst 51: 1449–1459
5. Eder M (1984) Magentumoren. In: Eder M, Gedigk P (eds) Lehrbuch der allgemeinen Pathologie und pathologischen Anatomie, 31st edn. Springer, Berlin Heidelberg New York Tokyo, pp 534–538
6. Evans RW (1956) Histological appearances of tumours. Livingstone, Edinburgh, pp 426–452 (Chap 21: Epithelial tumours of the alimentary canal)
7. Hermanek P (1982) Surgical pathology. The TNM system. Langenbecks Arch Chir 358: 57–63
8. Imai T (1968) Some comments on the geographical-pathologic aspects of gastric carcinogenesis. Gann Monogr 3: 123–127
9. Ishii T, Ikegami N, Hosoda Y, Koide O, Kaneko M (1981) The biological behaviour of gastric cancer. J Pathol 134: 97–115
9a. Japanese Pathological Society (ed) (1982) Annual of the autopsy cases in Japan. Vol 24 (Jan–Dec 1981) (in japanese)
10. Japanese Research Society for Gastric Cancer (1981) The general rules for the gastric cancer study in surgery and pathology. Jpn J Surg 11: 127–145
11. Järvi O, Nevalainen T, Ekfors T, Kulatunga A (1974) The classification and histogenesis of gastric cancer. Excerpta Med Int Congr Ser 6: 228–234
12. Järvi O, Laurèn P (1952) On the pathogenesis of gastric cancer. Acta Unio Int Contra Cancrum 8: 393–394
13. Kajitani T (1981) The general rules for the gastric cancer study in surgery and pathology. Part I. Clinical classification. Jpn J Surg 11: 127–139
14. Kajitani T (1976) Surgical treatment for gastric cancer. Their contribution to improvement in the five-year survival rate. Asian Med J 19: 915–935
15. Kato Y, Kitagawa T, Nakamura K, Sugano H (1981) Changes in the histologic types of gastric carcinoma in Japan. Cancer 48: 2084–2087
16. Kennedy BJ (1970) TNM classification for stomach cancer. Cancer 26: 971–983
17. Kim KH, Chi CH, Lee SK, Lee D, Kubo T (1972) Histologic types of gastric carcinoma among Koreans. Cancer 29: 1261–1263
18. Kubo T (1974) Geographical pathology of gastric carcinoma. Acta Pathol Jpn 24: 465–479
19. Kubo T, Imai T (1971) Intestinal metaplasia of gastric mucosa in autopsy materials in Hiroshima and Yamaguchi districts. Gann 62: 49–53
20. Kuru M, Sano R (1967) Histopathological study of gastric carcinoma in the Japanese. UICC Monogr Ser 10
21. Laurèn P (1965) The two histological main types of gastric carcinoma, diffuse and so-called intestinal type carcinoma. An attempt at a histo-clinical classification. Acta Pathol Microbiol Scand 64: 31–49
22. Ming SC (1977) Gastric carcinoma. A pathological classification. Cancer 39: 2475–2485
23. Ming SC (1973) Tumours of the esophagus and stomach. Atlas of tumor pathology 2, sect 7. AFIP, Washington
24. Morson BC, Dawson IMP (1972) Macroscopic features and topography. Gastrointestinal pathology. Blackwell, Oxford
25. Mulligan RM, Rember RR (1954) Histogenesis and biologic behavior of gastric carcinoma. Study of one hundred thirty-eight cases. Arch Pathol 58: 1–25
26. Muñoz N, Connelly R (1971) Time trends of intestinal and diffuse types of gastric cancer in the United States. Int J Cancer 8: 158–164
27. Muñoz N, Correa P, Cuello C, Duque E (1968) Histologic type of gastric carcinoma in high- and low-risk areas. Int J Cancer 3: 809–818

28. Nagata T, Ikeda M, Nakayama F (1983) Changing state of gastric cancer in Japan. Histologic perspective of the past 76 years. Am J Surg 145: 226–233
29. Nagayo T, Yokoyama H (1978) Recent changes in the morphology of gastric cancer in Japan. Int J Cancer 21: 407–412
30. Nevalainen T, Järvi O (1977) Ultrastructure of intestinal and diffuse type gastric carcinoma. J Pathol 122: 129–136
31. Oota K, Tanaka N (1952) Histological types of gastric carcinomas and their topographical incidence. Gann 43: 367–370
32. Stalsberg H (1972) Histological typing of gastric carcinoma. A comparison of surgical and autopsy materials and of primary tumours and metastases. Acta Pathol Microbiol Scand 80: 509–514
33. Stout AP (1953) Tumors of the stomach. Atlas of tumor pathology, sect 6. AFIP, Washington
34. Sugano H, Nakamura K, Kato Y (1982) Pathological studies of human gastric cancer. Acta Pathol Jpn [Suppl 2] 32: 329–347
35. Takeda K (1955) Cancer of the stomach in Japan from the viewpoint of pathological anatomy. Schweiz Z Pathol Bakteriol 18: 538–550
36. Takizawa N (1972) Histopathological classification of gastric carcinoma for standard reporting system used in Japan. Acta Pathol Jpn 22: 11–18
37. Tsukamoto K, Gaitan-Yanguas M (1973) A system for registration and classification of the stomach cancer for WHO International Reference Center. Jpn J Clin Oncol 12: 117–128
38. UICC/AJC (1973) TNM classification of malignant tumors of breast, larynx, stomach, cervix uterii, corpus uterii. Arch Geschwulstforsch 41: 373–381
39. Wanke M (1971) Magen-Carcinome. In: Doerr W, Seifert G, Uehlinger E (eds) Spezielle pathologische Anatomie, vol 2/1. Springer, Berlin Heidelberg New York, pp 594–716
40. WHO-CC (1980) The present status of diagnosis and treatment of cancer in countries participating in WHO-CC for stomach cancer. Ichikawa H (ed) WHO-CC Monograph, no 3. National Cancer Center, Tokyo
41. Willis RA (1953) Carcinoma of the stomach. Pathology of tumours. Butterworth, London, pp 391–411
42. Yamamoto T, Kato H (1971) Two major histological types of gastric carcinoma among the fixed population of Hiroshima and Nagasaki. Gann 62: 381–387

4. Morphology of Early Gastric Cancer and Related Subjects

Definition of Early Gastric Cancer and its Significance

Early gastric cancer (EGC) is defined as a cancer whose growth is limited to the gastric mucosa (mucosal cancer) or invades the submucosa but not the muscularis propria (submucosal cancer), regardless of the size and shape of the cancer (Fig. 27).

Thus the definition is based on grades of invasion of the cancerous tissue into the layers composing the gastric wall. A definite diagnosis of EGC is therefore

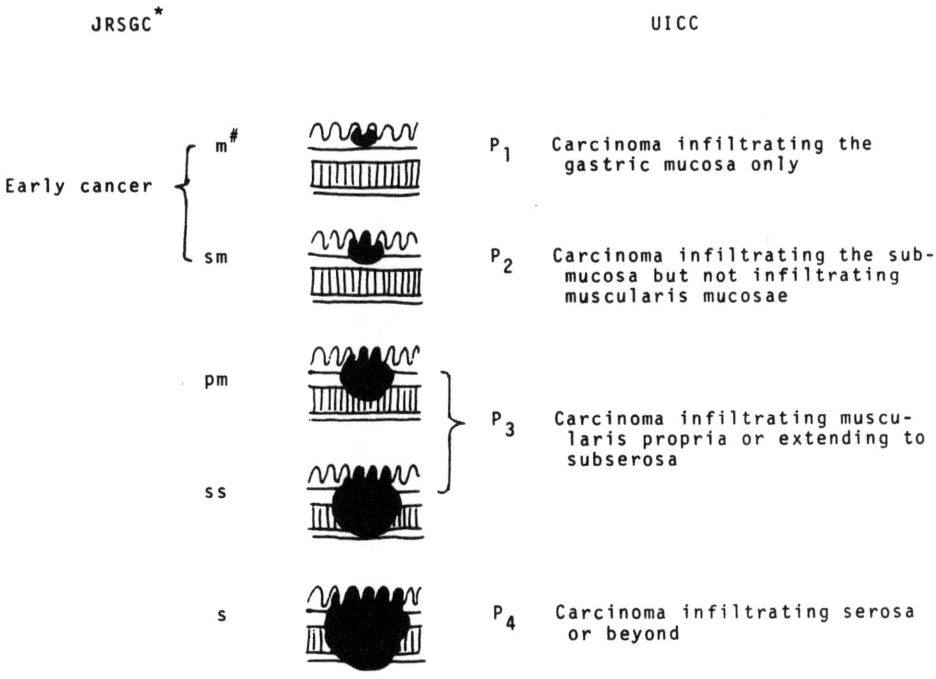

* Japanese Research Society for Gastric Cancer

Including muscularis mucosae

Fig. 27. Grading of degree of growth of gastric cancer (expressed in terms of the deepest layer invaded by cancer cells) not made without a histological examination of the resected stomach, but comparison of roentgenologic and endoscopic features of several stages and several types of gastric cancers, with the macroscopical and histological findings obtained in the resected stomachs, it can now be said that EGC is diagnosed with a fairly high degree of certainty not only by macroscopical examinations of resected stomachs but also by preoperative X-ray and endoscopic examinations.

The problem of whether submucosal cancer should be included in the category of EGC or not has been discussed from several aspects, mainly because metastases to the regional lymph nodes are not so rare in this group. But follow-up studies over more than 5 years in patients who had undergone surgical resection of the stomach revealed that complete recovery from this stage is highly likely except for a few types of submucosal cancer, which can recur even when the cancerous tissue and the lymph nodes have been completely extirpated. From these experiences and the results of examination, the definition of EGC came to be generally agreed upon among clinicians and pathologists throughout the world.

Grades and patterns of the cancerous invasion of the submucosa are various. In fact, there are some cases in which only a few, or small groups of, cancer cells infiltrate the upper layer of the submucosa, while in others large and well-demarcated cancerous masses occupy a large proportion of the submucosa and press the muscularis propria downwards while not invading it, owing to their expansive mode of growth. Some of these cases have gross appearances applicable to the macroscopical classification of AGC. The 5- and 10-year survival rates after surgical resection are lower in this type of EGC than the other type. For this reason, some investigators have stressed that the term "early gastric cancer" should be confined to mucosal cancer only, while others tried to subclassify submucosal cancer into two or three grades, including only its mildest grade under EGC, to make the term more specific, but neither this strict definition of EGC nor the subclassification of submucosal cancer has gained general acceptance, because of the difficulty of applying these criteria in routine work.

From the standpoint of linguistics, the name "early gastric cancer" is not correct and the concept would be more precisely expressed by "early/earlier stage of growth" of gastric cancer. I used to use this name in scientific papers as shorthand form for the concept. Some foreign investigators have preferred to use the name "superficial cancer" instead of EGC, but as will be described later on, superficial gastric cancer is a type of EGC and not synonymous with EGC. Anyway, it is more important to note here that the term early gastric cancer signifies that it is completely curable when it is clinically detected and surgically resected at this growing stage.

Age and Sex of Patients with EGC

The pattern of age and sex distribution in 1098 cases of EGC was similar to that in AGC. However, more precise comparison of the figures for EGC and AGC (Fig. 19) reveals that the relative frequency of patients aged 40–49 among all pat-

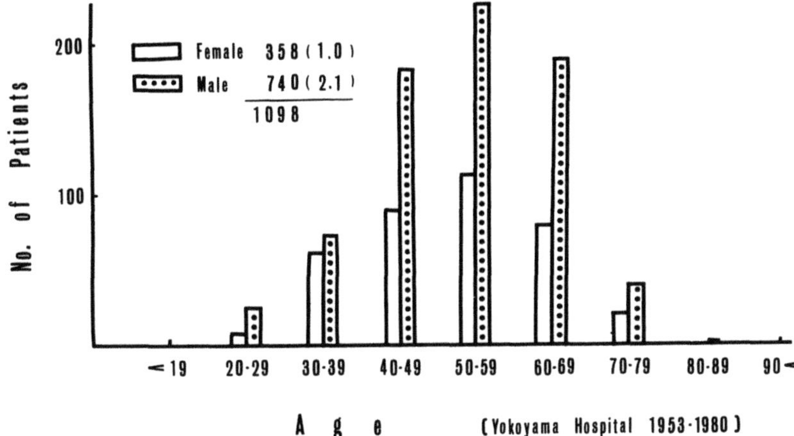

Fig. 28. Distribution of gastric cancer patients (EGC only) by age and sex. (Yokoyama Hospital, 1953–1980)

ients is significantly higher in EGC than in AGC. This means that the average age of patients is lower in EGC than in AGC (Fig. 28).

Gross Appearances and Histological Features of EGC

Owing to its several histological and histogenetic natures, gastric cancer takes various macroscopical forms even in its early stage. Some cases, for example, show a polypoid protrusion similar to adenomatous polyp of the stomach, and others are difficult to differentiate from a chronic peptic ulcer. Besides these cases, there are several types of EGC showing neither striking protrusion nor any ulceration of the affected mucosa, but with slight or superficial changes which might be overlooked on purely clinical examination.

Before 1955, cancerous lesions with such superficial changes were quite difficult to detect clinically, but since then, thanks to the remarkable progress made in diagnosis with double-contrast X-ray examination and fibergastroscopy [20], it has become feasible to detect even such slight cancerous lesions with no great technical difficulty. Owing to these newly developed diagnostic methods, the number of clinically detectable cases of EGC increased rapidly in the 1960s.

Under these circumstances, the Japanese Endoscopical Society asked those of its members who had had wide experience in gastric cancer, including myself, to establish new standard criteria for the macroscopical classification of EGC. After several discussion and deliberation with reference to photographs and slides, the macroscopical classification system for EGC was established in 1962 and the classification was adopted by Japanese Research Society for Gastric Cancer (JRSGC). Details of the proceedings were reported by MURAKAMI [34], Chairman of the Committee, and as he stressed in this report, the classification was

43

based exclusively on the macroscopical appearances of EGC, histogenetical considerations such as polyp cancer or ulcer cancer being eliminated from the classification (Fig. 29).

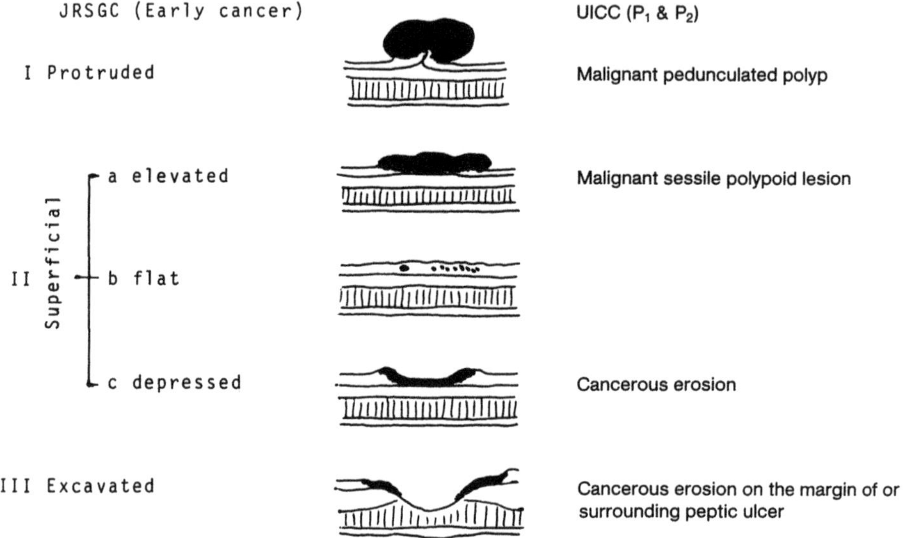

Fig. 29. Macroscopical classification of EGC adopted by JRSGC

The following classification of my own for EGC is not basically different from that proposed by the Committee, but from the standpoint of histology and histogenesis some modification has been made.

- Polypoid protruding type
- Broad-based, elevated type
- Focal depressed type
- Large eroded type
- Peptically ulcerated type

Polypoid Protruding Type

This type of EGC (type I in the Japanese classification) is characterized macroscopically by polypoid protrusion of the mucosa with a clear boundary from the surrounding mucosa (Figs. 30 and 31). The number, site, size, and shape of the protrusions vary in each case. No preferential site can be cited, in contrast to the other types. Rather, tumorous protrusions can be seen in any part of the stomach, even though the frequency is slightly higher in the antrum than in the angulus or in the corpus (Fig. 32).

Most of the tumors are not large, having a maximum diameter of less than 2 cm (Fig. 33). The shape of the protruding lesions is also not so irregular as in AGC,

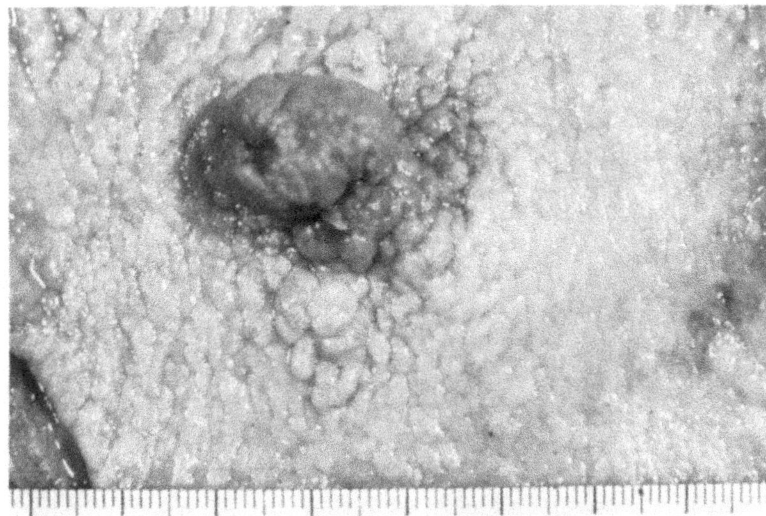

Fig. 30. EGC in form of hemispheric protrusion (type I in the Japanese classification) in the antrum. Surface of the protrusion is lobulated but relatively smooth. (Pt. no. 13 258, 68 years, m)

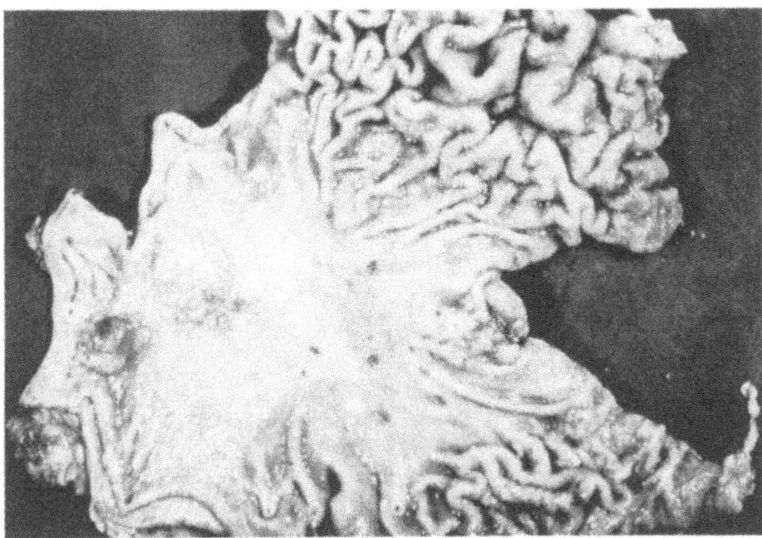

Fig. 31. Polypoid protruding type (type I) of EGC. Note the clear boundary from the surrounding mucosa. (Pt no. 12 286, 64 years, m)

and hemispheric and lobulated structures of the tumor can be seen in most cases. Most of the protrusions are sessile, the pedunculated form being quite rare. The surface of the polypoid protrusions is not so smooth as that of nonmalignant ones, but not so uneven as in AGC. It can assume a finely granular, an irregular nodular, a multilobular, a villous, or a cauliflower-like appearance: when a large

45

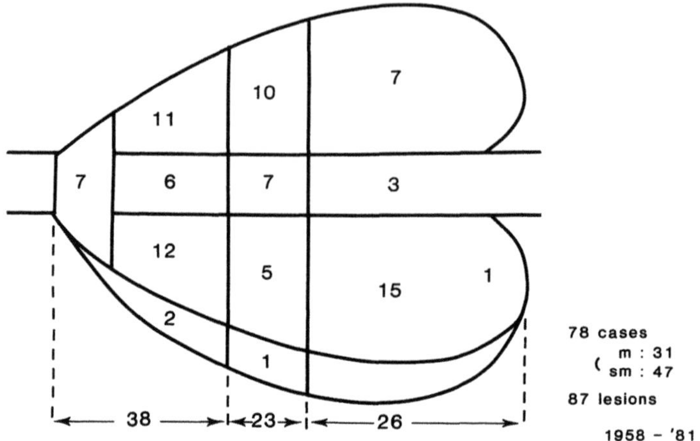

Fig. 32. Sites of development of polypoid protruding EGC (type I)

protruded mass has an irregularly nodular appearance, indentation of its surface may be seen in the central parts of the lesion but deep ulceration is seldom seen. Polypoid protrusions are not infrequently discolored by anemia, congestion, or hemorrhage.

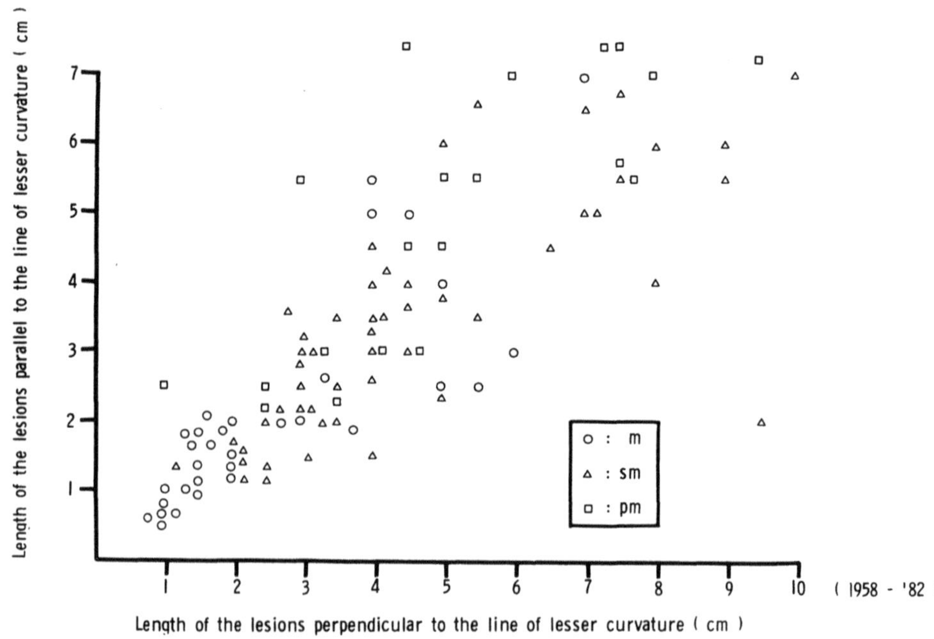

Fig. 33. Relationship between size and depth of type I cancerous lesions (polypoid mucosal protrusion)

46

About 87% of EGC cases of this type are unifocal in origin, but double or triple cancers are occasionally seen. In rare cases, malignant transformation of one or two polyps among multiple polyps is seen.

Most cases of EGC of this type show the histological picture of well-differentiated tubular or tubulopapillary adenocarcinoma, composed of tall columnar epithelial cells. This type is characterized by upward growth of foveolar epithelial

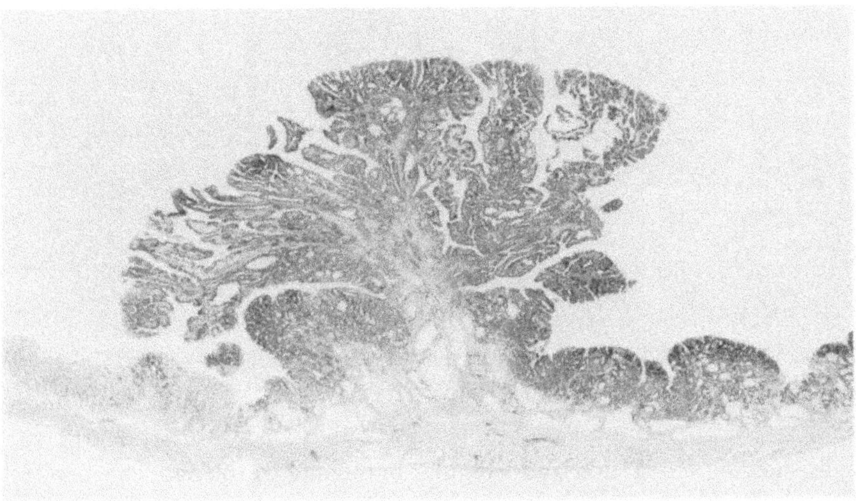

Fig. 34. Histological picture of the lesion shown in Fig. 30. Hemispheric protrusion shows adenomalike, well-differentiated tubular adenocarcinoma. Broad-based mucosal elevation is seen at the base of the protrusion. (Pt no. 13 258, × 4)

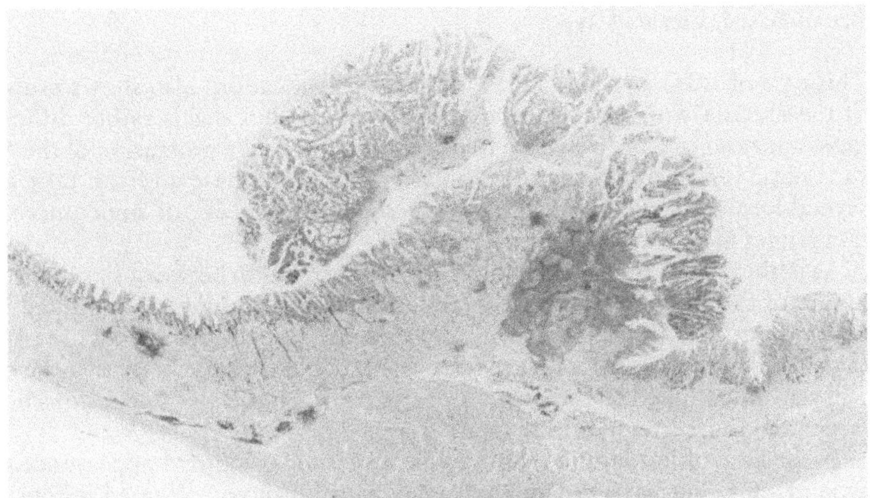

Fig. 35. Histological picture of the lesion shwon in Fig. 31. Hemispheric protrusion adjacent to the duodenum shows tubulopapillary adenocarcinoma with submucosal invasion. (Pt no. 12 286, × 6)

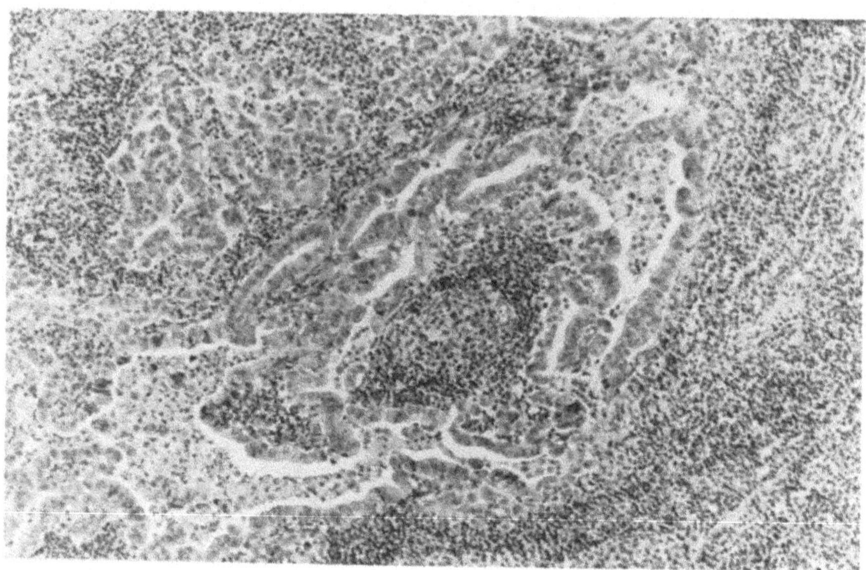

Fig. 36. Higher magnification of a part of the submucosal invasion shown in Fig. 35. Invaded cancerous tissue is surrounded by intense lymphoid reaction. (Pt no. 12 286, × 100)

cells showing elongation and irregular branching of the papillary projections of the tubules. Connective tissue stroma of the cancerous tissue is sparse in general and made up mostly of capillaries. Lymph node metastasis is not uncommon, especially when the cancerous tissue invades into the submucosa, but is never seen in cases of mucosal cancer (Figs. 34–36).

Broad-Based, Elevated Type

This type of EGC (type II a in the Japanese classification) also shows protrusion of the mucosa with a well-demarcated boundary, but this is rather different in gross appearance from polypoid mucosal protrusion: the protrusion of the mucosa is not hemispheric but relatively flat with a broad base and can take any of several forms, resembling plateaus, flowerbeds, coral reefs, or sometimes mountain ranges in appearance (Figs. 37 and 38).

As in the case of the previous type, a close correlation between size and surface nature of the elevated lesion and grade of the cancerous invasion is noted in this type. About 62% of the cases with intramucosal cancer occupy an area smaller than 3 cm^2, and their surfaces are relatively flat, but the possibility that the cancer will remain confined to the mucosa decreases when the elevated lesions become larger and more irregular in shape (Fig. 39).

In the case of borderline lesions, which are similar in gross appearance to this type of EGC but have no apparent malignant histology, elevated lesions occupying more than 2 cm^2 are exceptional and the surface is relatively smooth and grayish-white.

48

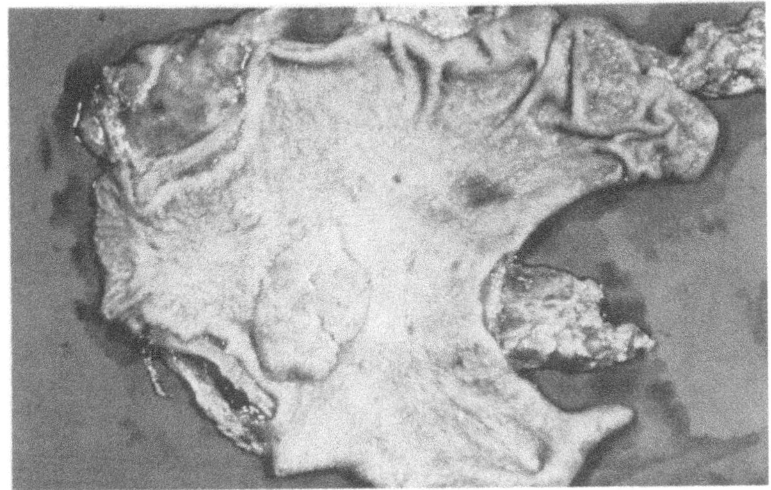

Fig. 37. EGC with large flat mucosal elevation (type IIa, m) in the antrum. The surface of the mucosa is relatively flat but is composed of irregularly shaped nodules. (Pt no. 13 219, 59 years, m)

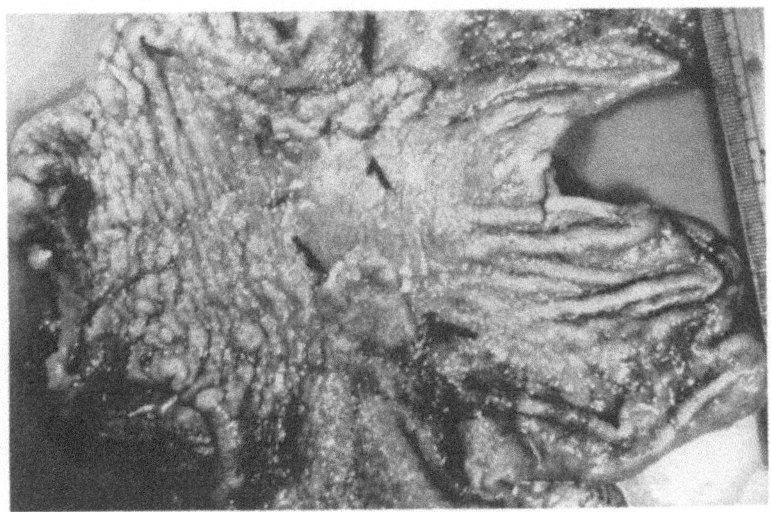

Fig. 38. Flat mucosal elevations (type IIa, sm) in anterior and posterior part of the angulus (arrows). Surface of the mucosa is slightly indented. (Pt no. 4230, 59 years, m)

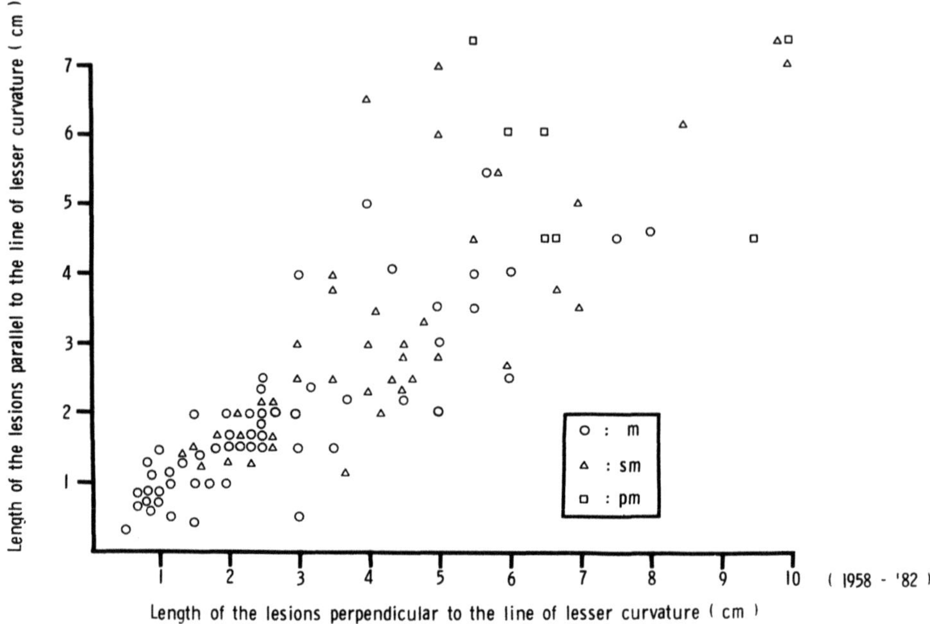

Fig. 39. Relationship between size and depth of type II a cancerous lesions (broad-based mucosal elevation)

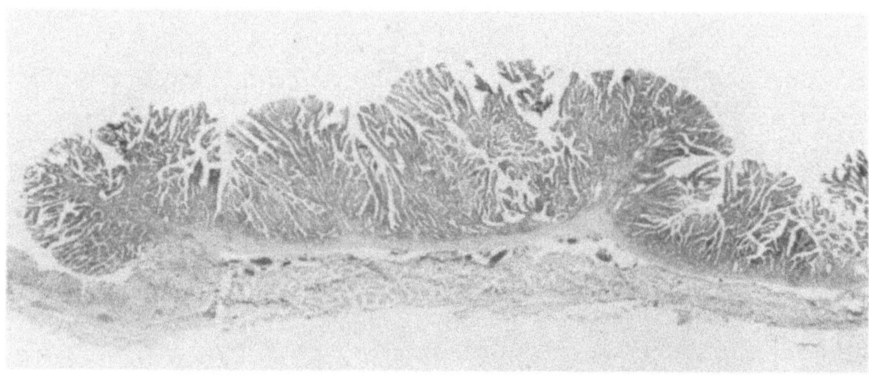

Fig. 40. Histological picture of the lesion shown in Fig. 37. Elevated mucosa is composed entirely of tubular adenocarcinoma with few connective tissue stroma. (Pt no. 13 219, × 3.5)

50

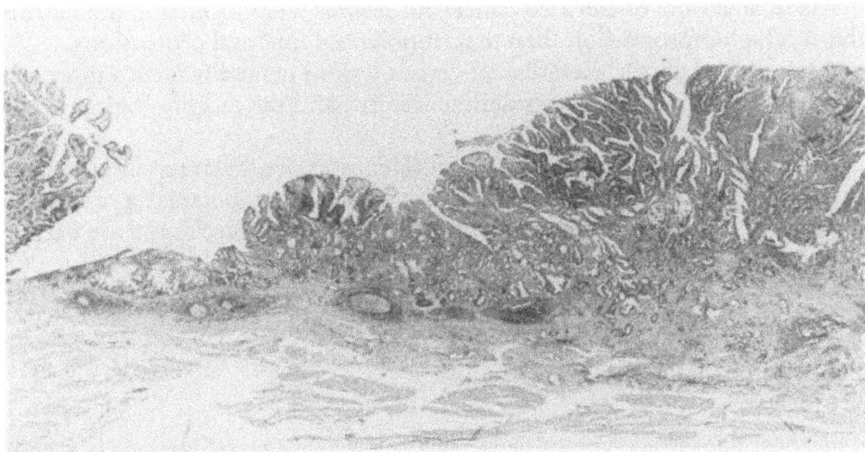

Fig. 41. Histological picture of the anterior side of the mucosal elevation in Fig. 38. Elevated but partly indented mucosa shows tubular adenocarcinoma. Submucosal invasion is seen in right half of the picture. (Pt no. 4230, × 10)

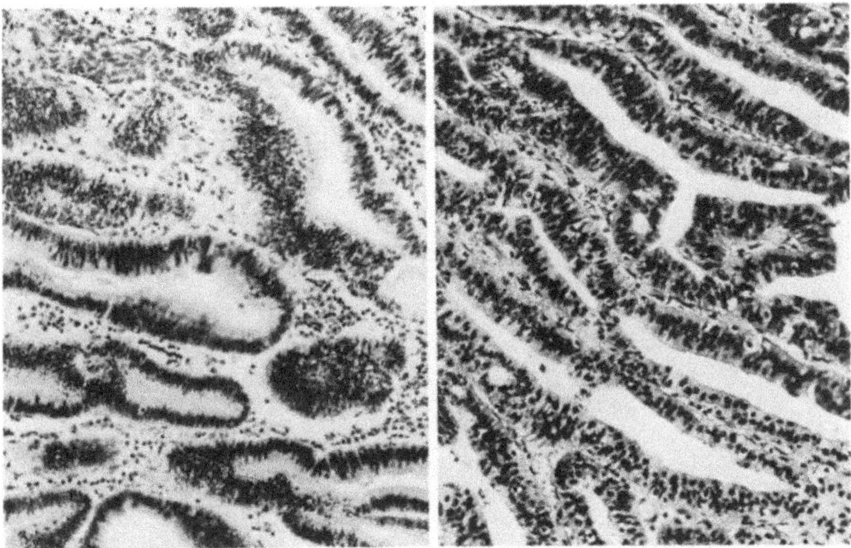

Fig. 42. Higher magnification of the view shown in Fig. 41. Most of the elevated mucosa shows obvious tubulopapillary adenocarcinoma *(right half)*, but its peripheral part shows highly differentiated tubular adenocarcinoma, which is difficult to differentiate from adenoma *(left half)*. (Pt no. 4230, × 100)

More than 60% of elevated cancerous lesions were located in the antrum, and this is a higher proportion than that of polypoid mucosal protrusions.

As described above, elevated cancerous lesions generally have a more irregular shape and surface than do borderline lesions, and the morphological irregularity is indicative of malignancy.

Most EGC of this type has histological features of tubular or villotubular adenocarcinoma surrounded by severe grades of intestinal metaplasia, and cases with features of moderately to poorly differentiated adenocarcinoma are exceptionally rare (Figs. 40–42).

Focal Depressed Type

The focal depressed type (type II c in the Japanese classification) is seen macroscopically as a circumscribed mucosal depression less than 2 cm in diameter; when the depression reaches a certain size and depth the mucosa around the lesion is elevated to a varying degree and forms a slight marginal wall. This change is expressed as type II c (superficial depressed type) or type II c + II a (surrounded by mucosal elevation) in the Japanese endoscopical classification. On X-ray and endoscopical examinations the lesion is sometimes classified as type II a + II c (mucosal elevation accompanied by central depression), as the elevated lesion looks like a major change in the living stomach. The lesion is found most frequently (56.8%) in the mucosa of the antrum, especially of its anterior or posterior wall without convergency of the mucosal folds (Figs. 43–45).

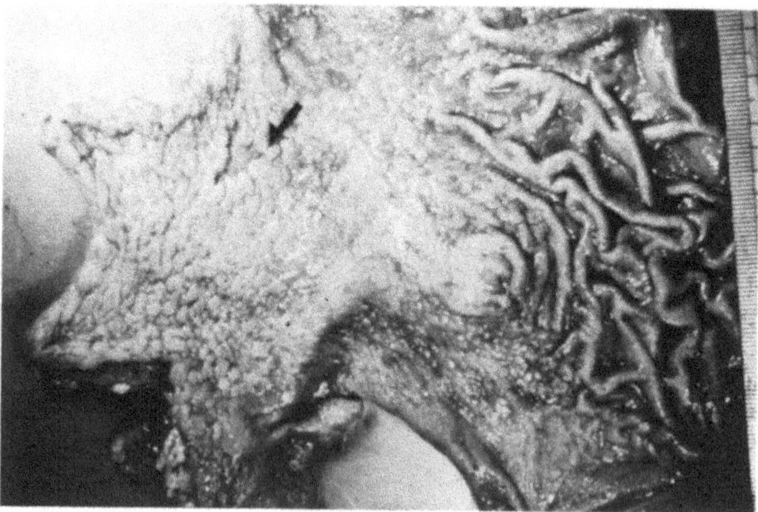

Fig. 43. EGC of focal mucosal depression with irregular contour (type II c′, m) in the anterior wall of the antrum (arrow). The small and shallow depression is surrounded by a slight mucosal elevation. (Pt no. 2762, 46 years, m)

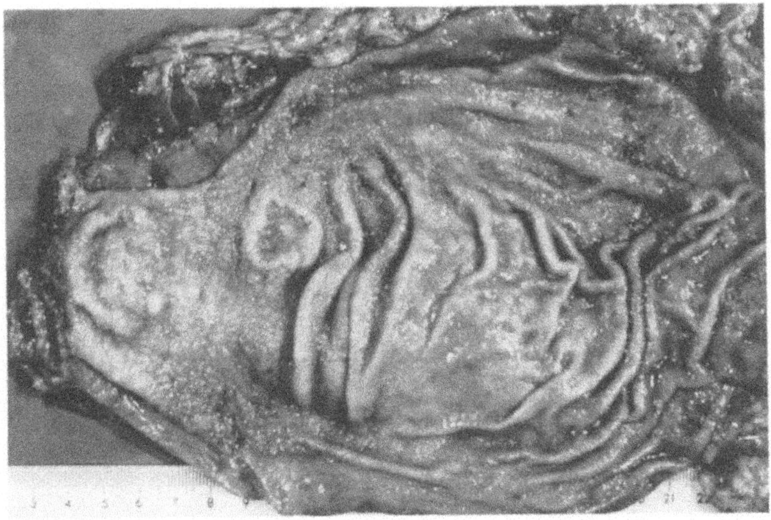

Fig. 44. EGC of focal mucosal depression with marginal elevated mucosa (type II c′ + II a, sm) in the antrum near the greater curvature. (Pt no. 16 547, 62 years, f)

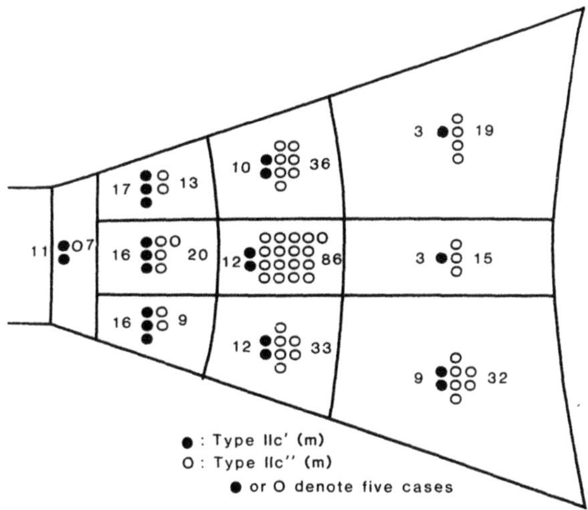

Fig. 45. Locations of superficial depressed-type lesions (type II c′, mucosal cancer alone)

Histologically the depressed lesion is occupied entirely by well-differentiated tubular adenocarcinoma, or intestinal-type cancer according to the Laurèn-Järvi classification, in most cases (Table 12). The boundary of the cancerous lesion from the surrounding mucosa is always well defined, and marginal mucosa adjacent to the cancer is elevated to a varying degree owing to reactive hyperplasia of the mucosa as a result of the depressed lesion. It is noteworthy that the inner side of the marginal elevated mucosa is always occupied by tubular adenocarcinoma but its surface and outer side are mostly free of cancer (Figs. 46–48).

53

Table 12. Number of cases, average age and sex ratio of
EGC of focal depressed type (type IIc′)

| | Grade of differentiation of adenocarcinoma | | |
	Well	Moderate	Poor
No. of cases	183	47	13
Av. age (years)	58.4	51.1	50.6
Sex ratio (m/f)	5.1	1.9	2.1

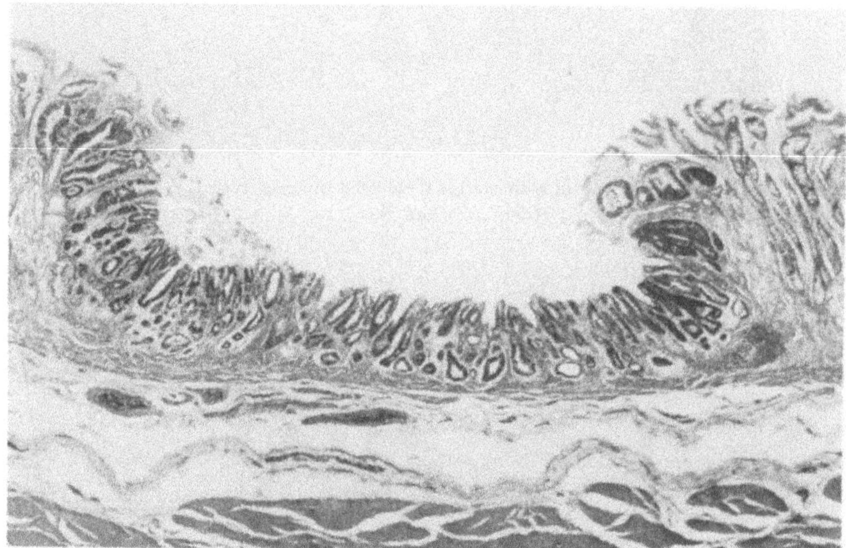

Fig. 46. Histological picture of the lesion shown in Fig. 43. The depressed mucosa is occupied entirely
by well-differentiated tubular adenocarcinoma. Same histology is seen in the inner half of the marginal elevated mucosa. (Pt no. 2762, × 20)

Mucosa surrounding the cancerous lesion is almost always affected by diffuse
and severe intestinal metaplasia. Pyloric or pseudopyloric glands, however, may
be seen near the basal layer of the marginal elevated mucosa. In general, size and
depth of the cancerous depression are proportional to each other and are indicative of the grade of cancerous invasion. When the depressed lesion reaches a certain size and depth the probability of cancerous invasion beyond the submucosal
layer is quite high (Fig. 49).

The thickness of gastric mucosa is always maintained at the same level in normal stomach by well-balanced changes in the epithelial cells, owing chiefly to
regulation of the proliferative and differentiating activities of the generating cells,
but in the cancerized mucosa this regulation is entirely lost, even though mitotic
cells are seen scattered randomly through the mucosa. This is why the cancerized
mucosa is thinner than the surrounding nonmalignant mucosa.

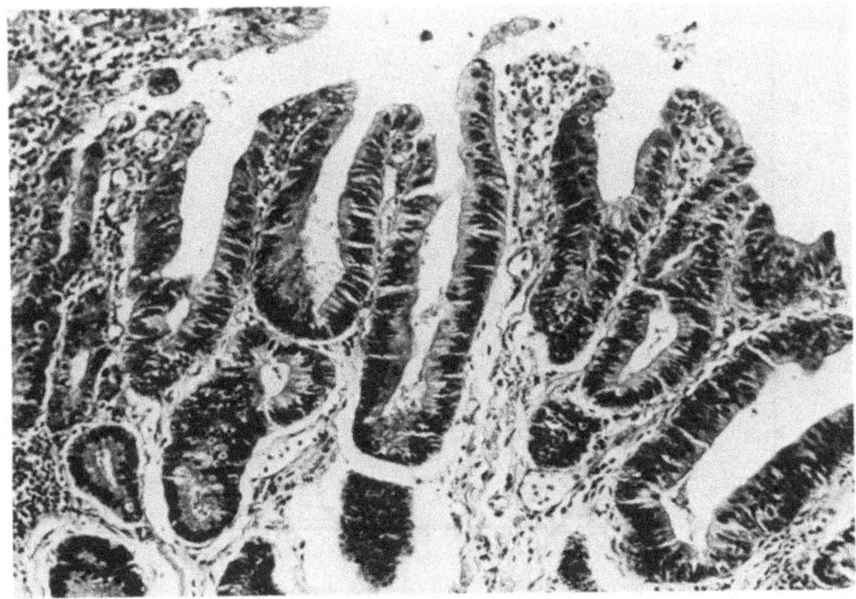

Fig. 47. Higher magnification of a part of the depressed mucosa shown in Fig. 46. The cancerous tubules are composed of tall columnar epithelial cells with elongated, hyperchromatic and piled-up nuclei, but pleomorphy is hardly visible among them. (Pt no. 2762, × 100)

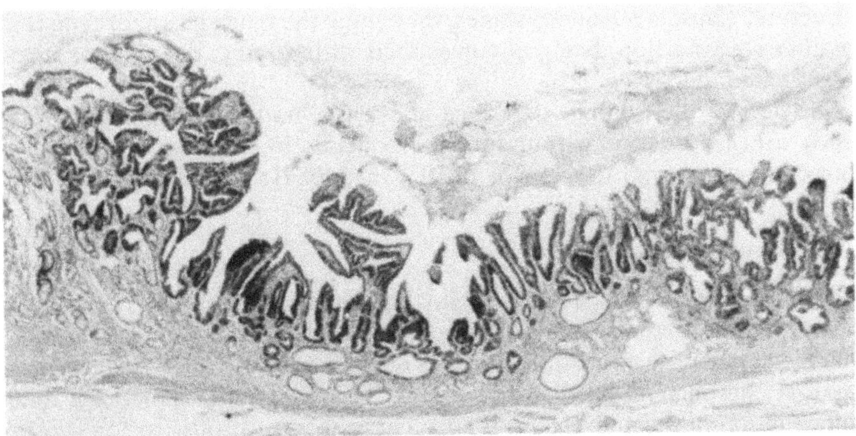

Fig. 48. Similar appearance to that in Fig. 46. Boundary of cancerous tissue to the surrounding mucosa is clear-cut. Nonmalignant cystically dilated glands are visible in basal layer of the depressed cancerous lesion. (Pt no. 13 962, × 20)

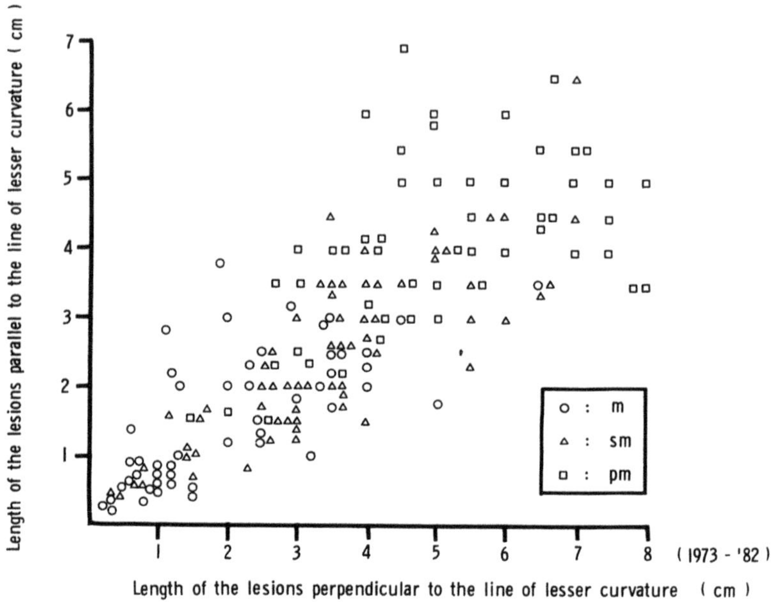

Fig. 49. Relationship between size and depth of type II c' cancerous lesions (focal mucosal depression)

When cancerous lesions of this type are not detected on routine examination, they definitely grow into larger and deeper lesions without losing their original structure. Thus, in advanced stages, they show the typical form of type II in Borrmann's classification, being circumscribed with a large, deep crater surrounded by elevated mucosa.

In view of the findings described above it is understandable that this type of early cancerous lesion is found more frequently in elderly persons, especially in men. I have referred to this type of EGC as type II c' in previous papers [38–40].

Large Eroded Type

This type of EGC (type II c also in the Japanese classification) is characterized by the superficial nature of the cancerous lesion. The affected mucosa shows a fairly extensive but shallow erosion, which is recognizable by rough surface, its serrated margin encroaching on the surrounding flat mucosa and the abrupt thinning or interruption of the mucosal folds adjacent to the cancerous erosion (Figs. 50–52).

The eroded mucosa is completely or partly covered by grayish-white, fibrin-containing exudate, and for this reason its hyperemic or hemorrhagic rough surface is often not apparent by endoscopy.

Unlike inflammatory erosions, the eroded lesion is mostly unifocal and often occupies certain area of the mucosa. When the erosion is fairly extensive, tiny noneroded mucosa can be seen within the erosin, like islands in the sea.

Another characteristic of this type is that the eroded mucosa is quite often accompanied by peptic ulceration, chiefly in the central parts of the erosion. This

56

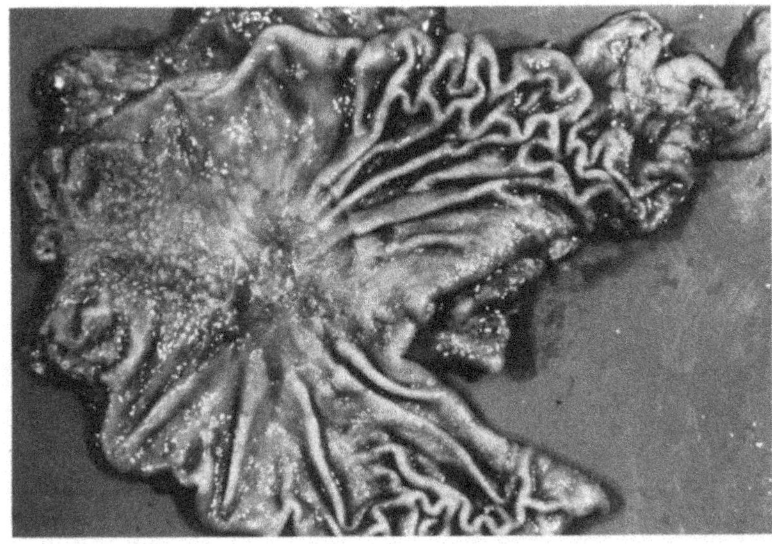

Fig. 50. EGC of large cancerous erosion (type II c″, m) in the angulus. Abrupt thinning of the convergent mucosal folds is visible in the peripheral part of the erosion. (Pt no. 14766, 43 years, m)

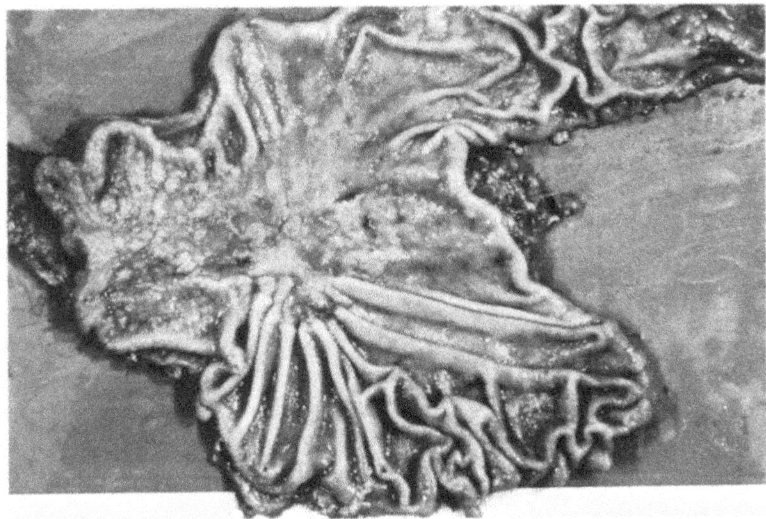

Fig. 51. EGC in form of large cancerous erosion (type II c″, sm) in the angulus. Convergency of the mucosal folds indicating presence of ulcer scar is seen in the posterior side of the erosion. Many small noneroded mucosae are visible within the erosion. (Pt no. 14167, 53 years, m)

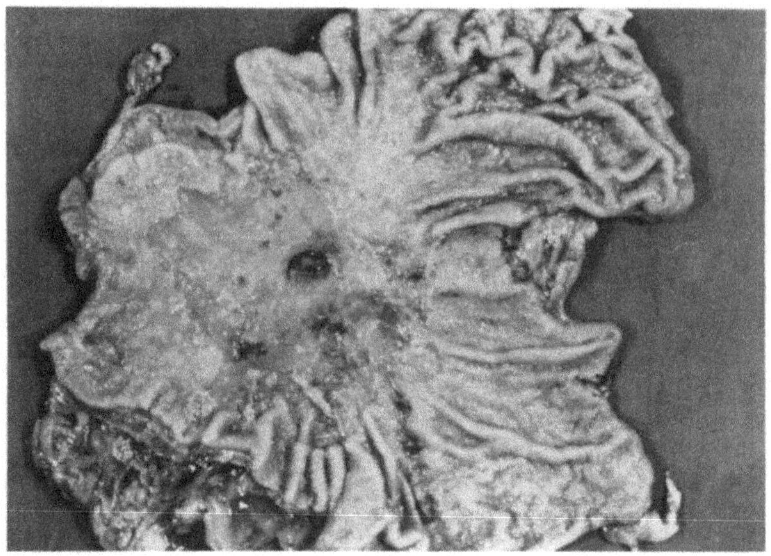

Fig. 52. EGC of large cancerous erosion (type II c″, m) in the angulus. Border of the erosion is zigzag but continuous. Convergency of the mucosal folds is weaker than in the previous case. (Pt no. 11 882, 56 years, f)

finding indicates that the mucosa affected by cancerous erosion is far more prone than the intact mucosa to ulceration by the peptic action of gastric juice. The status of the secondary ulceration varies in each case, from open and shallow ulcers to closed and fibrotic scars, but in most cases the presence of the secondary ulceration is shown by the convergence of the mucosal folds toward the center of the ulcer. Cancerous erosion without ulcer is noted merely as type II c, while erosion with small ulcer is noted as type II c + III in the Japanese classification. It is over 15 years since I named this type of EGC type II c″ (cancerous erosion).

The ratio of the frequency of cancerous erosion with to that without secondary ulceration was 4.5 : 1.0. The average age of the patients for both types was nearly the same (about 50 years), but the sex ratio (f : m) was significantly lower in the cases with ulcer (0.7) than in those without (1.2) (Table 13).

When frequencies of cancerous erosion with and without ulcer were analyzed from the aspects of site and size of the lesions, it became apparent that more than half (56.8%) were located in an area of the angulus and that the cases without ul-

Table 13. Number of cases, average age, and sex ratio for cancerous erosion by presence or absence of peptic ulcer

Cancerous erosion	Number of cases	Average age (years)	Sex ratio (female/male)
Without ulcer	82	50.1	1.2
With ulcer	367	49.0	0.7

58

cer were most often (54.9%) found in lesions bigger than 5×5 cm and most of these were female cases (68.9%), while in the cases with ulcer the erosion was mostly between 2×2 cm and 5×5 cm in area and the frequency was higher in male (74.3%) than in female patients (63.4%) (Table 14).

Table 14. Relationship between presence or absence of ulcer and size of cancerous erosions

Macroscopical appearance / Size of the lesion	Cancerous erosion						
	Without ulcer				With ulcer		
	Nos.	Frequency (%)			Nos.	Frequency (%)	
		m+f	m	f		m+f	m	f
Up to 2×2 cm	10	12.2	10.8	13.3	30	8.2	10.3	5.2
Up to 5×5 cm but more than 2×2 cm	27	32.9	51.4	17.8	256	69.8	74.3	63.4
Over 5×5 cm	45	54.9	37.8	68.9	81	22.0	15.4	31.4
Total	82 cases	(m:39, sm:43)			367 cases	(m:188, sm:179)		

It was seen from these results that the macroscopical features of cancerous erosion are fairly different between male and female patients.

Histologically, most (80%) cancerous erosion show the features of moderately to poorly differentiated adenocarcinoma lacking in evident glandular structure (Table 15), and signet-ring cells are quite often visible in the outer zone of the lesion. The central part of the eroded mucosa, which in most cases is the site of origin of the cancer, is always occupied entirely by the cancerous tissues, but in the peripheral parts pyloric or pseudopyloric glands are often visible in the lower half of the eroded mucosa. Cancer cells tend to infiltrate diffusely under the intact surface epithelium, and exfoliation of the surface epithelium resulting in erosion occurs when the upper layer of the affected mucosa is filled with infiltrating cancer cells. However, it is not uncommon to see nonmalignant mucosa composed of immature regenerative epithelium between the cancerous erosions (Figs. 53 and 54).

A brief mention of the nature of signet-ring type cancer cells must be made here (Figs. 55 and 56). In the mature state, these cells are characterized by cytoplasm filled with mucus and by this change the nucleus is pushed to the periphery of the cell, where it assumes a crescent-like appearance with routine H & E staining. It is known from our histochemical [25a] and electron microscopic [53] investigations that mature signet-ring cells are derived from an immature precursor, which is leucinaminopeptidase (LAP) positive and very poor in intracytoplasmic mucin granules, and are the only cells capable of neoplastic proliferation (Figs. 57 and 58).

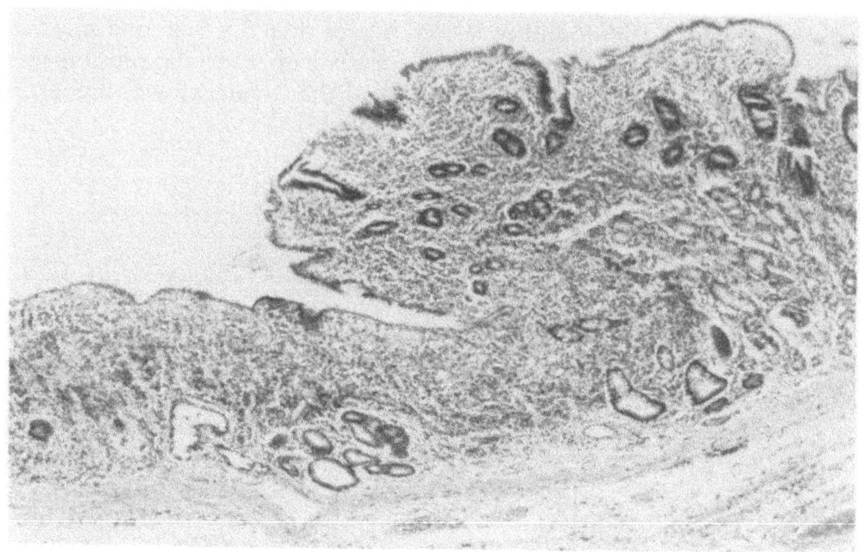

Fig. 53. Peripheral area of abrupt thinning of the mucosal folds shown in Fig. 50. Upper half of the eroded mucosa is diffusely infiltrated by poorly differentiated adenocarcinoma. (Pt no. 14766, × 40)

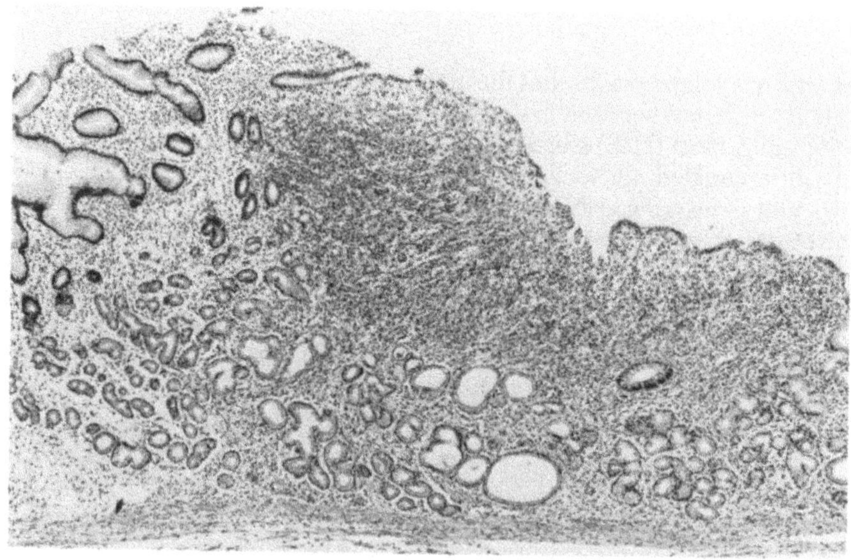

Fig. 54. Similar change to that shown in Fig. 53, seen in distal margin of the large cancerous erosion shown in Fig. 52. In the peripheral part of the eroded lesion cancer cells are infiltrating laterally into the upper half of the surrounding, slightly hyperplastic, mucosa. (Pt no. 11882, × 40)

60

Table 15. Number of cases, average age, and sex ratio for EGC of extensively eroded type (type IIc″)

| | Grade of differentiation of adenocarcinoma | | |
	Well	Moderate	Poor
No. of cases	91	140	296
Av. age (years)	57.3	49.8	46.2
Sex ratio (m/f)	4.4	1.9	0.8

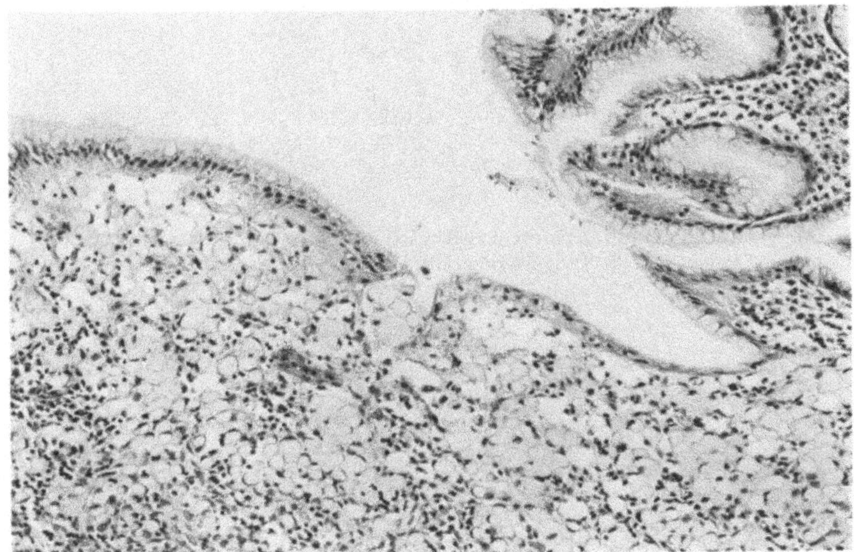

Fig. 55. Periphery of the cancerous erosion is occupied diffusely by matured type of signet-ring cancer cells. The eroded lesion is covered by regenerating nonmalignant epithelia. (Pt no. 16756, × 200)

Unlike the previous type of focal mucosal depression, intestinal metaplasia is generally absent or rare not only around the cancerous erosion but also in the cancer-bearing antral mucosa. This type of EGC is seen relative frequently in younger patients and in middle-aged women. It is evident from the analysis of several cases showing transitional or intermediate growing features that this type of EGC tends to develop into Borrmann's type III or IV AGC, which is characterized by diffuse thickening of the gastric wall with an ill-defined boundary.

The differences in macroscopical, histological, and other features between the focal depressed type and the large eroded type, both of which are classed under superficial depressed type (type IIc) in the Japanese Endoscopical Classification, are summarized (Fig. 59).

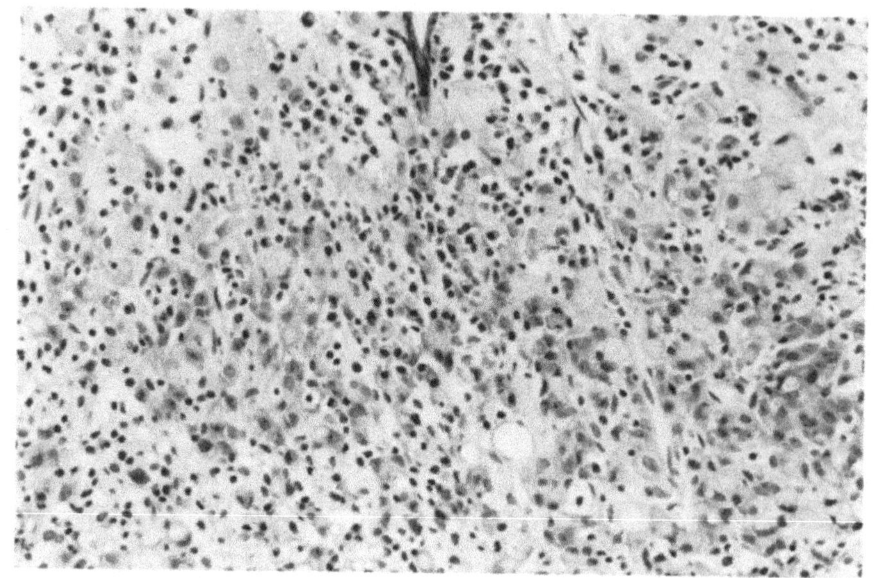

Fig. 56. Infiltrating poorly differentiated adenocarcinoma composed of immature (mainly lower half) and mature (mainly upper half) signet-ring cells; both types are transitional in nature. (Pt no. 11112, ×200)

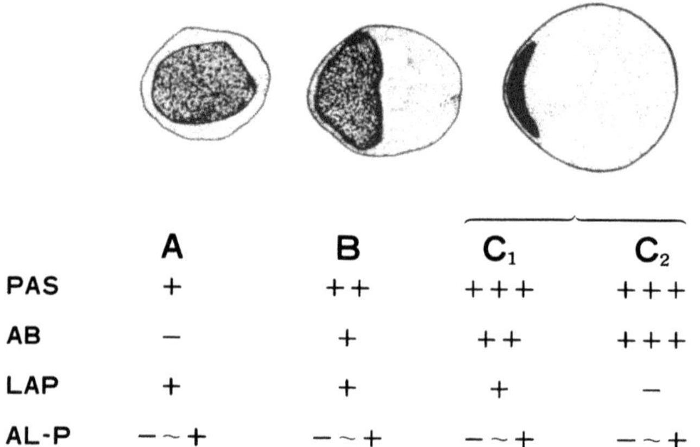

	A	B	C₁	C₂
PAS	+	+ +	+ + +	+ + +
AB	−	+	+ +	+ + +
LAP	+	+	+	−
AL-P	− ~ +	− ~ +	− ~ +	− ~ +

Fig. 57. Developmental phases of signet-ring type cancer cell. (Chap. 4 [25 a])

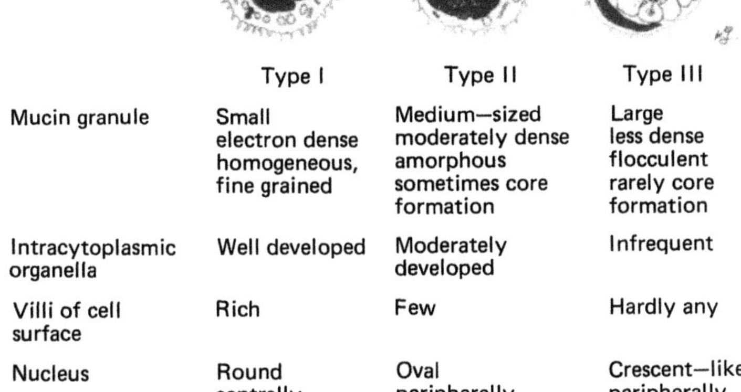

	Type I	Type II	Type III
Mucin granule	Small electron dense homogeneous, fine grained	Medium—sized moderately dense amorphous sometimes core formation	Large less dense flocculent rarely core formation
Intracytoplasmic organella	Well developed	Moderately developed	Infrequent
Villi of cell surface	Rich	Few	Hardly any
Nucleus	Round centrally located	Oval peripherally located	Crescent—like peripherally located

Fig. 58. Electron microscopical features of signet-ring-type cancer cell. (Chap 4 [53])

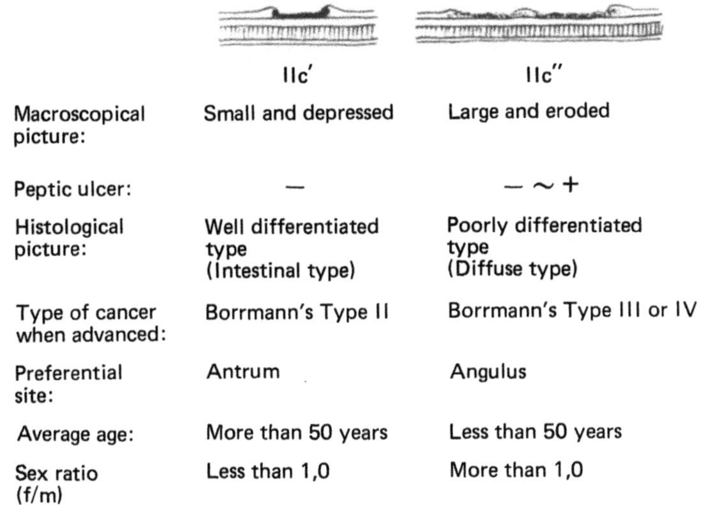

	IIc'	IIc''
Macroscopical picture:	Small and depressed	Large and eroded
Peptic ulcer:	—	— ~ +
Histological picture:	Well differentiated type (Intestinal type)	Poorly differentiated type (Diffuse type)
Type of cancer when advanced:	Borrmann's Type II	Borrmann's Type III or IV
Preferential site:	Antrum	Angulus
Average age:	More than 50 years	Less than 50 years
Sex ratio (f/m)	Less than 1,0	More than 1,0

Fig. 59. Subclassification of type IIc cancerous lesions (T. Nagayo)

Peptically Ulcerated Type

This type of EGC (type III in the Japanese classification) is similar in its gross appearance to nonmalignant peptic ulcer. Like ordinary peptic ulcer, the ulcerated lesion varies widely in morphology, from a shallow and nonfibrotic acute ulcer to a deep, fibrotic, and chronic one.

The most important finding differentiating these malignant ulcers from benign ones is the nature of the mucosa around the ulcer. For example, when the outline of the ulcer is regular and the mucosa adjacent to the ulcer is smooth a malignant basis for the ulcer is most unlikely, while when the edge of the ulcer is serrated or is surrounded by a narrow zone of erosion a malignant nature must be suspected. Fortunately, we now have a method of differentiating between a benign and a malignant nature of the marginal mucosa by histological examinations of the biopsied specimens with the aid of the endoscope (Figs. 60 and 61).

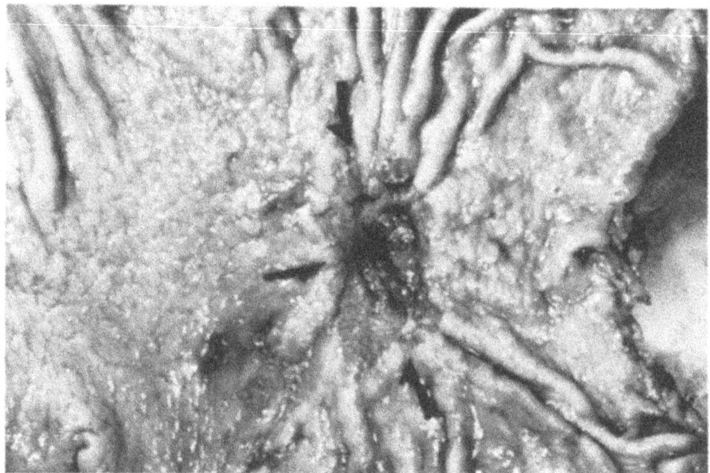

Fig. 60. Deep, chronic peptic ulcer in the angulus, surrounded by narrow zone of cancerous erosion (type III + II c″, m). Mucosal folds strongly converge to center of the ulcer and abrupt thinning or disruption of the convergent folds is visible. (Pt no. 3970, 46 years, m)

This type of EGC has various histological features, but nevertheless, it must be stressed at this point that the ulcerated lesion itself has basically the same nature and appearance as a nonmalignant peptic ulcer (Figs. 62–66). In the Japanese endoscopical classification, peptic ulcer surrounded entirely or partly by a narrow zone of cancerous erosion is classed as type III + II c and peptic ulcer without any macroscopically recognizable malignancy is classed as type III + II b after histological examination of the resected stomach. From the viewpoint of the histology and histogenesis of gastric cancer, however, I feel that type III + II c would better be expressed as UI + II c″ – major change of peptic ulcer is surrounded by minor change of cancerous erosion – and type II c + III, as II c″ + U1 – major change of cancerous erosion is accompanied by minor change of peptic ulcer. These

64

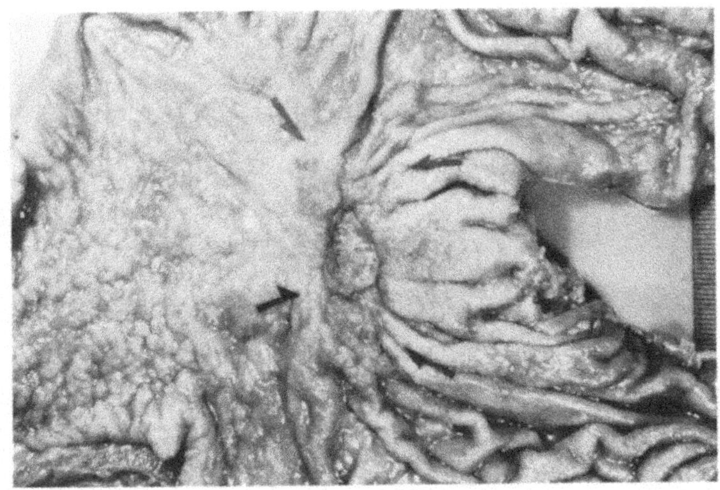

Fig. 61. Similar gross appearance to that in Fig. 60 (type III + II c″, m). The cancerous erosion extends to both anterior and posterior sides of the ulcer. (Pt no. 4260, 60 years, m)

designations seem to make the nature of EGC far more comprehensible for every doctor.

In contrast to the previous types, there is no recognizable histological trend in the cancerous tissue in this type, even though cases with poor differentiation are slightly more frequent (Table 16).

As described briefly in Chap. 1, original papers concerning the macroscopical and histological characteristics of EGC have been appearing since early in this century, but most of the early reports dealt with markedly protruding or deeply ulcerated cases. Another type of EGC – superficial cancer without prominent protrusion or deep ulceration – was then reported by several investigators, e.g., BORRMANN [5], KONJETZNY [24, 25], GUTMANN and BERTRAND [15], BERTRAND

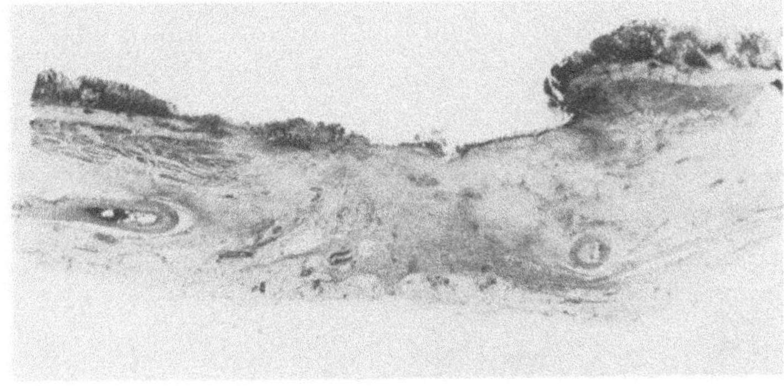

Fig. 62. Histological picture through center of the ulcer shown in Fig. 60. The ulcer shows basic structure of chronic peptic ulcer. Mucosa at anal *(left)* side of the ulcer is eroded. (Pt no. 3970, ×7)

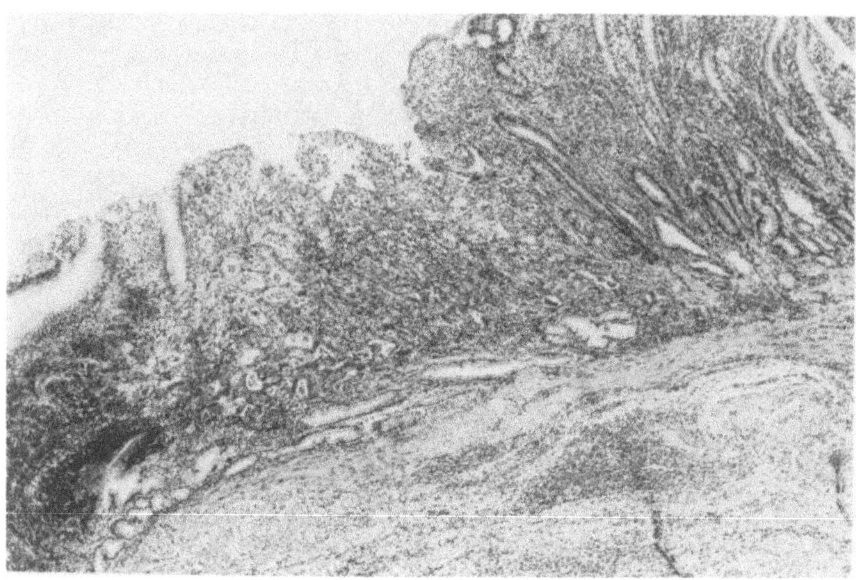

Fig. 63. High-power view of right-side mucosa shown in the previous figure. Upper part of the mucosa is infiltrated by moderately differentiated adenocarcinoma. (Pt no. 3970, × 40)

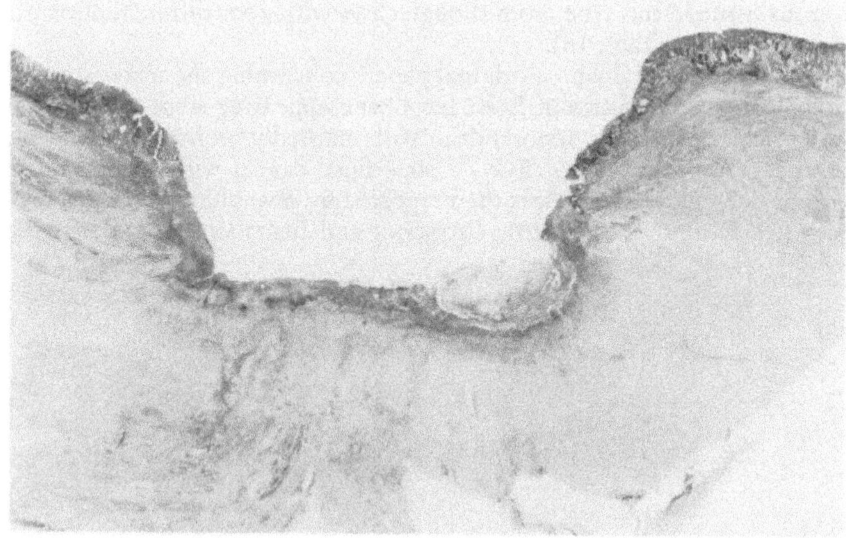

Fig. 64. Histological picture of section through center of the ulcer shown in Fig. 61. Oral *(right)*-side mucosa adjacent to the chronic peptic ulcer is atrophic and eroded. (Pt no. 4260, × 7)

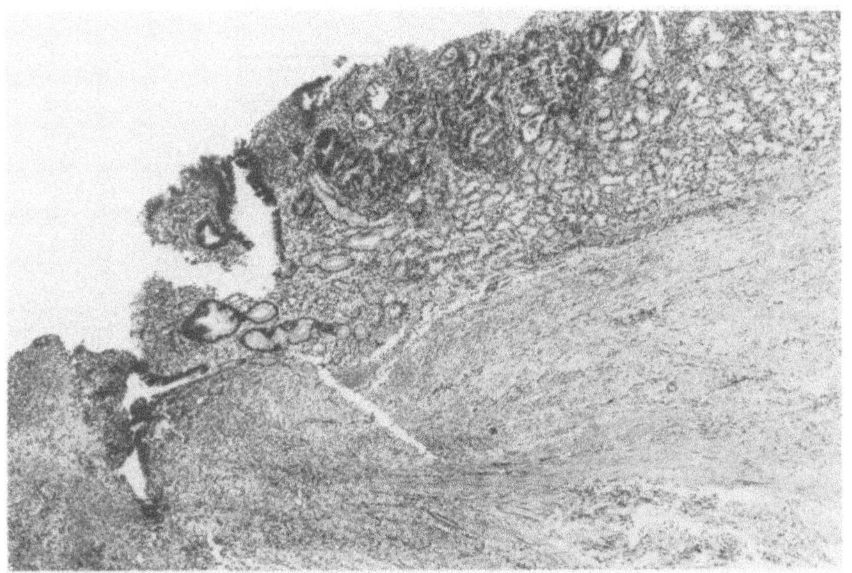

Fig. 65. High-power view of the atrophic mucosa shown in Fig. 64. Darkly stained adenocarcinomatous tissue is seen in upper half of the atrophic mucosa. (Pt no. 4260, × 40)

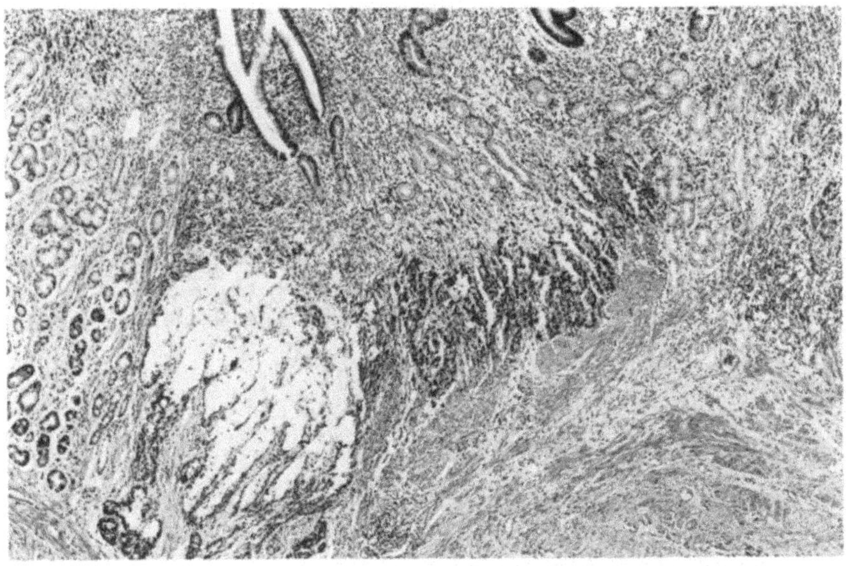

Fig. 66. Cancerous change with mucus-secreting small glandular cells is visible in deeper layer of the linear ulcer scar. In other parts of the linear ulcer scar no such change is visible. (Pt no. 4052, × 40)

Table 16. Relationship between macroscopical and histological types in EGC

Macro-scopical type	Histological type — Grade of differentiation		
	Well	Moderate	Poor
I	92.4%	5.7%	1.9%
II a	90.7%	9.3%	0%
II b	66.7%	27.8%	5.5%
II c′	72.7%	22.7%	4.6%
II c″	19.8%	33.2%	47.0%
III	37.2%	36.3%	26.5%

[3], EWING [9], MALLORY [29], GOLDEN and STOUT [11], STOUT [49, 50], RÖSSLE [46], during the 1930s and 1940s, under various similar but different terms, and since then the major interest in the histogenesis of EGC has tended to focus on this superficial type. In any case, it is important to note here that the basic principles of the macroscopical classification of EGC presently used throughout the world had already been set up by the pioneering investigators before the end of the 1940s.

Following the development of new diagnostic techniques, such as double-contrast radiography [20a, 48a] and endoscopic fibergastroscopy [46a, 52a], the number of cases of EGC detected in routine laboratory examinations increased rapidly in the 1960s. As a result of this great progress in clinical diagnosis, several kinds of EGC and the relative frequency of each type became recognizable in histological studies on resected stomachs [2, 4, 4a, 6–8, 10, 12, 15, 18, 22, 23, 26, 28, 30–32, 36, 44, 45, 48], and in this field of study Japanese investigators [1, 19, 21, 27, 34, 35, 37–43, 47, 52] played a leading and important role, even though the Japanese classification system based on the macroscopical classification of EGC has been criticized by some investigators [16, 17, 32, 33].

In 1974, GUTMANN [14] published a significant review dealing with the progress made in studies on EGC.

Frequency of Macroscopical Type of EGC

From 1953 to 1983, in all 1252 cases of EGC were surgically resected at Yokoyama Hospital, and after marcoscopical and histological examinations of these stomachs they were classified into several macroscopical types according to the criteria described above.

Among these 1252 cases, the most frequent type was cancerous erosion (type II c″) with 524 cases (41.9%), followed in declining order of frequency by peptic ulceration (type III) (283 cases or 22.6%), focal mucosal depression (type II c′) (242 cases or 19.3%), broad-based mucosal elevation (type II a) (101 cases or 8.1%), polypoid mucosal protrusion (type I) (78 cases or 6.2%), and superficial flat mucosa (type IIb) (24 cases or 1.9%). The relative frequency of type IIc" among all the cases of EGC was significantly higher in female than in male patients, while in types III and IIc' this situation was reversed (Fig. 67).

The statistics relating to a total 8334 cases of EGC treated by resection throughout Japan and registered with the WHO-CC·National Cancer Center in Tokyo from 1963 to 1973 yielded similar results on the relative frequency of each type of EGC, except for type III, the frequency of which was far lower in this sample than in that at Yokoyama Hospital (Fig. 68).

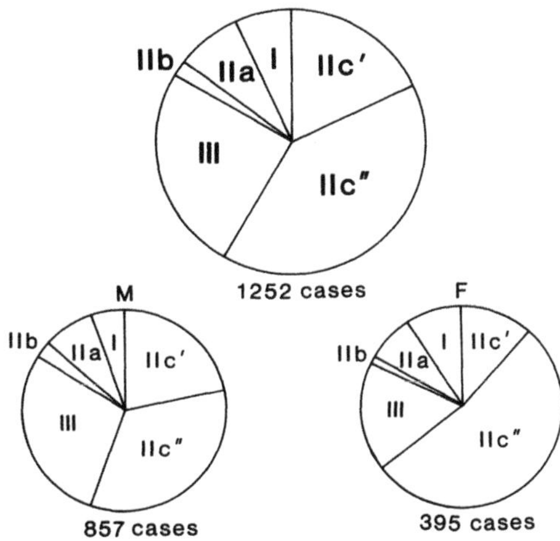

Fig. 67. Relative frequencies of different macroscopical types of EGC among cases seen at Yokoyama Hospital (1953–1983)

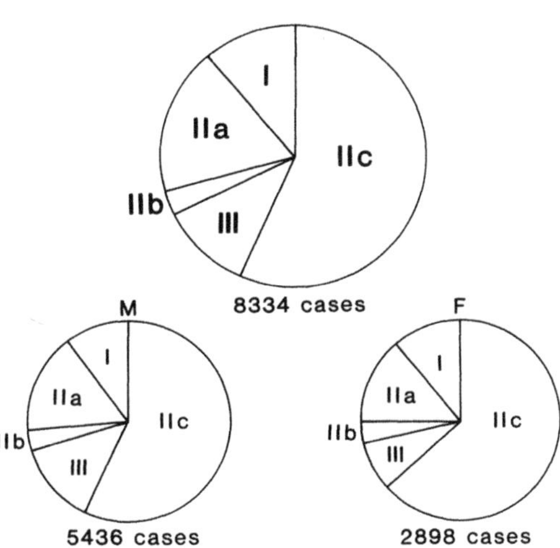

Fig. 68. Relative frequencies of different macroscopical types of EGC among cases registered with the Japanese Research Society for Gastric Cancer and the National Cancer Center, Tokyo (1963–1973)

The data from these samples show definitively that flat gastric mucosa with focal depression or shallow erosion accounts for more than half the recorded cases of EGC.

When macroscopical types of EGC were classified by age and sex of the patients, it became apparent that types I, IIa, and IIc', all of which are characterized by a clear boundary, increased in frequency with advancing age of the patients, while those of types IIc" and III, most of which had an ill-defined boundary, decreased in frequency with advancing age (Table 17).

Table 17. Average age of patients in each type of EGC

Type Grade	Protrusions (I)		Elevated lesions (IIa)		Depressed lesions (IIc')		Eroded lesions (IIc")		Ulcers (III)	
	No. of cases	Av. age (years)	No. of cases	Av. age (years)	No. of cases	Av. age (years)	No. of cases	Av. age (years)	No. of cases	Av. age (years)
m	31	60.7	53	59.1	104	54.5	253	47.5	170	50.8
sm	47	61.9	44	58.2	128	58.1	249	49.9	113	50.8
Total	78	61.4	97	58.6	232	56.5	502	48.7	283	50.8

m, mucosal cancer; sm, submucosal cancer

This conclusion was reinforced when the frequencies of macroscopical types of EGC in patients under 35 and over 65 of age were compared (Fig. 69).

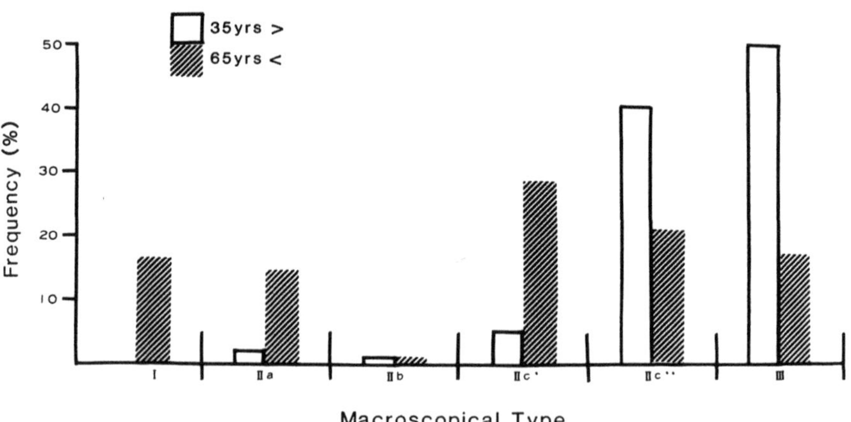

Fig. 69. Frequencies of different macroscopical types of EGC by patient age

Relationship Between Macroscopical Appearances
and Histological Features of EGC

As in AGC, the macroscopical and histological features of EGC are closely correlated. Owing to the relative simplicity of the histological features of cancer confined to the gastric mucosa alone, the correlation is more apparent in EGC than
in AGC. In the case of lesions that are seen to be well circumscribed lesions on
gross examination, such as polypoid mucosal protrusion, broad-based mucosal
elevation, and focal mucosal depression, cells characteristics of well-differentiated adenocarcinoma are predominant in numbers; in cases with ill-defined boundaries, in contrast, such as cancerous erosion, poorly differentiated adenocarcinoma (often accompanied by diffuse infiltration of signet-ring cancer cells) is the
major type, regardless of the presence or absence of peptic ulceration within the
eroded lesions. In the case of ulcerated lesions, which are similar in gross appearance to benign peptic ulcer, no such close correlation between macroscopical and
histological features is noted. In short, regardless of size, shape, and site of the lesion, lesions that are well demarcated on gross examination tend to have an intestinal-type histology according to the Laurén-Järvi classification, while lesions
with an ill-defined and serrated boundary more often have a diffuse-type histology (Table 18).

Table 18. Summary of relationship between EGC and AGC

Gross appearance	Well demarkated	Ill defined
EGC	Protruding (type I) Elevated (type II a) Depressed (type II c′)	Eroded (type II c″)
AGC	Borrmann's type I Borrmann's type II	Borrmann's type III Borrmann's type IV
Peptic ulceration	Rare	Frequent
Histology	Intestinal type	Diffuse type
Growth pattern	Extensive Expansive Penetrating	Spreading Infiltrative

As in AGC, intestinal-type histology is more frequently observed in elderly patients, especially with severe intestinal metaplasia, while diffuse-type histology is
seen more often in younger patients, most of whom have only slight intestinal
metaplasia or none at all.

In summary, there is a general tendency for the histological nature of EGC to
be determined by the nature of the affected gastric mucosa, especially by its grade
of intestinal metaplasia.

Changes in Frequency of EGC and its Macroscopical Types over Time

Owing to the great advances in clinical diagnosis, the frequency of detection and resection of EGC as a proportion of all cases of gastric cancer resected has increased in recent years and is now close to 40% (Fig. 70).

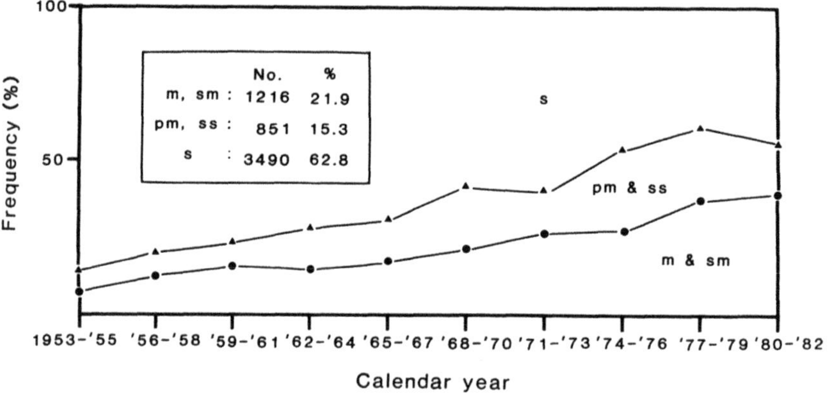

Fig. 70. Changes in frequency of resected gastric cancer over time by grade of cancerous invasion

As described already in Chap. 2, changes in the frequency of each macroscopical type of AGC over time are influenced a great deal by factors relating to the natural and social environments, while in the case of EGC, factors relating to advances in medical treatment seem to play more important part in changes over time. For example, before 1960 almost all gastric cancers were detected clinically by classic methods of X-ray examination, and for this reason most cases of EGC detected at that time involved prominent protrusion or profound ulceration. In these periods EGC of the superficial type was mostly observed by chance as secondary changes in the mucosa, adjacent to or apart from the main lesion of advanced cancer or peptic ulcer.

The most remarkable annual change observed during the period from 1955 to 1980 in our investigations was an increase in frequency of the superficially eroded type (type II c"), as opposed to a decrease in frequency of the focally ulcerated type (type III). The first signs of these changes date from the mid-1960s, when double-contrast X-ray examination and endoscopic fibergastroscopy were introduced into routine clinical examinations of the stomach. With these newly developed diagnostic methods, it became possible to detect superficial cancerous changes of the gastric mucosa with no great technical difficulty. Thus, the frequency of the eroded type, which was a minor form of EGC at the beginning of our study, increased every year thereafter. The tendency to increase was further accelerated by the introduction of the method of taking biopsies from areas in which malignancy was suspected under direct vision through the endoscope, which made confirmation of a preoperative diagnosis of EGC a more viable

72

proposition. In contrast, EGC of the ulcerated type, which was by far the most common around 1955, has gradually decreased in frequency over time and has become a minor form in recent years. Reason for this chronological change in the frequency will be discussed in Chapter 5 (Fig. 71).

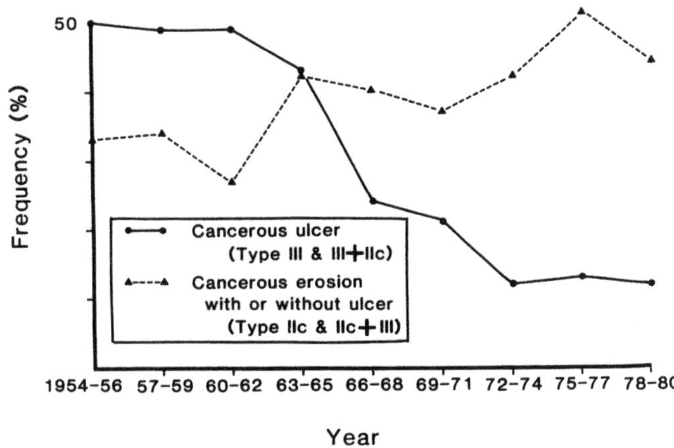

Fig. 71. Changes in frequency of cancerous ulcer (type III) and cancerous erosion (type II c") over time among cases of EGC treated by resection

Macroscopical Diagnosis of EGC

As described previously, a definite diagnosis of EGC is not possible without histological examination of the resected stomachs. In several studies, however, while most cases diagnosed roentgenologically, endoscopically, or macroscopically as EGC fulfilled the histological criteria for EGC, in some of these cases it became apparent from histological examination of resected stomachs that the cancer cell infiltration had already reached the serosa, and these cases had to be excluded from the final data on EGC. We have also had the experience that among the cases diagnosed macroscopically as EGC there were a few cases in which no malignant change could be detected at all on histological examination. Conversely, other cases were diagnosed macroscopically as benign lesions but cancerous change was found in the lesions on histological examination. Overestimation of the degree of growth of malignancy was also not exceptional. Thus, it has to be confessed that the macroscopical diagnosis of EGC does not always coincide with the histological diagnosis.

As shown in Table 19, among 1272 cases of EGC histologically confirmed during the 30 years of the study, in 915 cases (71.9%) EGC was correctly diagnosed at macroscopical examination but in 152 cases (12.0%) a diagnosis of gastric cancer in an intermediate or advanced stage was recorded. It has to be stressed here that there were 205 further cases (16.1%) of histologically confirmed EGC, in which the malignant nature of the lesions was not suspected at the time of the macroscopical examination. Retrospective analysis revealed that in most of these cases the gross appearance was suggestive of chronic peptic ulcer or its scar. As shown in Table 19, the frequency of incorrect diagnosis was relatively high in the years from 1953 to 1968, but it became lower thereafter and has accounted for only a few percent in the last 10 years. In contrast, among 1164 cases in which a macroscopical diagnosis of EGC was made, 105 cases (9.0%) did not fulfill the histological criteria of EGC, as the cancerous infiltration was already beyond the submucosal layer. A more important feature of this group was that there were 144 cases (12.4%) in which a diagnosis of EGC was made on macroscopical examination but no cancerous changes at all were observed on histological examination in the resected stomachs. Almost all these cases were seen in the early days of our experience and had the gross appearance of a large and deep ulcerated lesion with fibrosis, accompanied by inflammatory changes around the ulcer. Since the introduction of biopsying from suggestive areas of malignancy with the aid of a fibergastroscope, the number of such mistaken diagnoses has fallen remarkably (Table 19).

Table 19. Diagnostic features of EGC at Yokoyama Hospital (1954–1983)

Macroscopical diagnosis	Histological diagnosis	Number of cases (%)						
		1954–1958	1959–1963	1964–1968	1969–1973	1974–1978	1979–1983	1954–1983
EGC	EGC	62.1	63.9	64.6	69.4	79.2	82.5	71.9
AGC	EGC		4.5	10.3	14.3	16.1	14.0	12.0
BL	EGC	37.9	31.6	25.1	16.3	4.7	3.5	16.1
Total number of cases		58	158	243	320	236	257	1272
EGC	EGC	100.0	73.7	65.7	77.9	79.6	91.4	78.6
EGC	AGC		15.4	13.0	7.7	7.2	6.0	9.0
EGC	BL		10.9	15.3	14.4	13.2	2.6	12.4
Total number of cases		36	137	239	285	235	232	1164

BL, benign lesion

The statistical and morphological characteristics of EGC are briefly stated in the list below.

1) The frequency of EGC as a proportion of all gastric cancer resected has been increasing in recent years (Fig. 70).
2) The lesion detected with the highest frequency is type II c" (cancerous erosion), followed in declining order of frequency by type III, type II c', type II a, and type I. Most type II b lesions are found unexpectedly in resected stomachs (Figs. 67 and 68).
3) Type II c" is quite often accompanied by peptic ulceration and is relatively frequent in the younger and middle age groups, especially in female patients; the frequency declines with advancing age (Tables 13 and 15; Fig. 69).

4) In contrast, the frequency of type II c' (focal mucosal depression) increases with advancing age. Male patients significantly outnumber female patients in each age group (Table 12; Figs. 67 and 69).

5) Lesions of type I or type II a are found mostly in patients more than 50 years of age (Table 17 and Fig. 69).

6) Type III is relatively frequent in younger age groups, and in each age group there are more male than female patients (Table 17 and Fig. 69).

7) Gastric cancer with intestinal-type histology is predominant in types I, II a, and II c', while diffuse-type histology is far more frequent in type II c" (Tables 16 and 18).

8) Type III, whose main characteristic is the presence of peptic ulceration, has no apparent histological tendencies (Table 16).

9) The frequency of type II c" with or without ulceration among the cases of EGC resected has been increasing in recent years, while that of type III is decreasing (Fig. 71).

10) In a number of cases of EGC, macroscopical and microscopical diagnosis did not coincide (Table 19).

References

1. Ayabe S (1949) So-called mucosal carcinoma of the stomach (in Japanese). Rinsho to Kenkyu 26: 514–516
2. Bamforth J (1955) Early carcinomatous changes in the stomach. Br J Surg 43: 292–296
3. Bertrand I (1937) Diagnostic histologique précoce du cancer de l'estomac. 2nd International Congress au Gastroenterology, Paris
4. Bocian JJ, Geschke AE (1958) Carcinoma in situ of the stomach. Arch Pathol 65: 6–12
4 a. Bogomoletz WV (1984) Early gastric cancer. Am J Surg Pathol 8: 381–391
5. Borrmann R (1926) Makroskopisches Verhalten des Magenkrebses in seinen ersten Anfängen. In: Lubarsch O, Henke F (eds) Handbuch der speziellen pathologischen Anatomie und Histologie, vol 4/1. Springer, Berlin, p 139
6. Cain H, Kraus B (1973) Frühkarzinom des Magens. Morphologische Beobachtungen und Probleme. Dtsch Med Wochenschr 98: 1591–1596
7. Elster K, Thomasko A (1978) Histological classification of early gastric cancer in 300 cases-clinical significance. Leber Magen Darm 8: 319–327
8. Evans DM, Craven JL, Murphy F, Cleary BK (1978) Comparison of "early gastric cancer" in Britain and Japan. Gut 19: 1–9
9. Ewing J (1936) The beginning of gastric cancer. Am J Surg 31: 204–205
10. Friesen G, Dockerty MB, ReMine WH (1962) Superficial carcinoma of the stomach. Surgery 51: 300–312
11. Golden R, Stout AP (1948) Superficial spreading carcinoma of the stomach. AJR 59: 157–167
12. Grigioni WF, D'errico A, Milani M et al. (1984) Early gastric cancer. Clinicopathological analysis of 125 cases of gastric cancer. Acta Pathol Jpn 34: 979–989
13. Grundmann E (1975) Histologic types and possible initial stages in early gastric carcinoma. Beitr Pathol 154: 256–280
14. Gutmann RA (1974) Forty years of early diagnosis of gastric cancer. In: Grundmann E, Grunze H, Witte S (eds) Early gastric cancer. Current status of diagnosis. Springer, Berlin Heidelberg New York, pp 69–75
15. Gutmann RA, Bertrand I (1939) Le cancer de l'estomac au début. Le diagnostic du cancer d'éstomac à la periode utile. Paris

16. Hermanek P, Rösch W (1973) Critical evaluation of the Japanese "early gastric cancer" classification. Endoscopy 5: 220–224
17. Hermanek P, Rösch W (1973) Subclassification in early gastric cancer. Verh Dtsch Ges Pathol 57: 447
18. Hess R (1956) Early gastric cancer of the stomach. Gastroenterologia 86: 365–369
19. Hirota T, Itabashi M, Daibo M, Kitaoka H, Oguro Y et al. (1984) Chronological changes in the morphological features of early gastric cancer, especially recent changes in marcoscopical findings. Jpn J Clin Oncol 14: 181–199
20. Hirschowitz BI, Curtiss LI et al. (1958) Demonstration of a new gastroscope, the "fiberscope". Gastroenterology 35: 50–53
20a. Ichikawa H (1971) Detectability of early gastric cancer with indirect fluororadiography. In: Murakami T (ed) Early Gastric Cancer. Gann Monogr on Cancer Res. Univ of Tokyo Press, Tokyo (pp 27–43)
21. Inokuchi K (1984) Early gastric carcinoma – viewed from its growth patterns. 8th World Congress of CICD (Collegium Internationale Chirurgiae Digestivae). Amsterdam, pp 1–34
22. Iwanaga T, Kumano T (1972) Early pathological type of scirrhous cancer of the stomach and the clinico-pathological characteristics. Jpn J Clin Med 30: 1568–1574
23. Johansen AA (1981) Early gastric cancer. A contribution to the pathology and to gastric cancer histogenesis. Department of Pathology, Bispebjerg Hospital, Copenhagen
24. Konjetzney GE (1940) Der oberflächliche Schleimhautkrebs des Magens. Chirurg 12: 192–202
25. Konjetzney GE (1953) The superficial cancer of the gastric mucosa. Am J Dig Dis 20: 91–96
25a. Kubota K, Yamada S, Ito M, Nakamura W, Nagayo T (1977) Cytoplasmic leucine naphthylamidase activity expressed in signet-ring cell carcinoma. J Natl Cancer Inst 59: 1599–1604
26. Kuhlencordt F (1959) Das Carcinoma in situ des Magens und der kleinen Magenkrebs. Katamnestische Untersuchungen von 42 Fällen. Dtsch Med Wochenschr 84: 2111–2115
27. Kuru M (1967) Atlas of early carcinoma of the stomach. Nakayama Shoten, Tokyo
28. Machado G, Davies JD, Tudway AJC, Salmon PR, Read AE (1976) Superficial carcinoma of the stomach. Br Med J 2: 77–79
29. Mallory TB (1940) Carcinoma in situ of the stomach and its bearing on the histogenesis of malignant ulcers. Arch Pathol 30: 348–362
30. Marti MC, Cox JN, Widgren S, Bouzakoura C (1973) Carcinome intramuqueux et carcinome invasif de l'éstomac. A propos de 9 cas. Schweiz Med Wochenschr 103: 1458–1462
31. Mason MK (1965) Surface carcinoma of the stomach. Gut 6: 185–193
32. Miller G, Kaufmann M (1975) Das Magenfrühkarzinom in Europa. Dtsch Med Wochenschr 100: 1946–1949
33. Morson BC (1977) The Japanese classification of early gastric cancer. In: Yardly JH, et al. (eds) The gastrointestinal tract. William and Wilkins, Baltimore, pp 176–183
34. Murakami T (1971) Pathomorphological diagnosis. Definition and gross classification of early gastric cancer. Gann Monogr Cancer Res 11: 53–55
35. Murakami T (1952) Studies on the histogenesis of early gastric cancer. Acta Pathol Jpn 2: 10–22
36. Myhre E (1953) Superficial spreading type of carcinoma of the stomach. Acta Chir Scand 106: 392–398
37. Nagayo T (1975) Microscopical cancer of the stomach. A study on histogenesis of gastric carcinoma. Int J Cancer 16: 52–60
38. Nagayo T, Yokoyama H (1974) Early phases and diagnostic features (of gastric cancer). JAMA 228: 888–889
39. Nagayo T, Ito M, Yokoyama H, Komagoe T (1965) Early phases of human gastric cancer: Morphological study. Gann 56: 101–120
40. Nagayo T, Komagoe T (1961) Histological studies of gastric mucosal cancer with special reference of relationship of histological pictures between the mucosal cancer and the cancer-bearing gastric mucosa. Gann 52: 109–119
41. Nakamura K, Sugamo H, Takagi K, Fuchigami A (1967) Histopathological study on early carcinoma of the stomach. Some considerations on the ulcer-cancer by analysis of 144 foci of the superficial spreading carcinoma. Gann 58: 377–387
42. Nakamura K, Sugano H, Takagi K, Fuchigami A (1966) Histopathological study on early carcinoma of the stomach. Criteria for diagnosis of atypical epithelium. Gann 57: 613–620

43. Ostertag H, Georgi A (1979) Early gastric cancer: A morphological study of 144 cases. Pathol Res Pract 164: 294–315
44. Oota K (1976) Early phase of development of human gastric cancer. Gann Monogr Cancer Res 18: 77–83
45. Potet F (1977) Early gastric carcinoma. Superficial cancer of the stomach. The problem of early detection. Gastroenterol Clin Biol 1: 313–318
46. Rössle R (1944) Über einen frühen Oberflächenkrebs der Magenschleimhaut. Zentralbl Allg Pathol 82: 165–170
46a. Sakita T, Oguro Y (1971) Routine gastrocamera examination. In: Murakami T (ed) Early Gastric Cancer. Gann Monogr on Cancer Res. Univ of Tokyo Press, Tokyo (pp 145–157)
47. Sano R (1971) Pathological analysis of 300 cases of early gastric cancer with special reference to cancer associated with ulcers. Gann Monogr Cancer Res 11: 81–89
48. Schade ROK (1961) Cancerisierung und Frühkarzinom der Magenschleimhaut. Verh Dtsch Ges Pathol 45: 179–183
48a. Shirakabe H (1971) X-ray diagnosis of early gastric cancer. In: Murakami T (ed) Early gastric cancer. Gann Monogr on Cancer Res. Univ of Tokyo Press, Tokyo, (pp 105–111)
49. Stout AP (1953) Tumor of the stomach. Atlas of tumor pathology, sect 4, fasc 21. AFIP, Washington
50. Stout AP (1945) Superficial spreading type of carcinoma of the stomach. J Natl Cancer Inst 5: 363
51. Stout AP (1942) Superficial spreading type of carcinoma of the stomach. Arch Surg 44: 651–657
52. Takagi K, Someya M (1959) Histopathological study of mucosal carcinoma of the stomach. Gann [Suppl] 50: 147–148
52a. Tsuneoka K (1971) Diagnosis of early gastric cancer by fiberscope. In: Murakami T (ed) Early gastric cancer. Gann Monogr on Cancer Res. Univ of Tokyo Press, Tokyo, (pp 167–176)
53. Yamashiro K, Suzuki H, Nagayo T (1977) Electromicroscopic study of signet-ring cells in diffuse carcinoma of the human stomach. Virchow's Arch [A] 374: 275–284

5. Histogenesis

The histogenesis of gastric cancer can be separated into two categories: histogenesis of AGC and of EGC, which are described in that order.

Macroscopical and Histological Relationships Between EGC and AGC

Early gastric cancer (EGC) and advanced gastric cancer (AGC) are of course not separate entities, but the same entity at different stages of development, and therefore there is a sequential and transitional relationship between them. Regardless of the grade of the cancerous growth within the stomach, the lesions showing the histological picture of well-differentiated adenocarcinoma or gastric cancer of intestinal type have common marcoscopical characteristics, and the lesions showing poorly differentiated adenocarcinoma or gastric cancer of diffuse type have different characteristics common to all of them.

From these aspects, it can be assumed that one type of EGC is destined to grow into a certain type of AGC without changing its original nature, even though some modifications of the gross appearance and histological features may occur during intramural growth of the cancer owing to secondary changes in the tissue environment or heterogeneity of the original cancer itself.

Except in a few instances, it is impossible to follow such a transition from EGC to AGC over time in a single case, and the sequential changes have been observed by the indirect method of selecting a series of cancers with the same histological nature but at different stages of growth from many cases of surgically resected stomachs, and arranging these cases in order by grade of intramural growth.

In many cases of gastric cancer the cancer cells have already infiltrated beyond the submucosal layer but not to the serosal surface. They are similar in macroscopical appearance to EGC, but none of the criteria for macroscopical classification of AGC proposed by Borrmann really apply to them. After histological examination, the resected stomachs are grouped into the intermediate stage between EGC and AGC, and these cases are quite useful and important for understanding of the developmental course of EGC.

These methods allow a rough estimate of the relationship of each macroscopical type of EGC to the corresponding type of AGC. The developmental courses of each type of EGC are summarized (Fig. 72).

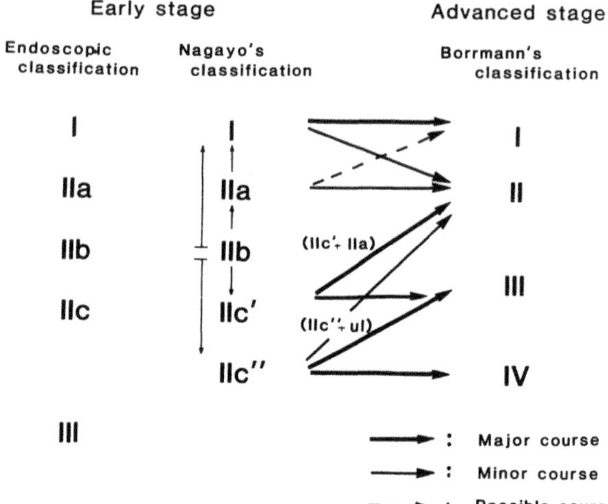

Fig. 72. Histogenesis of gastric cancer

Polypoid Protruding Type

It is obvious from the macroscopical and histological characteristics that protruding EGC (type I in the Japanese classification) can develop into a larger tumorous mass with a more irregular gross appearance when it progresses to the stage of AGC (polypoid protruding type or type I in BORRMANN's classification).

Shallow or multiple tiny erosions may be seen on the surface of the protrusion during the growth stage, but wide areas of deep ulceration owing to necrosis of the tumor, which results in transformation of the gross appearance into that of the excavating type, are infrequent, in contrast to colorectal cancer (Figs. 73–75).

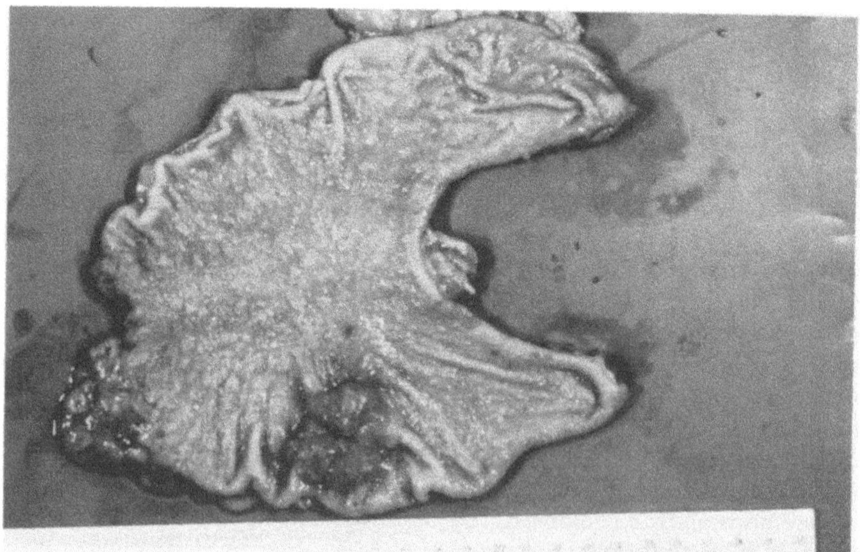

Fig. 73. Hemispheric protrusion of the mucosa in the posterior wall of the corpus (type I, sm). Surface of the protrusion is relatively smooth. (Pt no. 14 258, m)

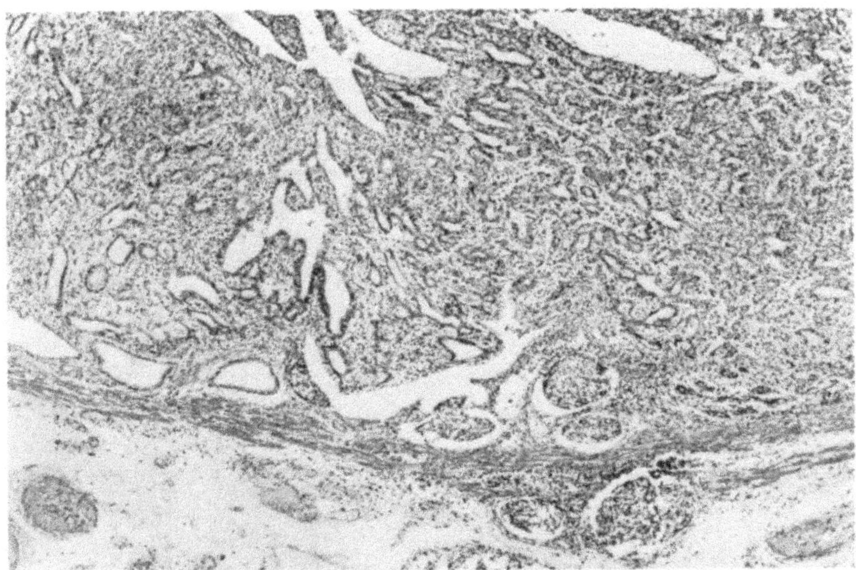

Fig. 74. Base of the hemispheric protrusion shown in Fig. 73. The protruded mucosa is composed of well-differentiated and medullary adenocarcinoma, but the lymphatics above and below the muscularis mucosae are already invaded by cancer cells. (Pt no. 14 258, × 40)

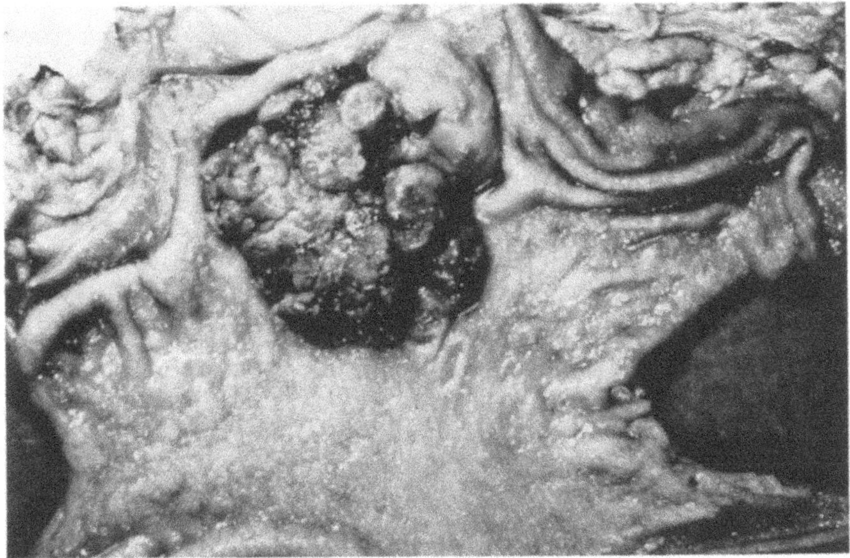

Fig. 75. Hemispheric and fragile protrusion of the mucosa in anterior wall of the angulus. Protrusion is larger and its shape and surface more irregular than in the case of the protrusion seen in Fig. 73 (Pt no. 4544, 54 years, f)

Broad-Based Elevated Type

As described previously, this type of EGC (type II a in the Japanese classification) is characterized by broad-based but slight mucosal elevation, with the histological appearance of well-differentiated tubular adenocarcinoma (Figs. 76 and 77). In advanced stages of this type the surface of the elevated mucosa becomes more uneven and its outline also becomes irregular as its upward growth progresses, giving rise to be macroscopical appearance of broad-based and large polypoid protrusion (type I in BORRMANN's classification) (Fig. 78).

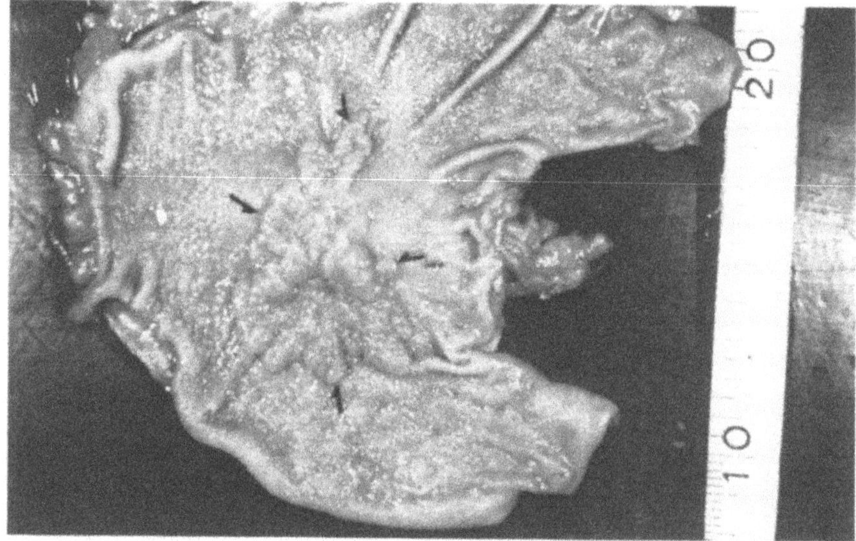

Fig. 76. Broad-based, coral-reef-like mucosal elevation in the angulus (type II a, sm) (arrows). Border of the elevated mucosa is well demarkated. (Pt no. 9772, 59 years, m)

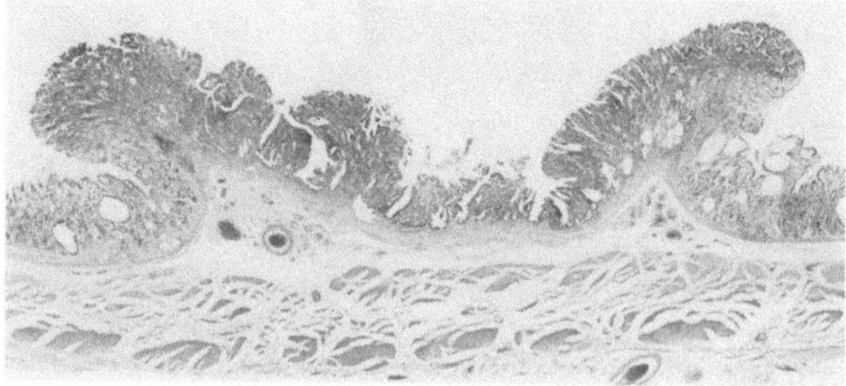

Fig. 77. Cross section through posterior wall of the elevated mucosa in Fig. 76. The cancerous mucosa is entirely occupied by tubular or tubulopapillary structure. Submucosal invasion of the cancer is not visible in this figure. (Pt no. 9772, × 2.5)

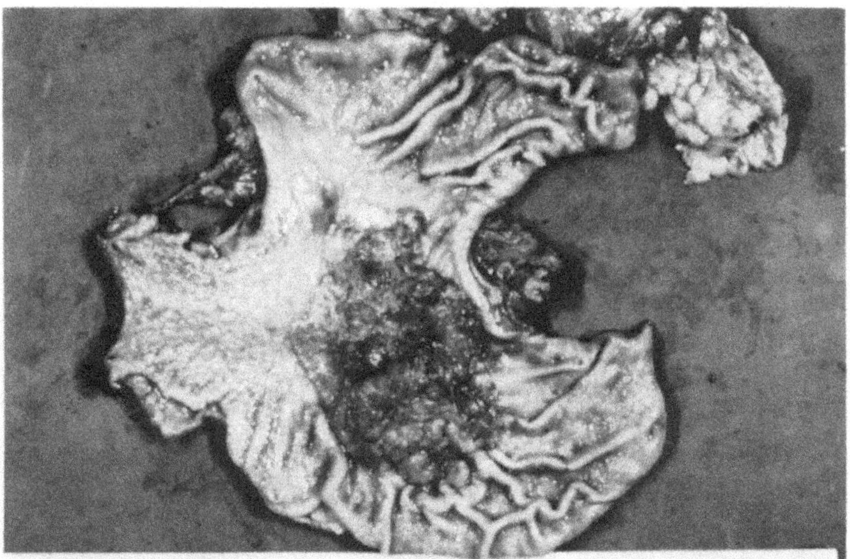

Fig. 78. Large, irregularly shaped mucosal elevation (type IIa, sm) at posterior side of the angulus. Surface of the elevation is also rough and partly destroyed. (Pt no. 15954, 50 years, f)

This type of EGC, especially with medullary stroma, is prone to ulceration over a large area from the central part of the elevated lesion, due to degeneration and necrosis of the cancerous tissues. Thus, some cases of this type may transform directly into the large excavating type with a well-defined boundary (type II in BORRMANN's classification), but the proportion undergoing this process seems to be low (Fig. 79).

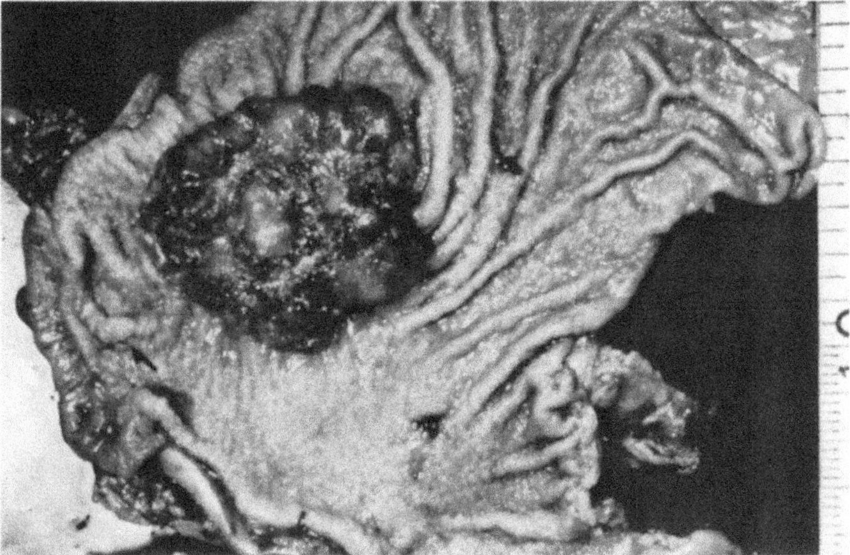

Fig. 79. Large and circumscribed mucosal protrusion in anterior wall of the antrum. Central part of the protrusion is heavily excavated and shows the features of Borrmann's type II, but cancerous growth is still limited to the submucosal layer. (Pt no. 9602, 63 years, m)

Focal Depressed Type

Not only the gross appearance but also the histological features of the lesion, including its surrounding mucosa, provide enough evidence to show that this type of EGC develops into the wider and deeper excavated type of AGC without losing its original well-demarcated structures (type II in BORRMANN's classification) (Figs. 80 and 81).

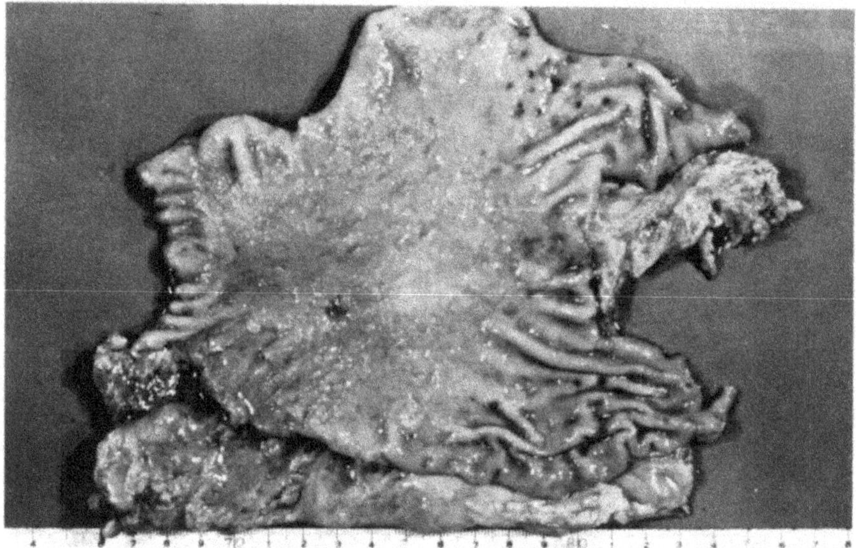

Fig. 80. Tiny but well-demarkated mucosal depression (type II c′, m) in posterior wall of the antrum. Depression is not round but star-shaped. (Pt no. 12633, 60 years, m)

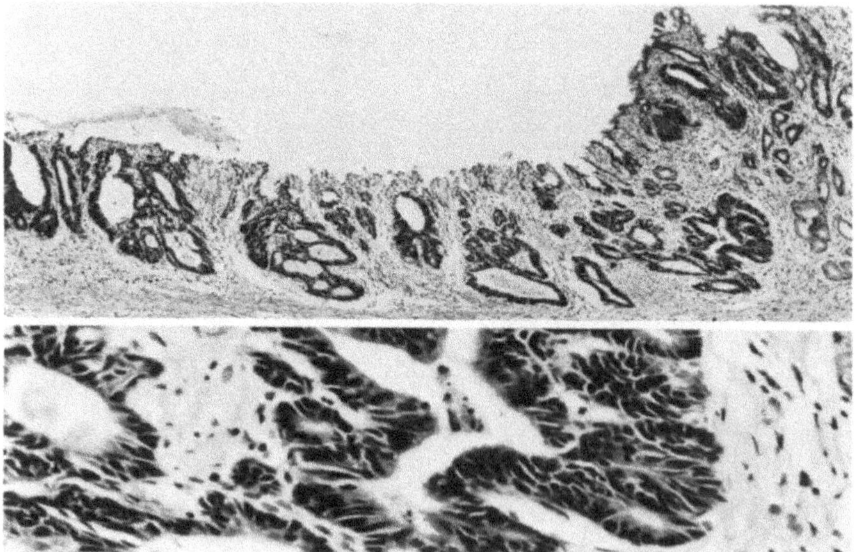

Fig. 81. Cross section through center of the depressed lesion shown in Fig. 80. The lesion is occupied entirely by differentiated-type adenocarcinoma (gastric cancer of intestinal type). The mucosa surrounding the lesion shows severe intestinal metaplasia. (Pt no. 12633, × 20 and × 120)

In general, the size and depth of the depressed cancerous mucosa are closely correlated with the grade of cancerous invasion. The larger and deeper the lesion is, the more probable it is that the cancerous growth will advance within the stomach. The degree of elevation of the marginal mucosa around the depressed lesion is also an another indicator of the grade of invasive growth (Figs. 82–84).

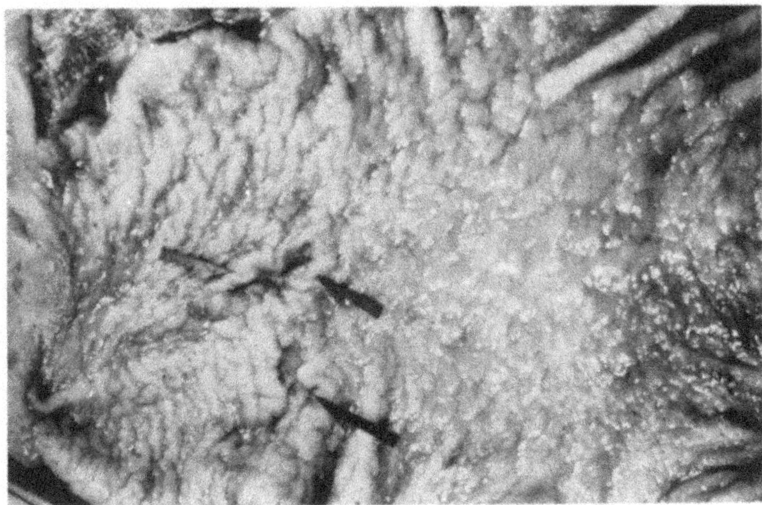

Fig. 82. Two small foci of a circumscribed mucosal depression (type IIc′, m and sm) (arrows). In the focus on the lesser curvature, showing deep depression, the cancer has already invaded the muscularis propria, while the focus on the posterior wall is restricted to the mucosa. (Pt no. 6025, 63 years, m)

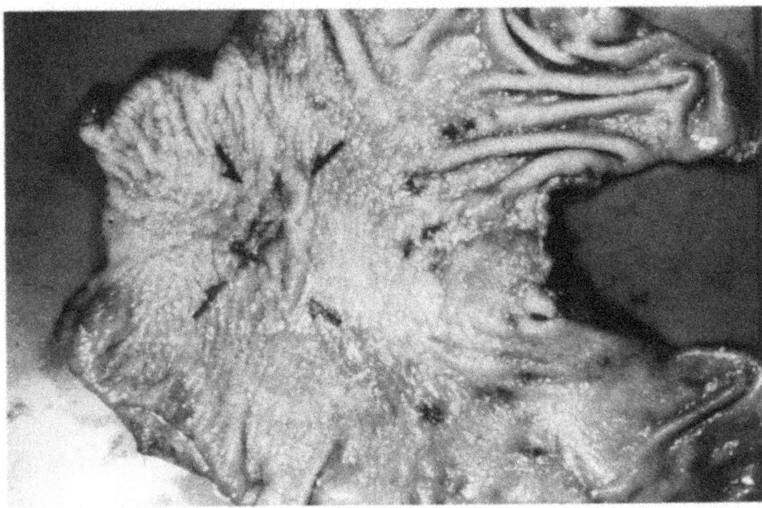

Fig. 83. Mucosal depression, larger and deeper than in the case shown in Fig. 82. and with more prominent elevation of the marginal mucosa (arrows). Cancerous tissue has invaded the submucosal layer (type IIc′, sm)

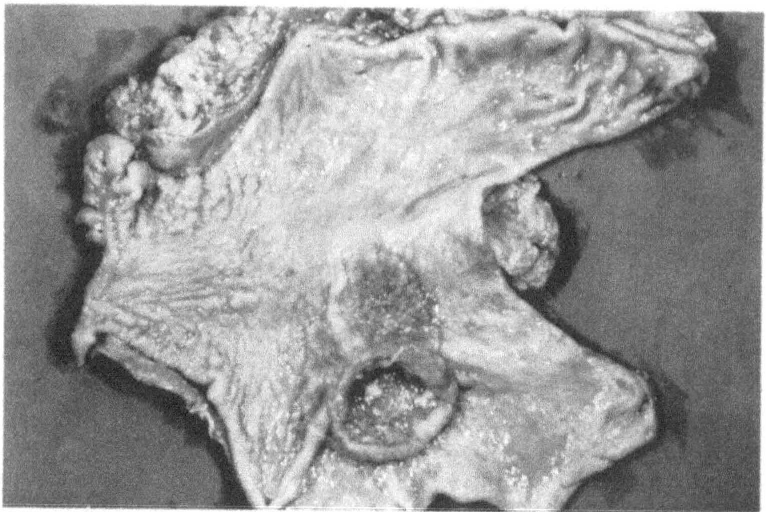

Fig. 84. Two large and circumscribed mucosal depressions situated side by side in the posterior wall of the stomach. In the deeper lesion, which has the gross appearance of Borrmann's type II, the cancer is already growing beyond the serosa, while in the shallow one (type II c′ + II a) the growth is limited to the mucosa. Both lesions show the same histology of well-differentiated adenocarcinoma. (Pt no. 13707, 65 years, m)

Large Eroded Type

In the early stage, this type of cancer shows only superficial changes in the affected mucosa: extensive erosion accompanied by serrated or ill-defined borders, regardless of the presence or absence of peptic ulcer within the erosion. Not infrequently, however, the same mucosal changes may be encountered, accompanied by slight induration of the gastric wall in the central parts of the eroded lesion. In these cases, infiltration of cancer cells is almost always seen not only in the submucosa but also in the deeper layers, together with fibrous connective tissue proliferation. In cases with such macroscopical findings the criteria used in BORRMANN's classification cannot be applied, and they are often called gastric cancer of intermediate stage.

These observations demonstrate that the eroded type of EGC showing poorly differentiated histology may grow into gastric cancer characterized by diffuse and scirrhous thickening of the gastric wall (type III or IV in Borrmann's classification) in the advanced stages (Figs. 85–90).

86

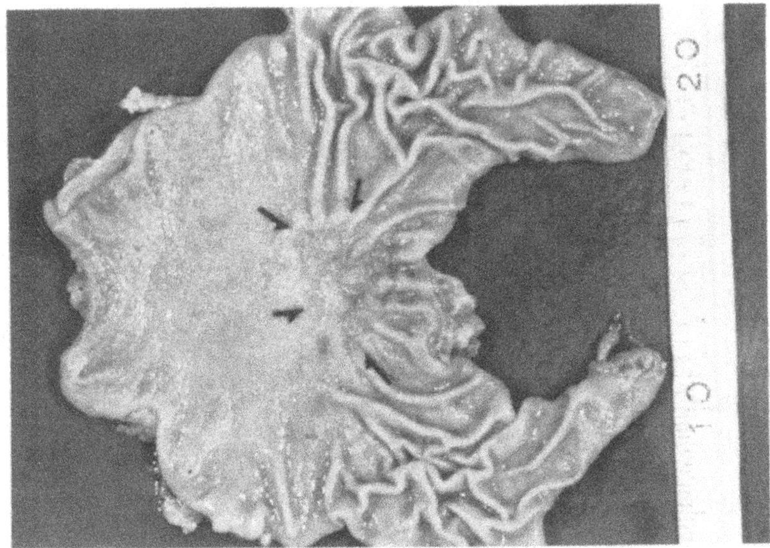

Fig. 85. Medium-sized cancerous erosion with central ulceration (type II c″ + III, sm) in the angulus (arrows). Interruption of the convergent mucosal folds is also apparent. (Pt no. 11 112, 27 years, m)

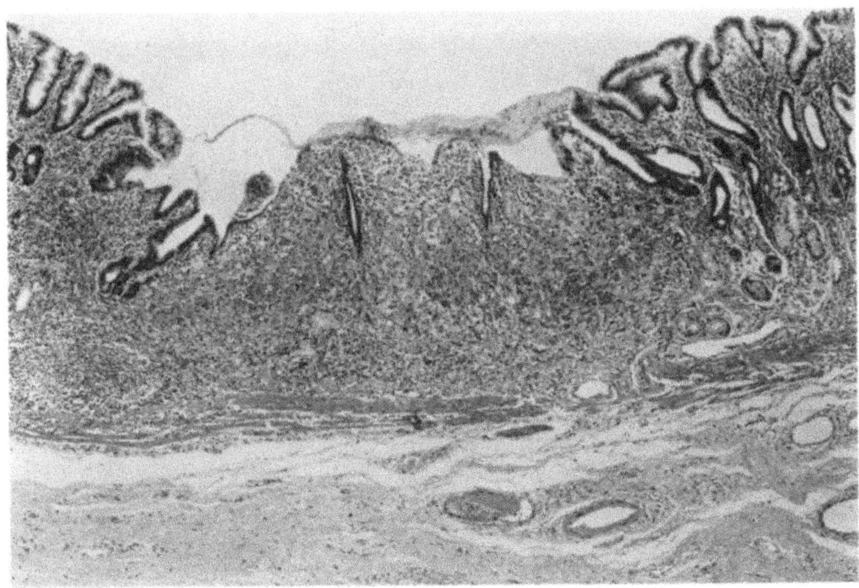

Fig. 86. Peripheral part of the cancerous erosion shown in Fig. 85. The eroded mucosa is covered with exudate and diffusely infiltrated by poorly differentiated adenocarcinoma. (Pt no. 11 112, × 20)

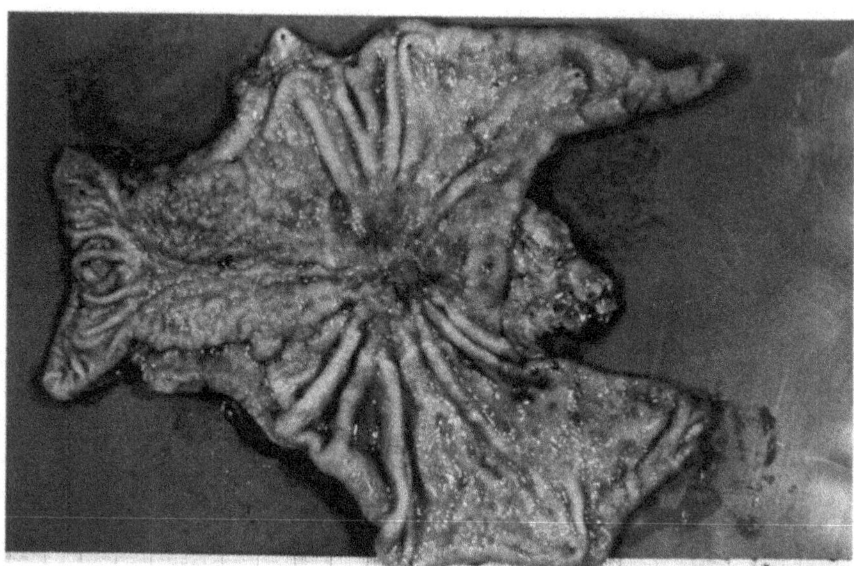

Fig. 87. Cancerous erosion with central ulceration (type II c″ + III, ss) in the angulus. Cancerous infiltration involves the subserosa but none of the criteria use in Borrmann's classification system are applicable. (Pt no. 13 532, 66 years, m)

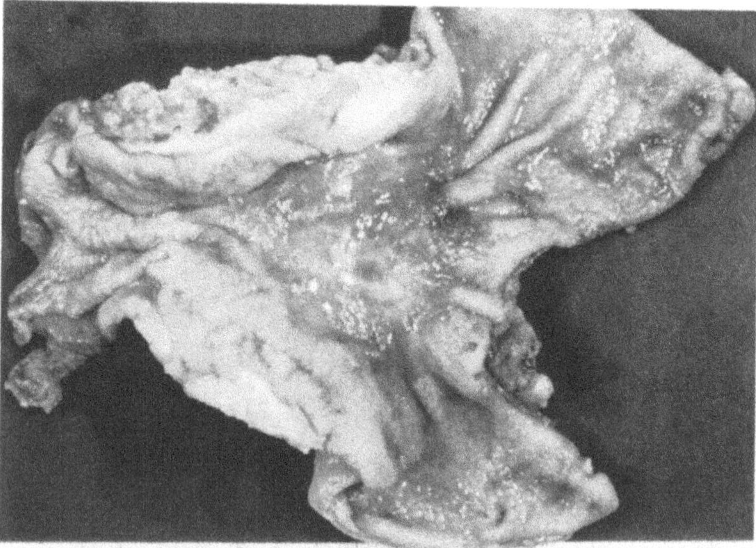

Fig. 88. Wall of the antrum diffusely thickened by scirrhous growth of cancer (Borrmann IV). Large cancerous erosion, as indicated by abrupt thinning of the mucosal folds, is still visible in the affected mucosa. (Pt no. 12 121, 48 years, m)

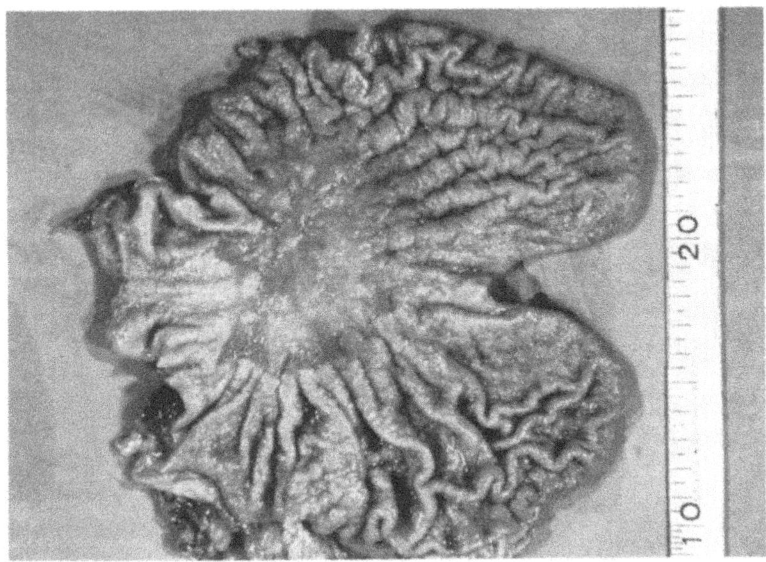

Fig. 89. Another example of Borrmann's type IV. Mucosal folds in anterior wall of the corpus are swollen due to intramural scirrhous infiltration of the cancer cells. (Pt no. 10021, 44 years, m)

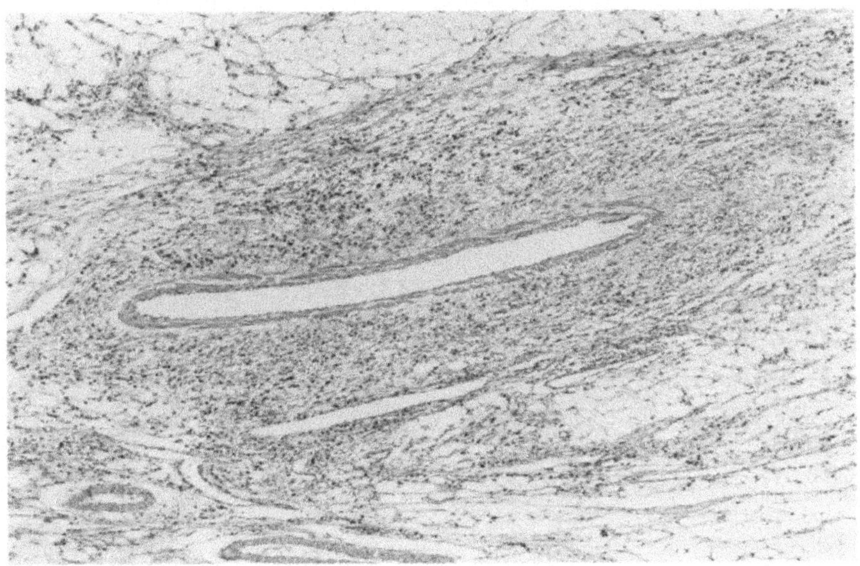

Fig. 90. Histological features of the serosa in the case illustrated in Fig. 89. The serosa is diffusely infiltrated by free cancer cells, and the infiltration is more intense in the tissue around blood vessels than in the adipose tissue. (Pt no. 10021, × 40)

Peptically Ulcerated Type

As described previously, EGC showing macroscopical changes similar to those seen in nonmalignant peptic ulcer is not characterized by any particular histological type. Because of this, there is no definite developmental course and various macroscopic appearances may be found in the advanced stages. The nature of the

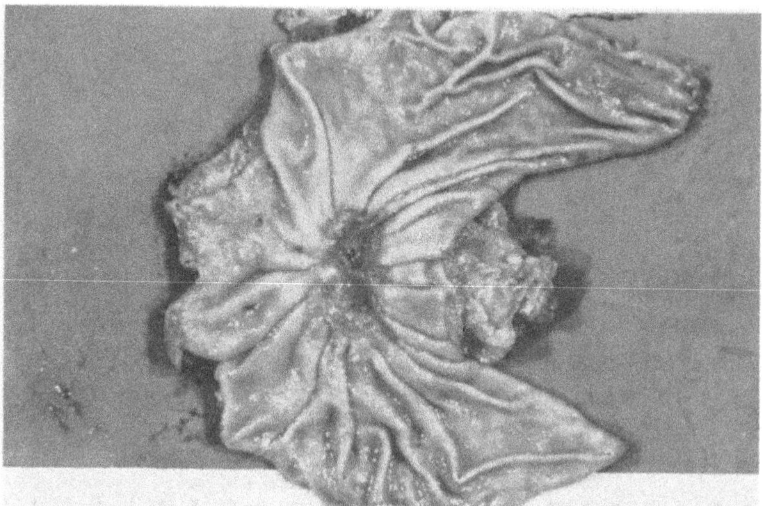

Fig. 91. Chronic peptic ulcer in the angulus is surrounded by a narrow zone of cancerous erosion (type III + II c″, pm). Grade of cancerous invasion cannot be determined by macroscopical examination alone. (Pt no. 15011, 47 years, m)

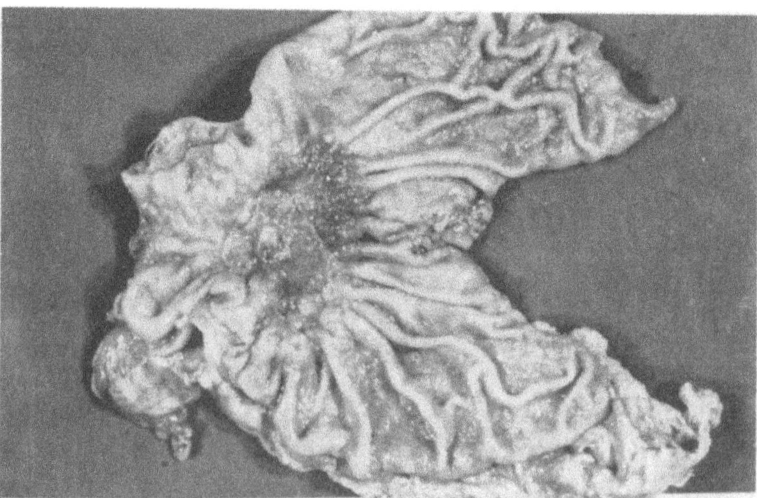

Fig. 92. More advanced stage of an ulcerated lesion (Borrmann III). Due to diffuse infiltration of the cancer cells into a deeper layer of the gastric mucosa, the wall of the antrum is already indurated and stenotic. (Pt no. 12288, 41 years, m)

90

cancer, whether it is histologically of the intestinal or the diffuse type, and the behavior of peptic ulcer, whether it is healing with scar formation, growing into a deeper and larger ulcer, or stationary forming an open chronic ulcer, may be some of the determining factors when the cancer progresses to the stage of AGC. Thus, during progression of their growth, the cases with intestinal-type histology may assume the gross appearance of BORRMANN's type II, while other cases with diffuse-type histology will develop into BORRMANN's type III and others with the same histology but with healing ulcer may assume the form of BORRMANN's type IV (Figs. 91–93).

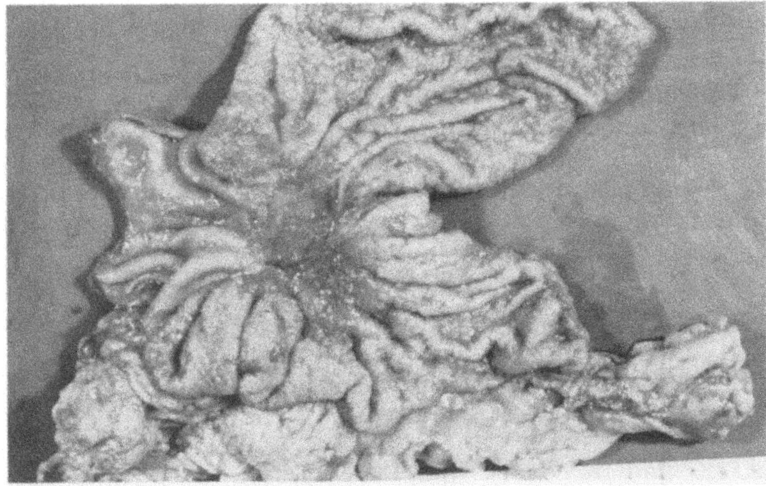

Fig. 93. Similar appearance to that seen in Fig. 92 (Borrmann III). Stomach wall around the ulcer is diffusely indurated and the border of the induration is indistinct. (Pt no. 13 047, 60 years, m)

Histogenesis of EGC

Before going into detail on the histogenesis, I should like to mention my own opinion as to the reason for the most remarkable changes over time in the relative frequencies of the different macroscopical types of surgically resected EGC during the past 30 years. In Chap. 4 it was stressed that the most prominent changes is the decrease in the frequency of the ulcerated type (type III + II c" or III + II b) that is similar in gross appearance to chronic peptic ulcer, contrasting with a gradual increase in the frequency of cancerous erosion both without (type II c") and with peptic ulceration (types II c" + III). This pronounced change over time can be explained on the basis of the following factors: from the viewpoint of histogenesis, EGC of types III + II c" and of type III + II b has two entirely different courses of development, one of which is preceded by chronic gastric ulcer or gastric cancer showing histological evidence of the ulcer-cancer sequence (marked with an arrow pointing to the right), while the other is due to secondary peptic ulceration and its exacerbation in the area of cancerous erosion without perceptible enlargement of the erosion in a limited period of time (marked with an arrow pointing to the left (Fig. 94).

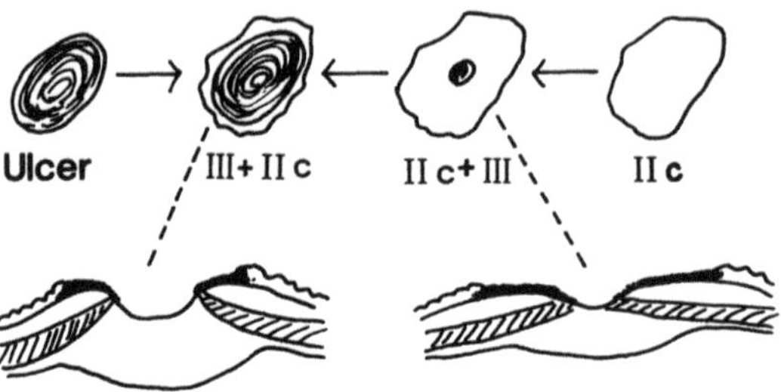

Fig. 94. Histogenesis of ulcerated type of EGC (type III + II c)

EGC of type III + II c" is decreasing in frequency owing to a drastic decrease in the number of cases of chronic gastric ulcer (Fig. 95) in the resected stomachs in one hand, and also to earlier detection and resection of cancerous erosion in its developmental course in another hand. According to recent studies, however, the latter factor seems to play a major role in the declining frequency of type III EGC.

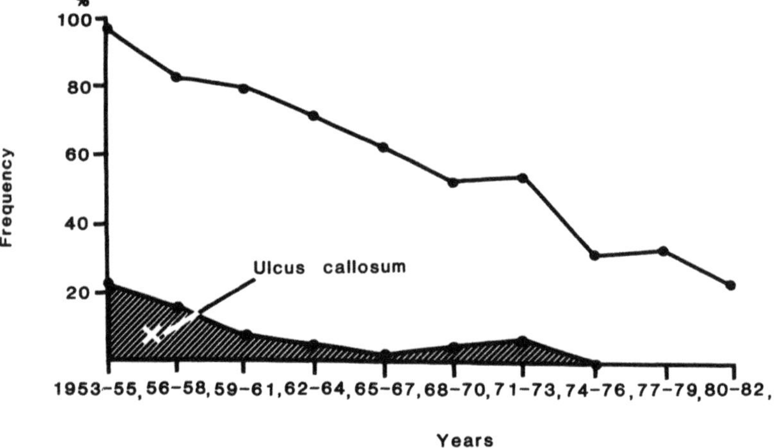

Fig. 95. Changes in frequency of chronic gastric ulcer over time among a total of 7254 cases of all types of gastric ulcers treated by surgical resection

Knowledge of the histogenesis of EGC means determination of the earliest change initiating the development of gastric cancer. This is by no means easy, especially in the stomach without any prominent polypoid protrusion or focal ulceration, as detection of minute or superficial mucosal cancer in routine clinical examinations is quite difficult, and sometimes almost impossible. In the Japanese endoscopical classification the slightest change of a cancerous lesion is classified, after histological examination of the resected stomachs, as "superficial flat" type (type II b). Indeed, at present most of the earliest cancerous lesions are found by chance in resected stomachs as accessory or unexpected changes apart from the

92

main lesion of peptic ulcer or gastric cancer. Two types of precursors of EGC will be described.

Minute Focal Cancer

From the standpoint of histogenesis, it is certain that minute cancerous foci less than 5 mm in diameter, most of which are hardly recognizable on naked-eye examination, represent the earliest stage in the development of gastric cancer. In earlier periods of our study, such foci were found unexpectedly in the mucosa apart from the main lesion of AGC or EGC or peptic ulcer. Owing to the great progress in diagnosis by X-ray and/or endoscopy, minute cancerous foci also became detectable with the aid of biopsy, and for these reasons the frequency of recorded cases with minute cancer alone among patients undergoing gastric resection is increasing slowly but steadily.

Up to 1973, a total of 87 minute cancerous lesions had been found in 70 patients. Among them 50 lesions were found in the mucosa incidental to peptic ulcer as main lesion, 30 were found incidental to gastric cancer, and only 7 lesions (3 patients) were themselves the reason for the resection (Table 20).

Table 20. Cases with minute cancerous lesions

Main lesion	No. of cases	No. of lesions
Ulcer	43	50
Cancer	24	30
Minute cancer	3	7
Total	70	87

Table 21. Macroscopical changes in minute cancerous lesions

Main lesion	Macroscopical changes		
	Erosion	Depression	Not recognizable
Ulcer	25	3	22
Cancer	10	7	13
Minute cancer	6	1	0
Total	41	11	35

Retrospective examination of these cases on the basis of the macroscopical photographs taken after surgical resection revealed that more than half (59.8%) the lesions showed tiny erosions or tiny mucosal depressions, but no macroscopical changes could be recognized in the other 35 lesions (Table 21 and Fig. 96).

The minute lesions were mostly unifocal and were found more frequently in the mucosa of the antrum than of the corpus, as in the cases of EGC and AGC (Fig. 97).

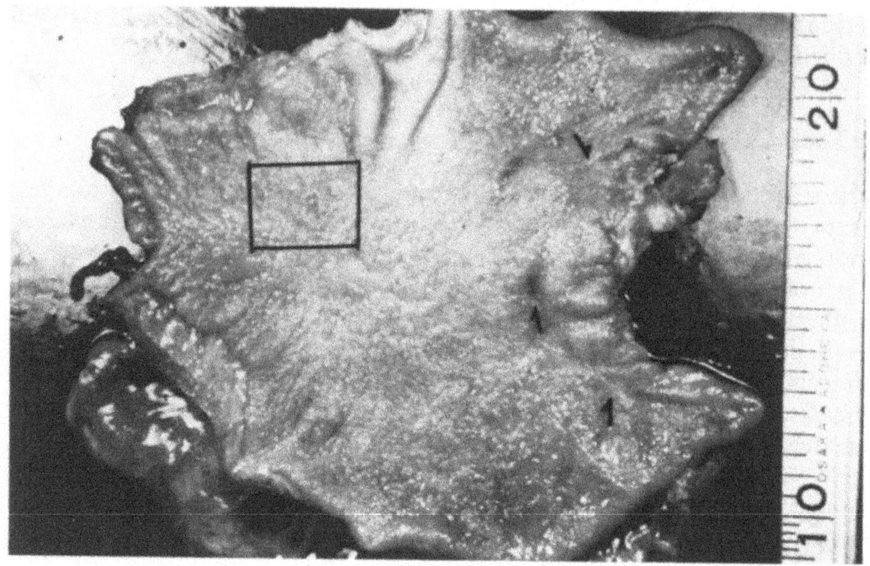

Fig. 96. Apart from three linearly arranged ulcer scars *(arrows)* and a small polyp in posterior wall of the angulus, tiny but well-defined mucosal depression (surrounded by *square*) is seen in the antrum. (Pt no. 9453, 54 years, f)

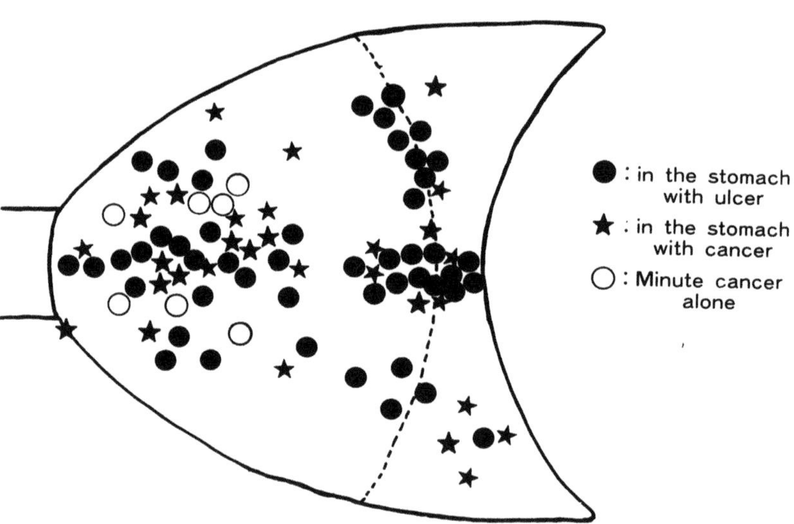

Fig. 97. Sites of minute cancerous lesions

The minute cancerous lesions also vary in their histological features, ranging from well-differentiated tubular adenocarcinoma to infiltrative poorly differentiated adenocarcinoma containing signet-ring cells, and regardless of histological type the center of the minute cancerous lesions is mostly situated in the grooved area between area gastricae (Figs. 98–100).

94

A close correlation between the histology of minute cancerous tissue and the grade of intestinal metaplasia of the cancer-bearing gastric mucosa was confirmed by several investigators [4, 8–16, 19]. Similar to these reports, all cases of well-differentiated adenocarcinoma synonymous with gastric cancer of intestinal

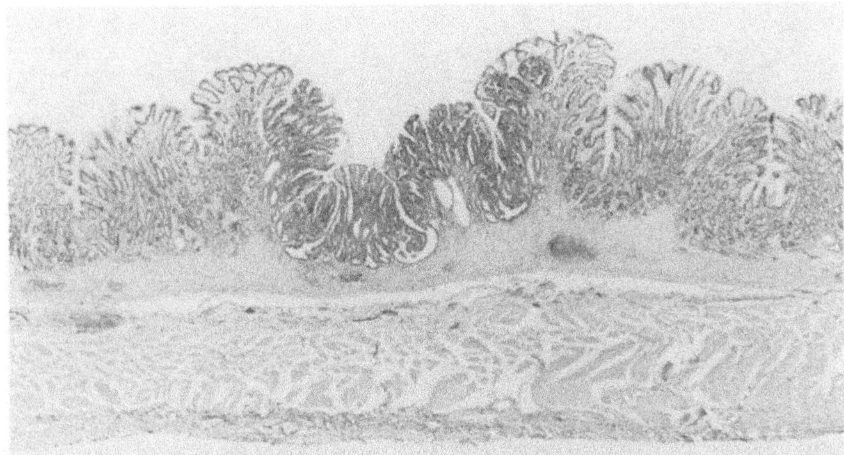

Fig. 98. Histological section through center of the tiny mucosal depression shown in Fig. 96. The depressed mucosa is composed of well-differentiated tubular adenocarcinoma with clear border from surrounding metaplastic mucosa. (Pt no. 9453, × 10)

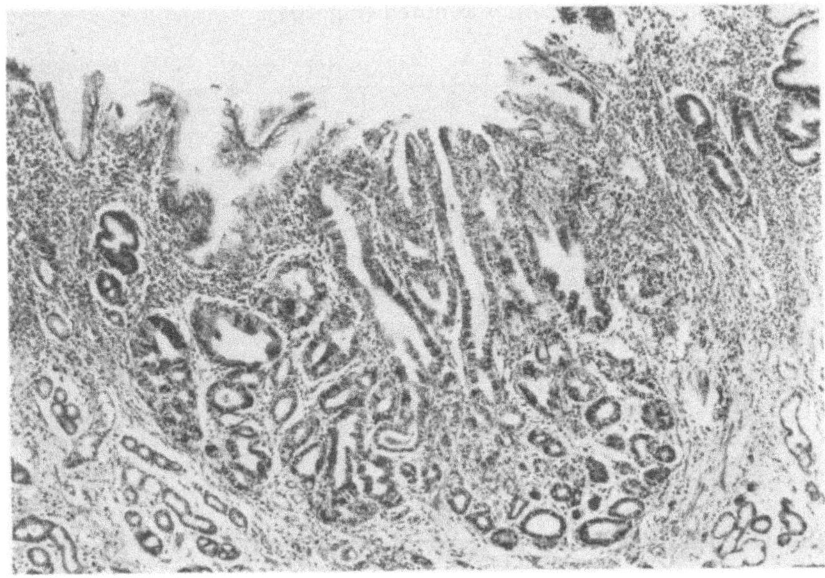

Fig. 99. Grooved area of the nonmetaplastic mucosa is occupied by tiny lesion of tubular and glandular adenocarcinoma composed of columnar and cuboidal epithelial cells. Border of the lesion is well defined. (Pt no. 8516, × 40)

95

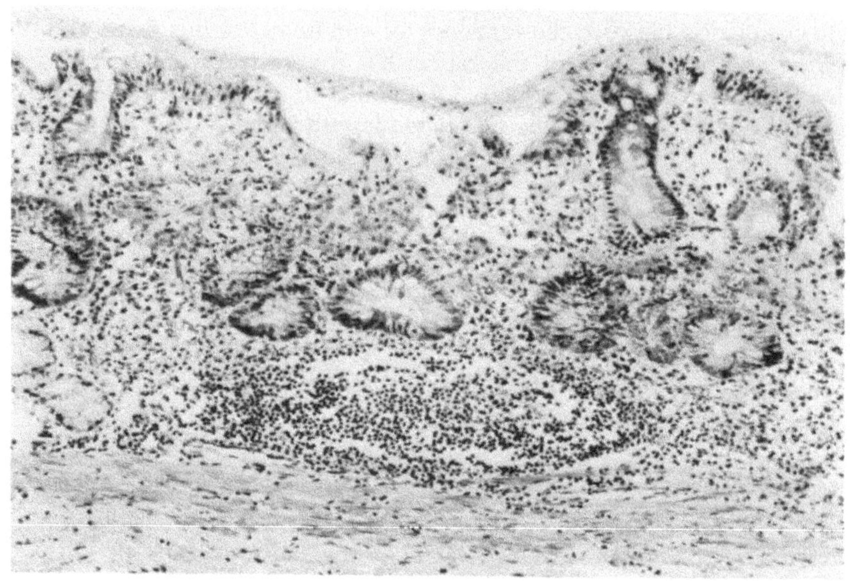

Fig. 100. In the grooved area of the atrophic and metaplastic mucosa, minute cancerous tissue infiltrated by poorly differentiated cancer cells is visible. Surface of the grooved mucosa is covered by fibrin. (Pt no. 2315, × 40)

type showed a high grade of intestinal metaplasia, while in the case of poorly differentiated adenocarcinoma almost equal to gastric cancer of the diffuse type no such histological inclination was noted (Fig. 101).

Histological types \ Grade of metaplasia		╫	╪	+	−	Total
Grade of differentiation	well	●▲▲▲▲▲ ●▲▲▲▲○ ●▲▲▲○ ●▲▲▲○	●●●●● ●●●▲ ●●● ●●●			3 4
	moderate	● ▲ ▲	●●●▲ ●●●▲ ●●●▲ ●●●▲	●● ●● ●▲ ●		2 2
	poor	●●	●●●	●●●●● ●●	▲▲▲	1 4
Total		2 5	2 9	1 3	3	7 0

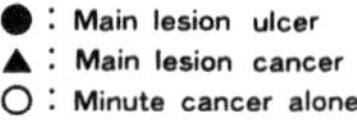

Fig. 101. Relationship between histological types of minute gastric cancer and grades of intestinal metaplasia in cancer-bearing stomachs

Superficial Cancer Without Perceptible Macroscopical Change

In the days when cases of EGC with widespread cancerous erosion were increasing in number, the eroded lesion was thought to be characterized by a recognizable border from the surrounding mucosa, by a shallow serrated configuration in

96

an area of antrum, or by abrupt thinning of the mucosal folds in an area of the corpus. But recently we have quite commonly encountered cases in which the erosion is quite extensive but its boundary cannot be clearly seen owing to the flat, gradual, and atrophic nature of its periphery (Figs. 102 and 103).

Histological specimens taken from these areas often show cancer cell infiltration containing signet-ring cells in the upper layer of the atrophic mucosa while the surface epithelium remains intact, or in other cases, the affected mucosa is composed entirely of cancerous tissues in situ and they show a fine network or anastomosing glandular structures composed of small and cuboidal cancer cells without any erosive changes at the surface and infiltrative growth within the mucosa (Figs. 104 and 105).

From the findings described above, the changes seem to be in the earliest stage or incipient phase of cancerization of the gastric mucosa, which corresponds to the "superficial flat type" (type IIb) of EGC in the Japanese endoscopical classification. Even though some endoscopists cite discoloration and/or roughness of the surface of the affected mucosa, the lesion shows no elevation or depression at all, and is really almost imperceptible on naked-eye examination. For such reasons, few papers deal with EGC of this type, and most lesions reported are found unexpectedly in the resected stomachs apart from or adjacent to the clinically detectable main lesion of cancer or ulcer [2, 5, 6, 17].

The histogenesis of this type of EGC, whether it develops from the superficial spread of a unifocal minute cancer, results from the coalescence of multiple minute foci occurring in a certain limited area, or is preceded by an extensive precancerous lesion, is not yet fully elucidated.

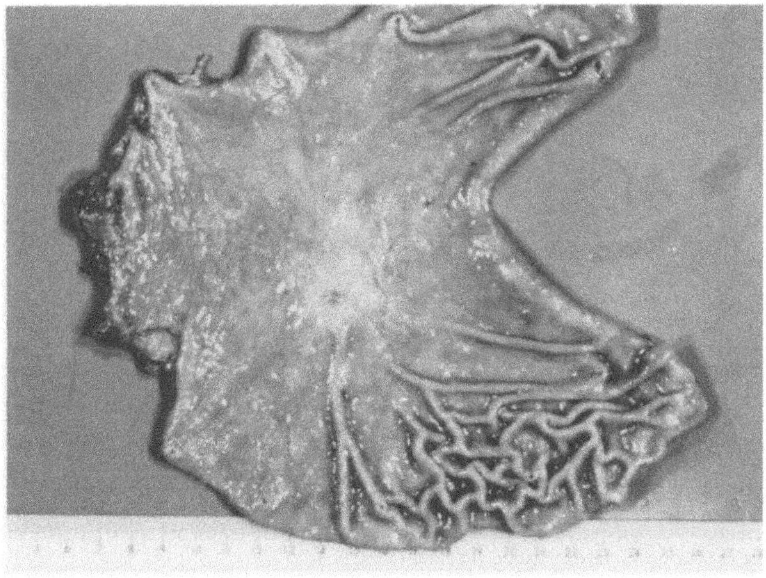

Fig. 102. Medium-sized cancerous erosion in the angulus. Periphery of the erosion is well defined at the posterior wall side but ill defined at the anterior wall side. (Pt no. 18 055, 32 years, f)

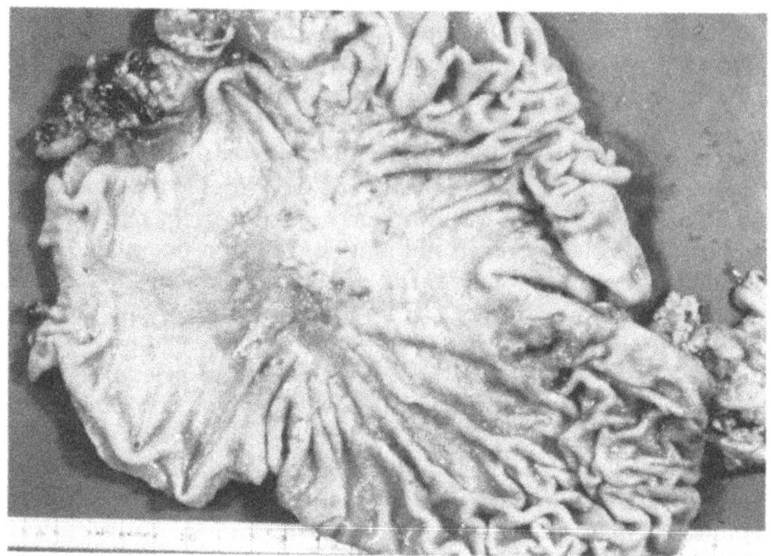

Fig. 103. Large and shallow cancerous erosion located in the angulus. Most of its periphery is clearly recognizable as a zigzag contour or as disruption of the mucosal folds, but the oral side periphery of the lesion is somewhat obscure. Another smaller cancerous erosion is seen in posterior wall of the corpus. (Pt no. 12 983, 61 years, m)

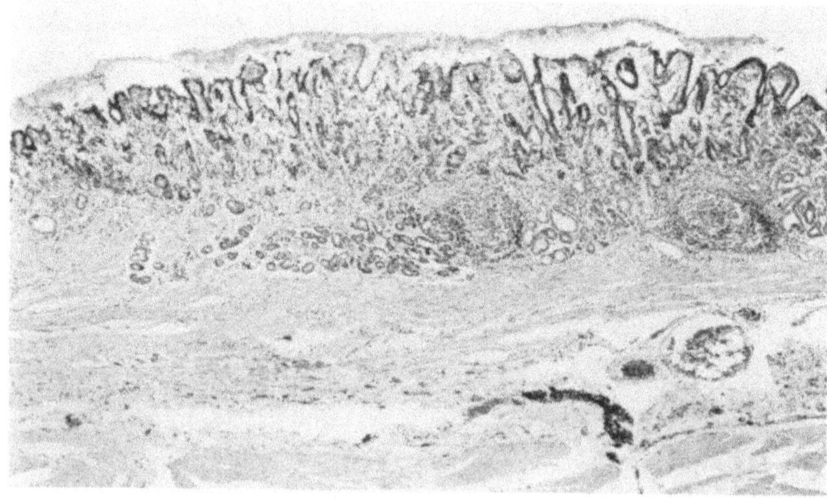

Fig. 104. Histological features of the mucosa, showing obscure periphery in macroscopical examination. The eroded and regenerated mucosa covered by fibrin coat is diffusely occupied by poorly differentiated adenocarcinoma composed of small cuboidal epithelial cells, but no infiltrative growth of the cancerous glands is visible. (Pt no. 14 529, × 40)

98

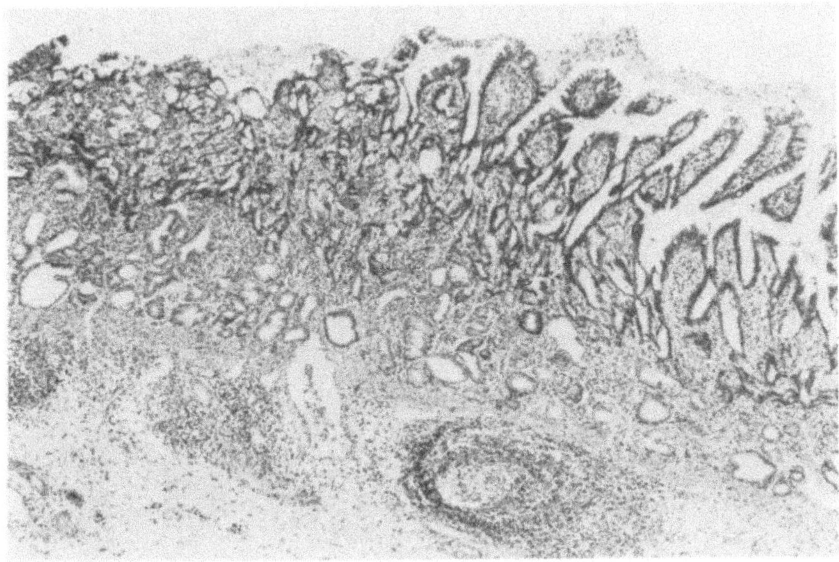

Fig. 105. Another example of cancerous erosion with no clear boundary. The atrophic mucosa is made up of small carcinomatous glands forming a reticular or anastomosing structure. The malignant change is more obvious at the left of the figure, but a gradual transition to the right side change is recognizable. (Pt no. 13 320, × 40)

Double or Multiple Foci of EGC

As reported by several investigators, cases showing double or multiple cancerous foci in a stomach are not infrequent. There is no doubt that gastric cancer can occur in two or more sites apart from each other (Fig. 106), but the frequency of double or multiple cancers among all the surgically resected stomachs is lower than 10% in almost all papers [1, 3, 7, 18, 20]. It is also known from the reports that the frequency rises with advancing age of the patients (Fig. 107).

Size, shape, and grades of double, triple, and multiple cancerous foci vary from case to case, but in cases of AGC a second or third focus is far smaller than the original one and often in a stage of EGC, while in EGC the size and grade of a second focus are not very different from those of the primary one. From the viewpoint of histogenesis of EGC, the multiple occurrence of cancer in a certain limited area is possible. As described earlier in this chapter, it is not unusual for the gastric mucosa to contain two or more minute cancerous lesions but most of these foci are found some distance apart in the mucosa. It is possible that such minute cancers develop close together and fuse during growth to form a single macroscopical focus. This seems more likely in diffuse-type histology than in the intestinal type, according to the superficially spreading nature of the former. However, without serial sectioning of the paraffin-embedded blocks such detailed histogenetical studies cannot be achieved. Among 5510 surgically resected stomachs, those with double cancerous foci accounted for 259 (4.7%): of these, 158 were affected by AGC + AGC or AGC + EGC (3.6% of all the AGC resected) and 101 by double lesions EGC (8.3% of all the EGC resected) (Table 22).

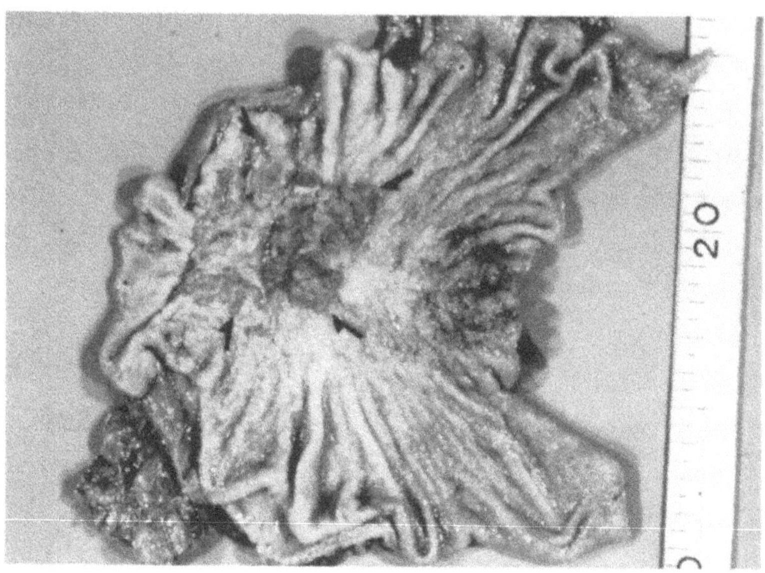

Fig. 106. Triple EGC in a stomach: Polypoid protrusion (type I, m) adjacent to well-demarcated mucosal depressions (type IIc + IIa) in anterior side of the angulus; in addition, small but deep mucosal depression (type IIc′, m) with slight convergency of the mucosal folds is visible near proximal cut end of the stomach. (Pt no. 9816, 48 years, f)

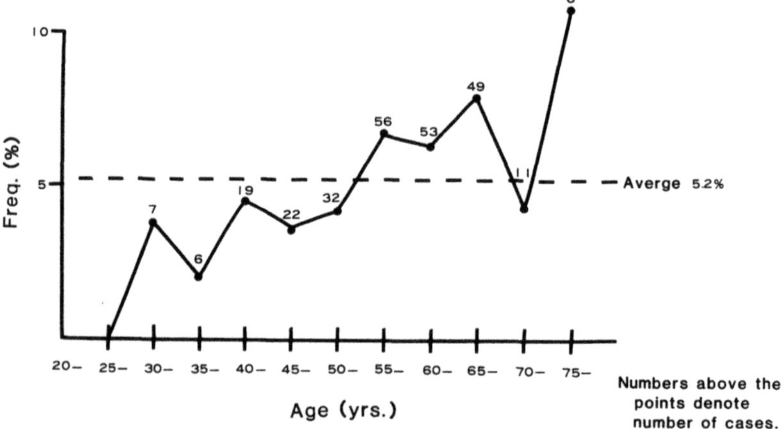

Fig. 107. Frequency of double gastric cancer by patient age

Table 22. Double gastric cancer

Type of coexistence	No. of cases	Frequency (%)
AGC – AGC	56	3.6[a]
AGC – EGC	102	
EGC – EGC	101	8.3[b]
Total	259	4.7[c]

[a] Among cases of AGC
[b] Among cases of EGC
[c] Among all cases of gastric cancer

100

Double or multiple cancerous lesions in a single stomach are dealt with in this chapter because some of these cases, where the same type of morphology but at different stages of cancerous growth, yield important information on the developmental course of EGC, example of which is illustrated in Fig. 84.

References

1. Collins WT, Gall EA (1952) Gastric carcinoma: A multicentric lesion. Cancer 5: 62–72
2. Elster K, Kolaczek F, Shimamoto K, Freitag H (1975) Early gastric cancer – experience in Germany. Endoscopy 7: 5–10
3. Grundmann E, Schlake W (1982) Histological classification of gastric cancer from initial to advanced stages. Pathol Res Pract 173: 260–274
4. Hirota T, Itabashi M, Yoshida S (1980) Clinicopathologic study of minute and small early gastric cancer. Histogenesis of gastric cancer. Pathol Ann 5: 1–19
5. Johansen A (1981) The imperceptible EGC. Early gastric cancer. A contribution to the pathology and to gastric cancer histogenesis. Department of Pathology, Bispebjerg Hospital, Copenhagen, pp 70–75
6. Miller G, Kaufmann M (1975) Das Magenfrühkarzinom in Europa. Dtsch Med Wochenschr 100: 1946–1949
7. Moertel CC, Bargen AA, Soule EH (1957) Multiple gastric cancers. Review of the literature and study of 42 cases. Gastroenterology 32: 1095–1103
8. Murakami T (1960) On the point of the development of stomach cancer. Proc Jpn Cancer Assoc 19: 305–312
9. Murakami T (1953) On the histogenesis of adenocarcinoma of the stomach. Gann 44: 33–37
10. Murakami T (1952) Studies on the histogenesis of early gastric cancer. Acta Pathol Jpn 2: 10–22
11. Nagayo T (1975) Microscopical cancer of the stomach – A study on histogenesis of gastric carcinoma. Int J Cancer 16: 52–60
12. Nakamura K, Sugano H (1983) Microcarcinoma of the stomach less than 5 mm in the largest diameter and its histogenesis. 13th International Cancer Congress, Seattle, pp 107–116
13. Nakamura K, Sugano H (1983) Microcarcinoma of the stomach measuring less than 5 mm in the largest diameter and its histogenesis. Prog Clin Biol Res 132: 107–116
14. Nakamura K, Sugano H, Kato Y (1978) Histogenesis of microcarcinoma of the stomach measuring less than 5 mm in the largest diameter (Abstr). 12th International Cancer Congress, Buenos Aires, p 238
15. Oohara T, Aono G, Ukawa S et al. (1984) Clinical diagnosis of minute gastric cancer less than 5 mm in diameter. Cancer 53: 162–165
16. Oohara T, Tohma H, Takezoe K et al. (1982) Minute gastric cancer less than 5 mm in diameter. Cancer 50: 801–810
17. Rösch W, Kock H (1976) Magenfrühkarzinom: Makroskopie und Biopsie. Erfahrungen bei 50 Fällen. Aktuel Gastrol 5: 238–246
18. Schlake W, Grundmann E (1979) Multifocal early gastric cancer of mixed type. Pathol Res Pract 164: 331–341
19. Taki K, Kuwabara N (1981) Studies on histogenesis of the gastric carcinoma using minute cancers. Pathol Res Pract 172: 176–190
20. Wiendl HJ, Piger A (1971) Multizentrische Frühkarzinom des Magens. Endoscopy 4: 210–211

6. Precursors of Early Gastric Cancer

Before any detailed discussion, it seems necessary to define the term "precursor," because casual use of this term can lead to serious difficulties owing to misunderstanding. In the author's opinion, the term precursor includes two different concepts – precancerous condition and precancerous lesion. "Precancerous condition" is a clinical term or clinical concept meaning merely that the condition is attended by a higher risk of cancerization than other diseases of the stomach, while "precancerous lesion" is a histological term and means that the presence of the dangerous lesion can only be detected by histological examination. Thus, the two terms are by no means synonymous, but it is also true that all precancerous lesions are found in gastric diseases that can be described as precancerous conditions (Fig. 108).

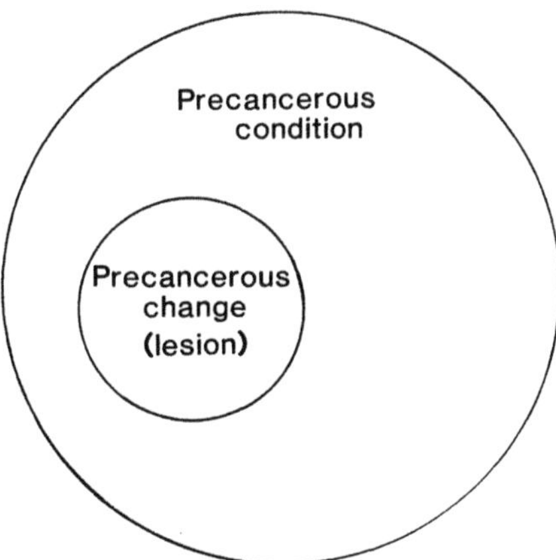

Fig. 108. Relation between precancerous condition and precancerous change (lesion)

Several types of precancerous conditions, e.g., gastric polyp, chronic peptic ulcer, chronic gastritis, will be described at first and then the concept of precancerous lesions will be explained.

Gastric Polyp

Regardless of size, shape, and number, gastric polyps are defined macroscopically as hemispheric, pedunculated, or sessile protrusions of the gastric mucosa. Some polyps have a smooth or lobulated surface, while others have a granular, or strawberry-like, appearance. The number and size of polyps also vary from single, large polyps to multiple, smaller ones, but they are mostly unifocal and less than 2 cm in diameter. The site or the polyps is also random and there is no preferential site. Small polyps are not uncommonly seen in the stomach without any clinical symptoms.

When the real frequency of malignant transformation of epithelial gastric polyps is sought, the method should not be based on surgically resected stomachs but on endoscopically detectable polyps, because of the highly restricted surgical resectability of the polyps. For these reasons, biopsy specimens taken from consecutive patients with polyps over certain periods of time were used for the study.

On basis of their histological nature, the biopsied gastric polyps were classified into two main types:

a) hyperplastic and
b) adenomatous polyps.

Tiny and often multiple regenerative polyps, such as gastritis verrucosa, were excluded from the statistics, owing to their regenerative and hyperplastic nature.

A hyperplastic polyp is characterized essentially by focal hyperplasia of the gastric mucosa, and especially of foveolar epithelial cells, without loss of its original structures even though secondary changes such as edema and congestion of the stroma or superficial inflammation or erosion, etc. may be seen. Intestinal metaplasia of the surface and foveolar epithelia is seldom seen, except when the polyp has grown to more than 2 cm in diameter (Table 23; Figs. 109–112).

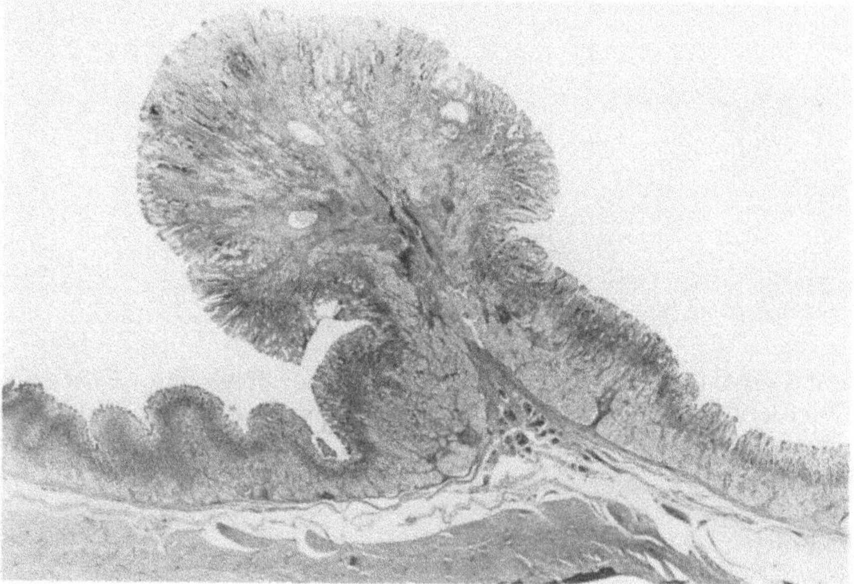

Fig. 109. Pedunculated and hyperplastic polyp of the stomach. The polyp is composed of hyperplasia of both foveolae and gastric glands with a few cysts. Core of the polyp is apparent. No intestinal metaplasia is visible in the polyp. (Pt no. 11 300, × 10)

104

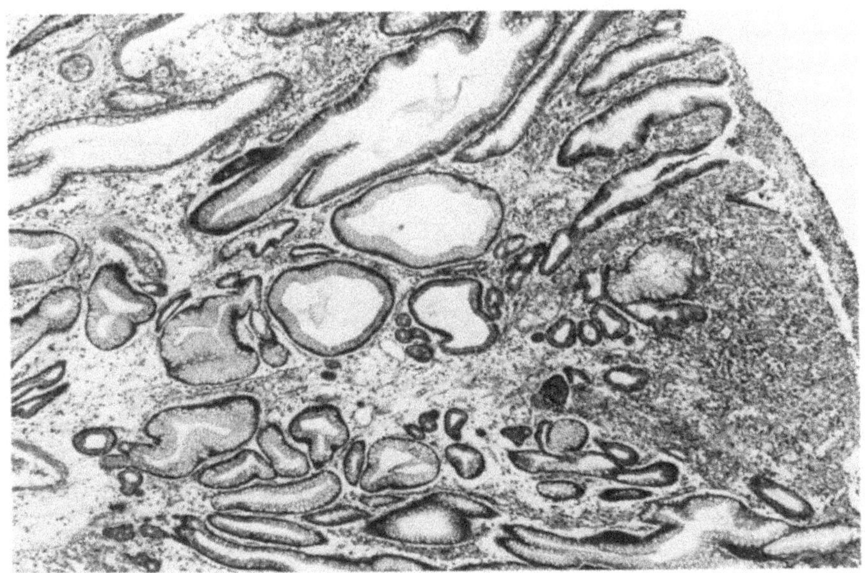

Fig.110. Higher magnification of a part of upper layer of the hyperplastic polyp of Fig. 109. Foveolae forming tubules are elongated, twisted, and branched. Focal inflammation due to erosion is visible on *right* of figure. (Pt no. 11 300, × 40)

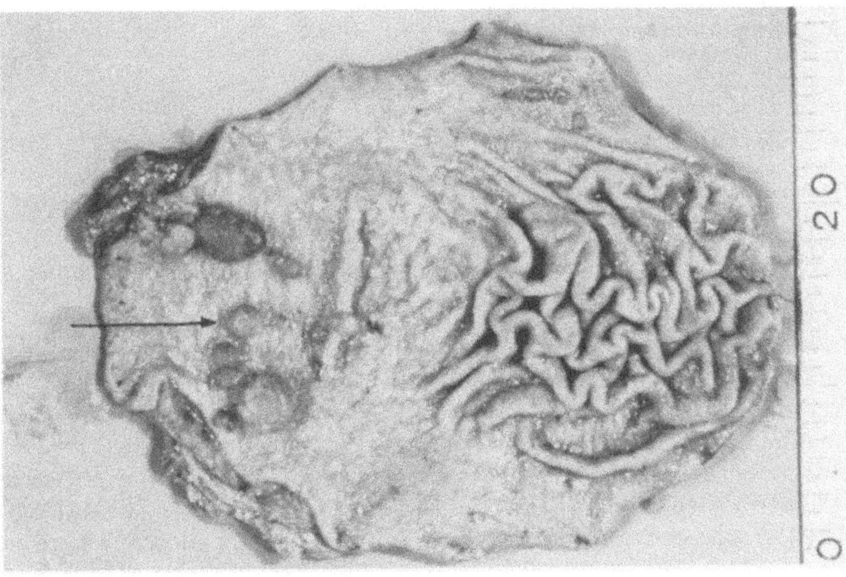

Fig.111. Multiple polyps of various sizes and shapes in the antrum. Larger polyps are pedunculated but smaller ones are hemispheric. (Pt no. 10 153, 66 years, m)

105

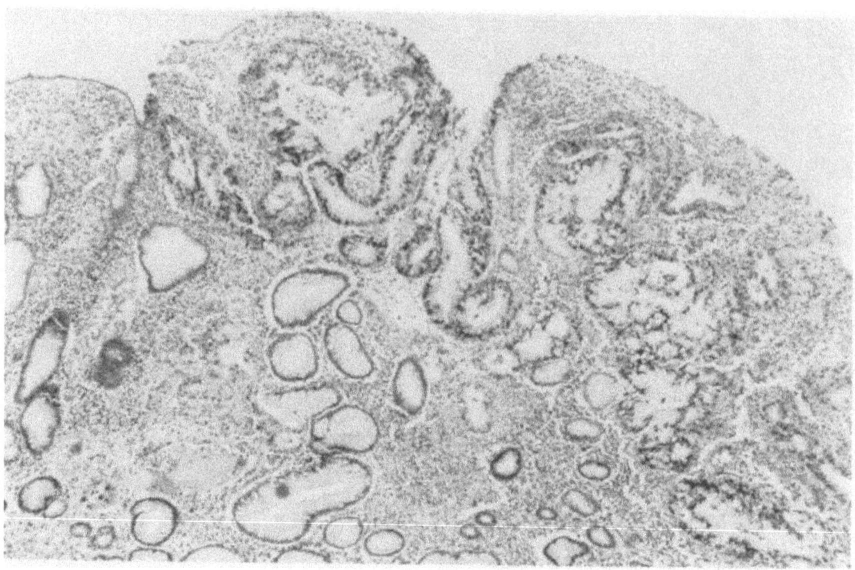

Fig. 112. Surface of the small polyp indicated by the *arrow* in Fig. 111 is transformed into adenocarcinoma with clear cytoplasm. Basic structure of the polyp is hyperplastic. In the other polyps no such cancerous change was visible. (Pt no. 10 153, × 40)

Table 23. Characteristics of hyperplastic polyp

Balanced proliferation of constituents of gastric mucosa
1. Elongation and branching of foveolar tissue
2. Proliferation of pyloric or fundic glands
3. Proliferation of stromal connective tissue
4. Fountain-like contour of muscularis mucosae

Other changes often present
a. Edema of the stroma
b. Erosion of mucosal surface
c. Cystic dilatation of the glands
d. Increase of mucus production

In contrast, the basic structure and histological features of the protruding gastric mucosa are greatly modified in the case of adenomatous polyp. In particular, the lesions are composed mainly of irregularly proliferated tubules or glands with the nature of neoplastic, intestinal metaplastic epithelium, and pyloric or fundic glands have almost always disappeared from the lesion. From every aspect, it looks like an adenomatous colorectal polyp (Table 24 and Figs. 113–116).

The 198 consecutive cases of gastric polyp detected by endoscopy were biopsied during the 8 years from 1966 to 1974. Among them 174 cases (87.8%) were diagnosed histologically as hyperplastic polyp, while 13 cases (6.6%) were diagnosed as adenomatous polyps and in another 10 cases classification into either type was impossible owing to insufficient evidence. Malignant changes were seen in only 1 case of the first type, which was exceptionally large (more than 2 cm in

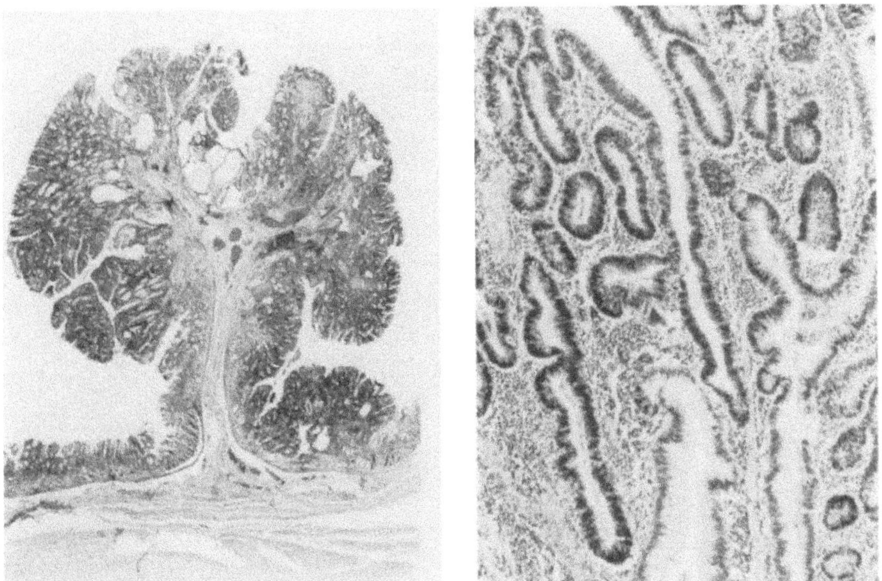

Fig. 113. Pedunculated and adenomatous polyp of the stomach. The polyp is lobulated and composed entirely of elongated and hyperchromatic foveolar tubules made up of tall columnar epithelial cells with the nature of intestinal metaplasia. (Pt no. 3149, ×7 and ×40)

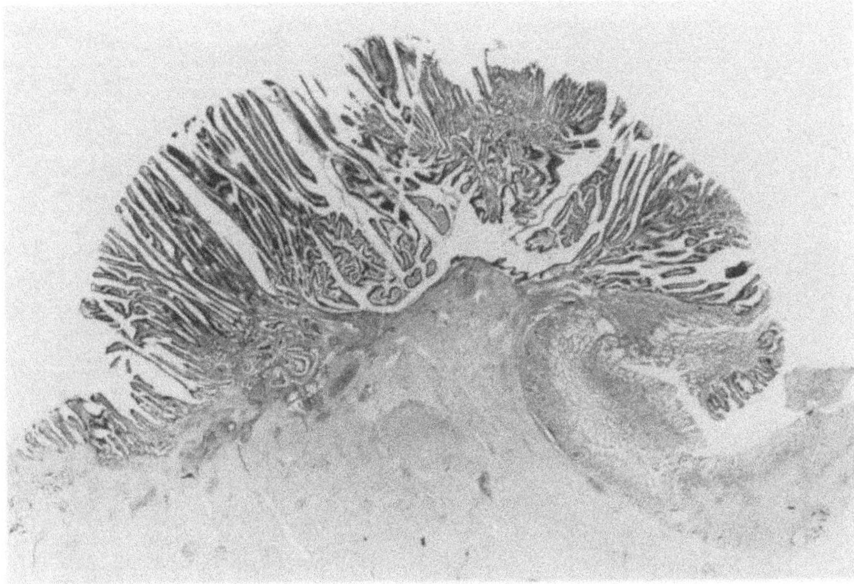

Fig. 114. Hemispheric protruded mucosa composed entirely of adenocarcinoma similar in appearance to villous adenoma of the colon. Submucosal invasion of the cancer is seen in the *left* half. (Pt no. 6833, ×10)

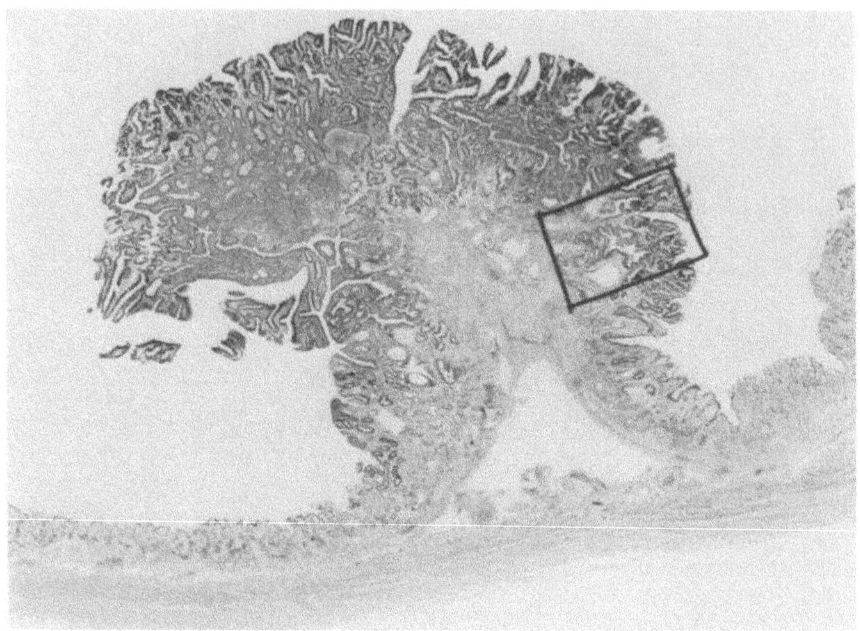

Fig. 115. Pedunculated polyp composed mostly of tubular adenoma. No malignant change is obvious in this low-power view. Atrophic mucosa with severe intestinal metaplasia is seen in the mucosa on the *left*. (Pt no. 13 147, ×7)

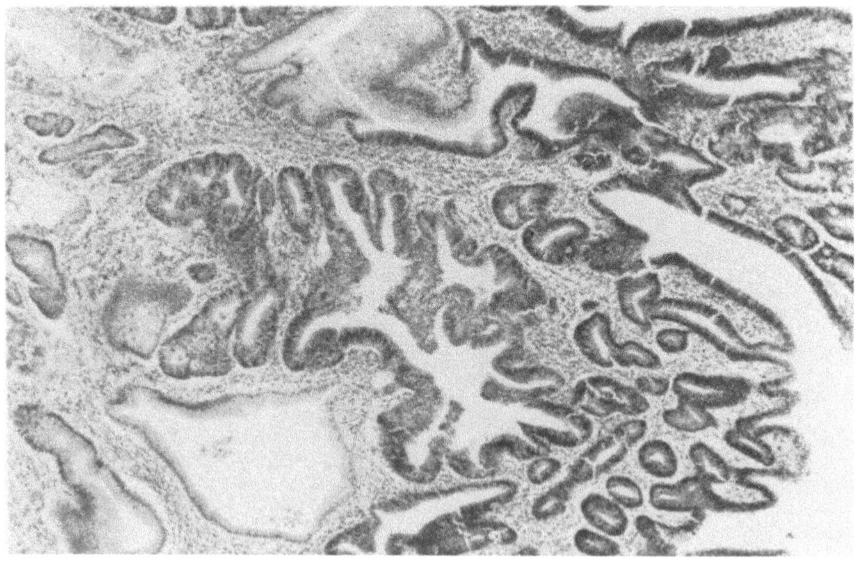

Fig. 116. High-power view of part of the polyp shown in Fig. 115 *(square)* allows detection of well-differentiated tubular adenocarcinoma with branching structure (*central* part of figure) (Pt no. 13 147, ×40)

Table 24. Characteristics of adenomatous polyp

Adenomatous proliferation composed solely of foveolar tissue
1. Irregular growth of metaplastic foveolar tissue
2. Atrophy of pyloric or fundic glands
3. Compression of stroma by the epithelial growth
4. Fountain-like contour of muscularis mucosae

Other changes often present
a. Decrease in number of goblet cells
b. Cystic dilatation of tubulus or glands
c. Appearance of atypical epithelia
d. Appearance of cancerous epithelia

Table 25. Frequencies of hyperplastic and adenomatous polyps and rate of association with cancer as detected by histological examination of biopsies. (Aichi Cancer Center Hospital 1966·4–1974·4)

Diagnosis	No. of cases	%
Hyperplastic polyp (HP)	174	87.8
Adenomatous polyp (AP)	4	2.0
Unclassified	10	5.1
Cancer in polyp	$10 < {}^{1\ (\mathrm{HP})}_{9\ (\mathrm{AP})}$	5.1
Total	198	100.0

$$\text{Hyperplastic polyp} \quad \frac{1}{174+1} \times 100 = 0.6\%$$

$$\text{Adenomatous polyp} \quad \frac{9}{4+9} \times 100 = 69.2\%$$

$$\frac{10}{198} \times 100 = 5.1\%$$

Table 26. Calculated rate of malignant transformation of hyperplastic and adenomatous polyp (findings in resected stomachs)

$$\text{Hyperplastic polyp} \quad \frac{6}{349+6} \times 100 = 1.7\%$$

$$\text{Adenomatous polyp} \quad \frac{54}{16+54} \times 100 = 77.1\%$$

$$\text{Total} \quad \frac{60}{425} \times 100 = 14.1\%$$

diameter) and in 9 cases of the second type. From these results, the rate of coexistence of malignancy in gastric polyp was calculated as 0.6% in the hyperplastic type, while it was 69.2% in the adenomatous type (Table 25).

Similar results were also obtained in the histological examination of polyps in resected stomachs. That is, among 425 cases of gastric polyps, 355 (83.5%)

showed the basic changes typical for hyperplastic polyp and 70 cases (16.5%), those typical for adenomatous polyp. In polyps of the hyperplastic type, cancerous changes were noted in 6 cases (1.7%), while in adenomatous polyps such changes were seen in 54 cases (77.1%) (Table 26).

In the case of adenomatous polyp, it is known that the larger the polyp the higher the frequency of malignant transformation (Fig. 117).

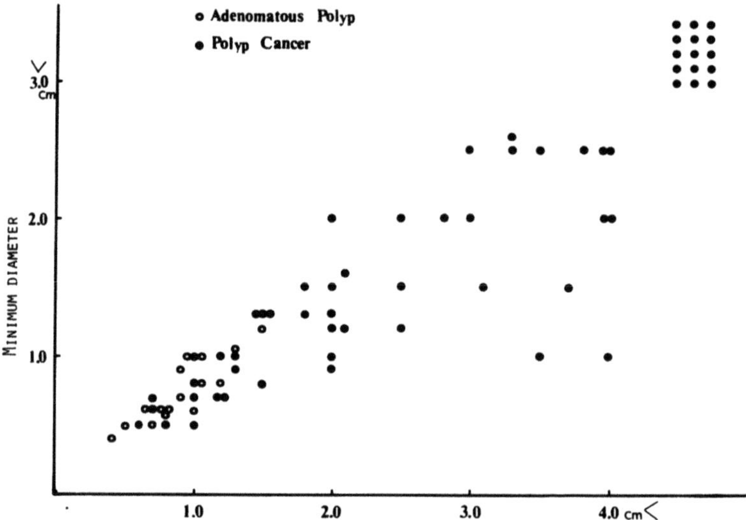

Fig. 117. Sizes of adenomatous polyps with and without cancer

With reference to the gross appearance in these cases, gastric polyps with hyperplastic histology were slighthly more frequently pedunculated in form, while among the polyps with adenomatous histology the sessile form was much more frequent (Table 27).

Table 27. Form of gastric polyps

Form	Hyperplastic		Adenomatous
	Total	Single	
Sessile	35.8%	40.9%	93.7%
Pedunculated	64.2%	59.1%	6.3%

It can therefore be said that most of the focal lesions diagnosed by means of X-ray and/or endoscopy as gastric polyps are hyperplastic in nature, and that this type of polyp rarely undergoes malignant transformation, except for large lesions more than 2 cm in diameter, while gastric polyps of the adenomatous type have a far higher risk of becoming malignant than the former, even when they are not large. In this sense, adenomatous polyps are not merely precancerous conditions, but rather an example of precancerous lesions (Fig. 118).

110

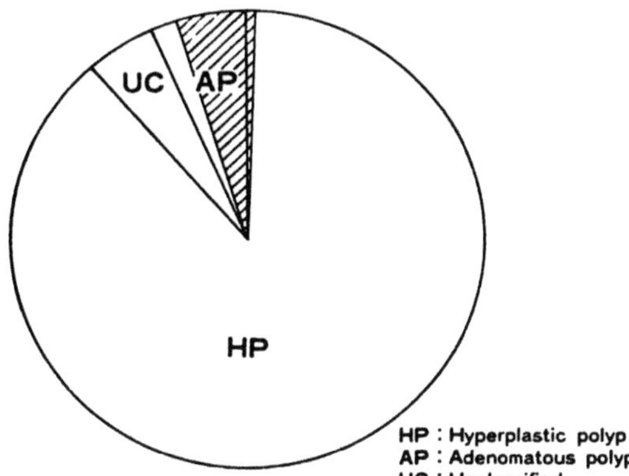

Fig. 118. Frequencies of both types of polyp
and their combination with cancer

The histological forms of gastric polyp have been discussed by several investigators [1–20], and most authors stress that adenomatous polyps are highly prone
to malignant transformation. A good method of polypectomy with the aid of endoscopy has been reported recently.

Chronic Peptic Ulcer and Ulcer Scar

Peptic ulcer is one of the commonest diseases of the stomach and shows various
macroscopical and histological features according to site, size, depth, and stage
of the ulcer. From the aspect of the histogenesis of gastric cancer, however, only
the chronic type of peptic ulcer is concerned. EGC of type III often assumes a
similar macroscopical appearance to that of peptic ulcer, but at present observations cases of EGC that have developed on the basis of preexisting peptic ulcer
became quite few in number. Histological examinations have revealed that most
of the peptic ulcerations seen in lesions of type III or type III + IIc occur as secondary phenomena in areas of cancerous erosion, as already described in Chap. 5.
Chronic peptic ulcer is characterized macroscopically by the presence of an
open, deep ulcer, accompanied by shortening of the lesser curvature and convergency of the mucosal folds toward the center of the ulcer due to intensive fibrosis
at the base of the ulcer. Even X-ray examination filled with barium allows recog-
nition of such changes with no great technical difficulty owing to its characteristic
deformity (Figs. 119–121).
In earlier periods of the study around 1955 such chronic peptic ulcers were by
no means rare, and indeed, this type of gastric disease was the commonest in the
resected stomachs. Among these ulcers, cases showing cancerous change in the
mucosa around the ulcer on routine histological examinations were not infrequently found, and many of these cases fulfilled the histological criteria for ulcer
cancer proposed by Hauser. On the basis of these experiences, the author came to
the opinion that cancerization can occur in the mucosa around chronic peptic ulcers (Figs. 122–125).

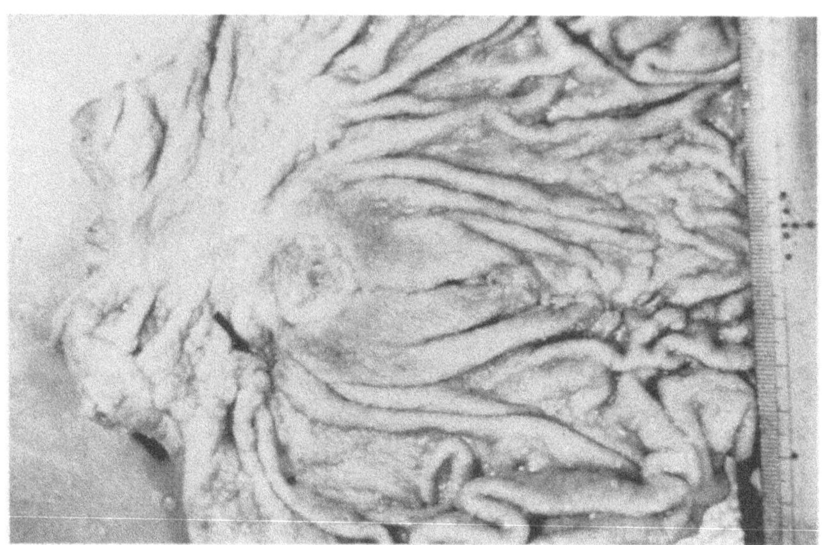

Fig. 119. Round, chronic peptic ulcer in the angulus. On both sides of the ulcer, linear ulcers accompanied by convergency of the mucosal folds are noticeable. (Pt no. 2516, 59 years, m)

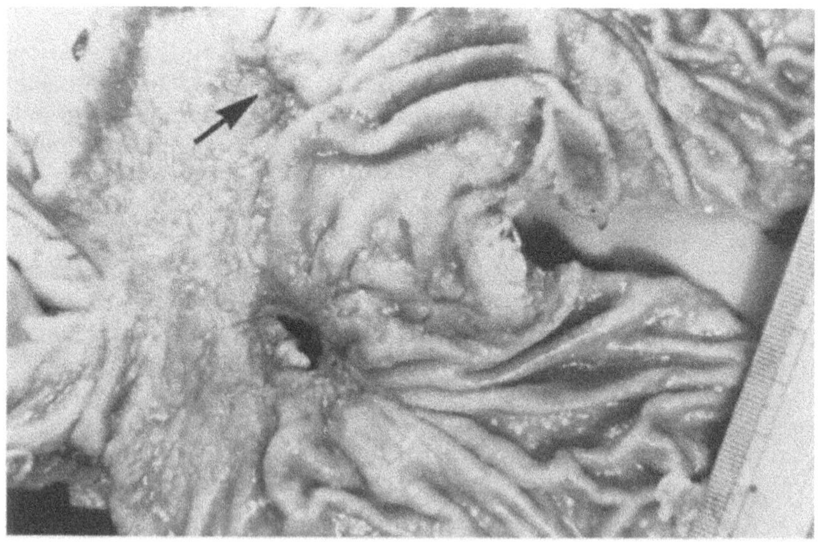

Fig. 120. Oval, chronic and perforated gastric ulcer in posterior wall of the angulus. Smaller, oblong and deep ulcer scar is visible also in anterior wall of the angulus. (Pt no. 3475, 69 years, m)

112

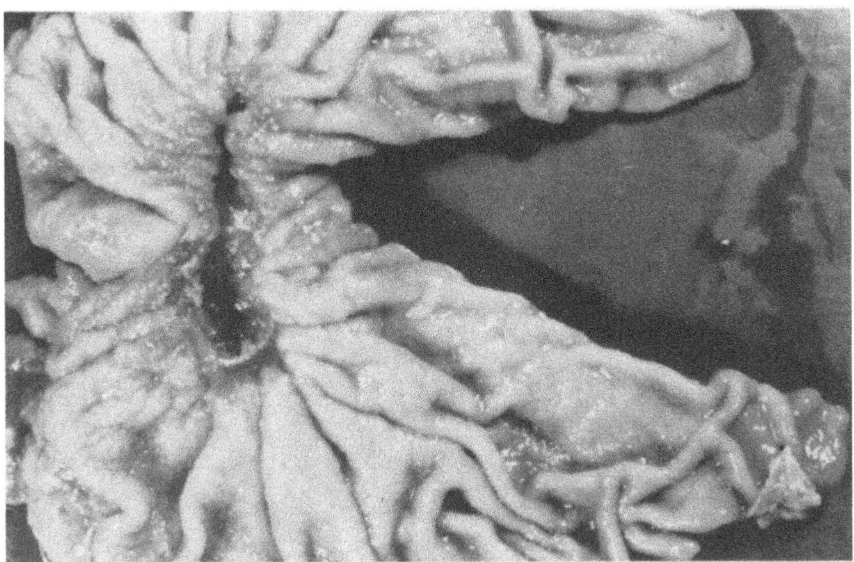

Fig. 121. Large, oblong and deep ulcer in the angulus resulted in shortening of the lesser curvature. Mucosa around the ulcer, especially on the posterior wall side, is eroded. In this case, the cancer that developed in marginal mucosa around the ulcer has already invaded the base of the ulcer. (Pt no. 9029, 43 years, m)

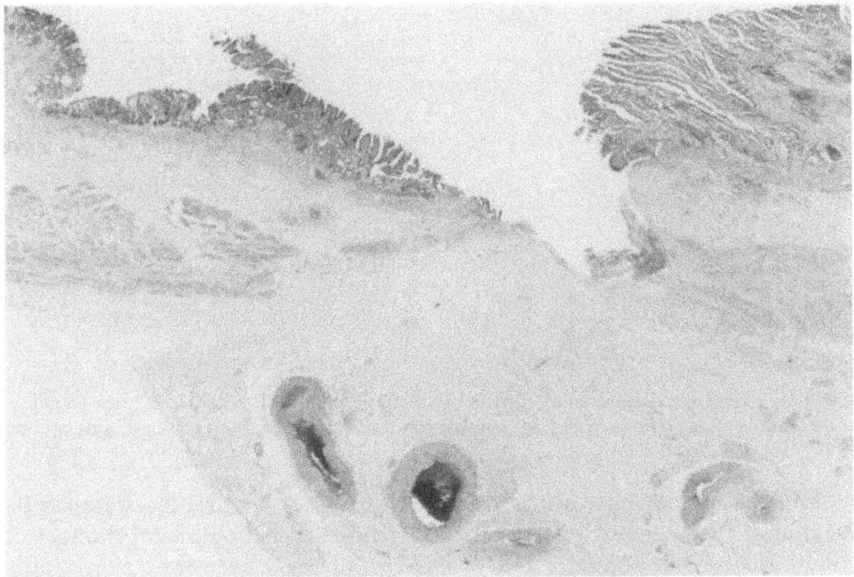

Fig. 122. Histological features of section cut through center of the scarred ulcer shown in Fig. 119 *(arrow)*. *Right* (oral)-side mucosa adjacent to the ulcer is simply hyperplastic, but *left* (anal)-side mucosa is focally depressed. (Pt no. 2516, ×7)

113

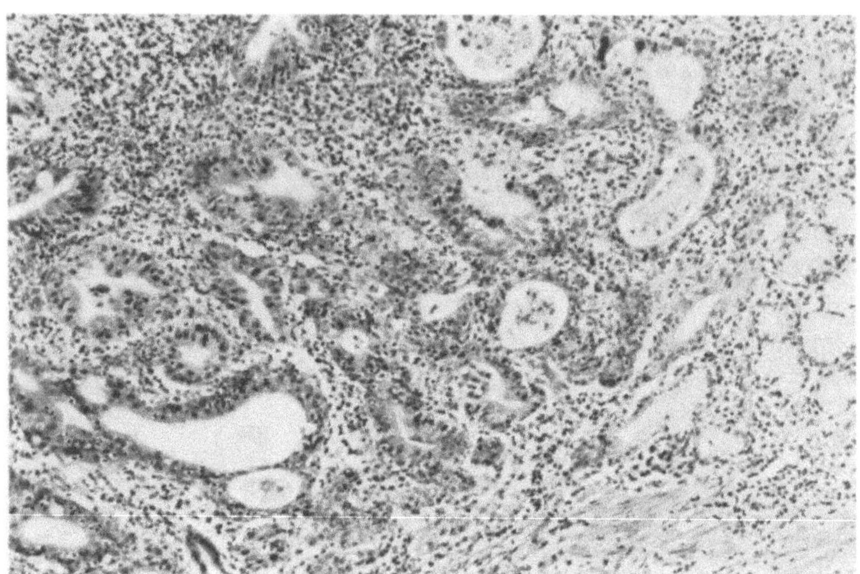

Fig. 123. High-power view of the depressed mucosa seen in Fig. 122. Adenocarcinomatous tissue is seen in the lower half of the depressed mucosa. (Pt no. 2516, × 100)

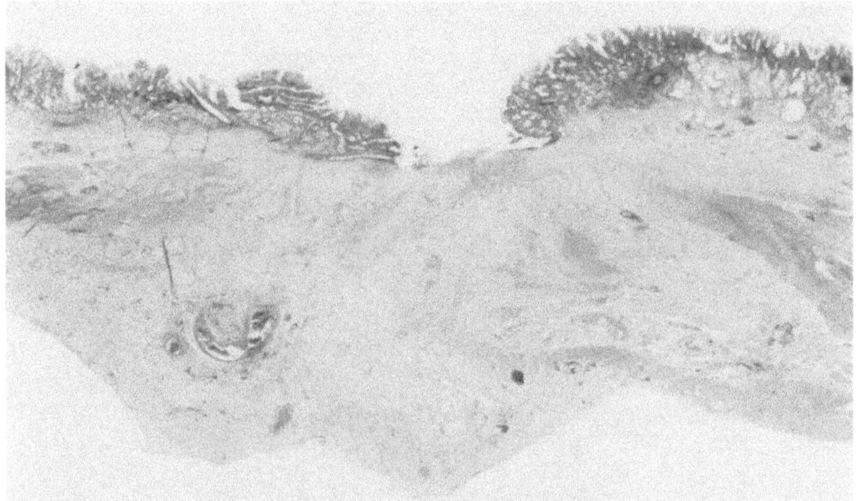

Fig. 124. Histological features of section cut through center of the scarred ulcer shown in Fig. 120 *Left* (anal)-side mucosa is rough, in contrast to intact nature of the *right* (oral)-side mucosa. (Pt no. 3475, × 7)

Since then, however, the incidence of EGC of type III has decreased year by year and it has become a minor form. With these chronological changes cases fulfilling the criteria for ulcer cancer have hardly ever been found on routine histological examination in recent years (Fig. 71). The main reason for this dramatic decline in number of Type III must be the marked decrease in the number of chronic peptic ulcers in recent times (Fig. 95).

114

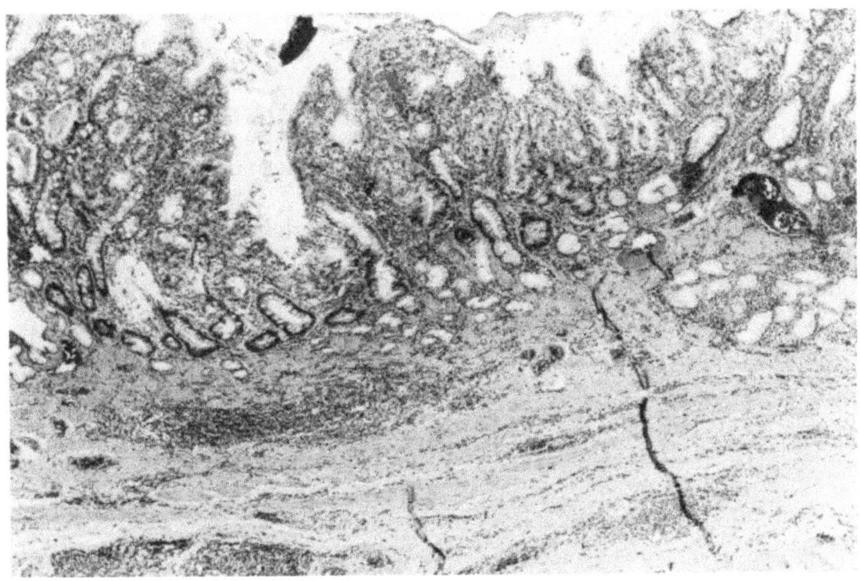

Fig. 125. High-power view of the rough mucosa seen in Fig. 124. Adenocarcinomatous change is seen in the upper half of the atrophic and metaplastic mucosa. (Pt no. 3475, × 40)

Over the whole 30-year study period, the frequency of EGC with histological evidence of the ulcer-cancer sequence among the total gastric ulcers resected was calculated as 1.4% (96/7023).

As described in Chap. 5, in a few cases of minute cancers cancerous changes were detected histologically in the mucosa quite close to the ulcer scar, while cancerous changes were never observed in the immature regenerating epithelium covering the scar itself. From these findings, it seems reasonable to suppose that this type of minute gastric cancer has the same histogenetic basis as that of large and open ulcer cancer.

There was much discussion involving lively controversy concerning the role of chronic peptic ulcer in the development of gastric cancer, and the conflict has not entirely disappeared even now. But owing to the great progress in histological studies on EGC, it has gradually become apparent that most cases of endoscopically detectable malignant ulcer are not preceded by chronic peptic ulcer, but rather followed by ulcers after development of the cancerous erosion. Several opinions on the role of peptic ulcer in the development of gastric cancer in the first half of this century were described in Chap. 1. In the articles and textbooks published in the second half of this century [21–46] almost all authors acknowledge the existence of ulcer cancer, but most estimate that its frequency is far lower than was once envisaged. Thus, chronic peptic ulcer is now counted as one of the less significant precancerous conditions in the stomach.

Chronic Atrophic Gastritis and Intestinal Metaplasia of Gastric Mucosa

As described in Chap. 4, among 1109 cases of EGC, conditions without prominent polypoid protrusions or deep excavations were by far the most frequent. When gastric polyp or gastric ulcer becomes malignant it will take on the gross appearance of type I or type III in the early stage. From studies on the histogenesis, the frequency of EGC having histological evidence of polyp-cancer or ulcer-cancer sequences among all the stomachs resected for EGC was calculated at less than 15%, as expressed by dark oblique lines in the figur (Fig. 126).

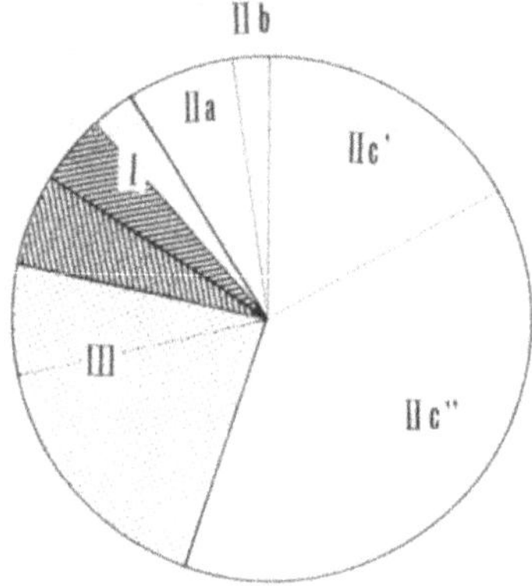

Fig. 126. Relative frequencies of different types of histogenesis in EGC

These results definitively confirm the importance of the role of a flat mucosa as a possible precancerous condition of the stomach. It has already been pointed out by many clinical investigators that most patients suffering from long-standing stomach discomfort have some degree of hypoacidity of the gastric juice, or sometimes achlorhydria, and that this is generally more frequent in elderly than in younger people. From the viewpoint of clinical pathology, hypoacidity results principally from the atrophy of acid-secreting parietal cells of the fundic gland, but atrophy of gastrin- and mucin-secreting pyloric gland cells is also involved, and this is quite often observed in the stomach affected by EGC. For these reasons, chronic atrophic gastritis has been cited as one of the most important precursors of gastric cancer.

When atrophy of the gastric glands, and especially of the phyloric glands, becomes intensive, the foveolar epithelium composing the upper layer of the mucosa always transforms into metaplastic intestinal epithelium characterized by tall columnar epithelial cells with a brush border, sporadically distributed goblet cells, and cells with Paneth's granules in the base of the foveolar tubules. The metaplastic changes usually appear in the mucosa of the antrum or of the angulus along the lesser curvature and then extend gradually to the surrounding mucosa. Microscopically, the metaplastic focus or foci commence(s) from the grooved area of the mucosa between area gastricae, extending to the surrounding mucosa by replacemental growth. Intestinal metaplasia of gastric mucosa is therefore a histological marker showing the grade of chronic atrophic gastritis (Figs. 127 and 128).

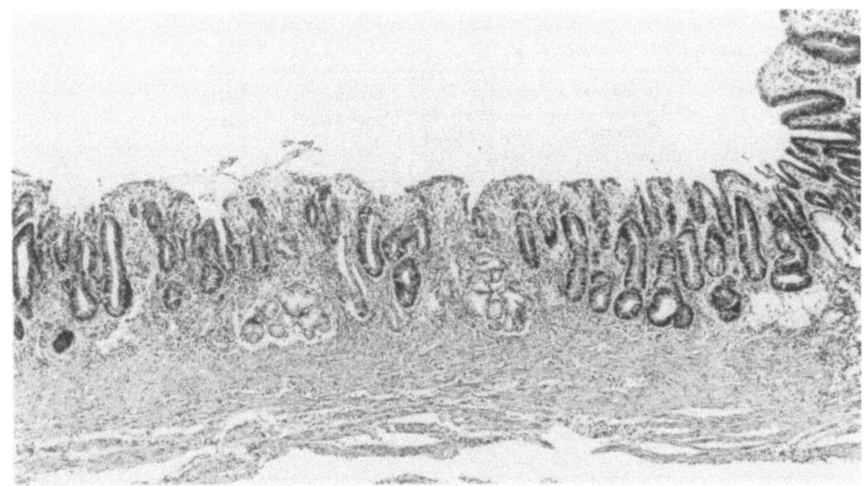

Fig. 127. Severe grade of intestinal metaplasia. Atrohpic mucosa of the antrum is occupied diffusely by metaplastic epithelial cells of foveolar nature. The pyloric glands are still seen sporadically among them. (Pt no. 12388, × 40)

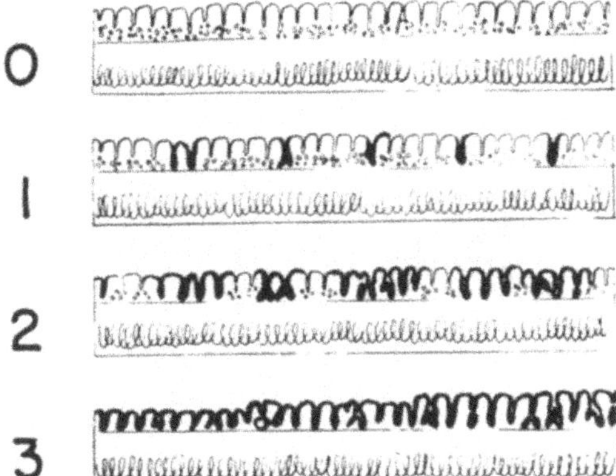

Fig. 128. Diagrams of four grades (0, 1, 2, 3) of intestinal metaplasia in pyloric mucosa

As described in Chap. 5, there is no doubt that intestinal metaplasia of gastric mucosa is closely correlated with the development of gastric cancer, especially with intestinal-type histology. However, owing to the limited conditions of the study a causal relationship between the two changes is still not clear. Recently, an incomplete type of intestinal metaplasia, in which goblet cells are decreased in number, Paneth's cells disappear from the metaplastic epithelium, and mucin and enzyme histochemistry reveal rather different attitudes than seen in the complete type, has been seen more frequently in the mucosa adjacent to the cancer and thus is more closely correlated to precancerous change of the stomach than metaplasia of complete type (Table 28).

Table 28. Differences between complete and incomplete type of intestinal metaplasia in stomach. (Matsukura et al. [91])

Marker	Intestinal metaplasia		Small Intestine	Large Intestine
	Complete type	Incomplete type		
Cell				
Goblet cell	+	+	+	+
Paneth cell	+	−	+	−
Mucus				
HID	−	+	−	+
Enzyme				
Succurase	+	+	+	−
Treharase	+	−	+	−
LAP	+	+	+	−
AIP	+	−	+	−

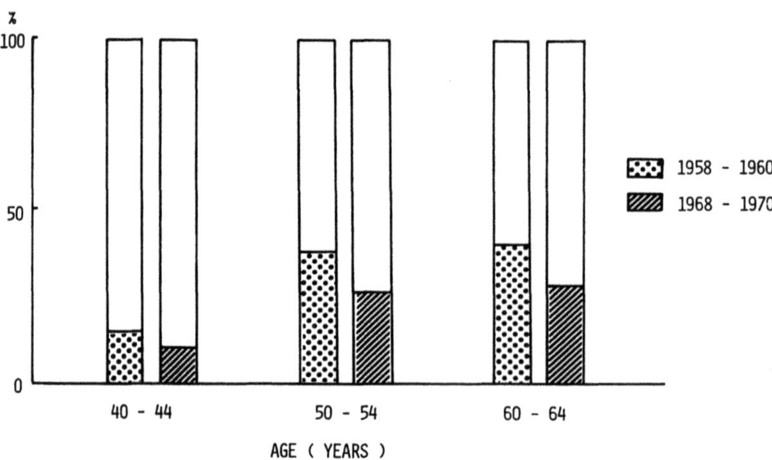

Fig. 129. Comparison of frequency of intestinal metaplasia of the gastric mucosa in three age groups in 1958–1960 and 1968–1970

Analytical approaches from several aspects are necessary for future study. At all events, a long-standing condition progressing toward the atrophy of gastric glands seems a necessary factor in the development of gastric cancer.

It has to be added here that complete-type intestinal metaplasia of the gastric mucosa is not uncommon in persons over 60 years of age; this ordinary metaplasia is considered to be merely a senile change of the stomach and cannot be counted as a precancerous change. Comparative examinations of 10 years interval have shown a declining frequency of intestinal metaplasia in stomachs resected for changes other than cancer in three age groups (Fig. 129).

Chronic atrophic gastritis is a clinical condition revealed mainly in functional disorders such as hypoacidity or anacidity of the gastric juice with vitamin C deficiency. Most of the papers concerning the nature of this disease, especially of its

118

relation to precancerous conditions of the stomach, have therefore emanated from physicians and endoscopists [47, 69, 83, 118, 119, 123, 125, 131, 141], and in this connection attention has been focused on a specific type of chronic atrophic gastritis, pernicious anemia. On the other hand, the presence or absence of intestinal metaplasia of gastric mucosa, a histological marker of chronic atrophic gastritis, is revealed chiefly by histological and histochemical examination of the stomach. Accordingly, most of the earlier papers on metaplasia emanated from pathologists [54, 57, 90, 130, 142, 144, 147].

Intestinal metaplasia in the gastric mucosa was known more than 50 years ago, and until the middle of this century a close correlation of these changes with the development of gastric cancer was assumed by most authors [52, 62, 64, 65, 68, 70, 81, 82, 90, 94, 129, 140, 142, 143] on the basis of histological examinations of stomachs resected for polyp, ulcer, or cancer.

Studies on the role of intestinal metaplasia in the histogenesis of gastric cancer have progressed since the 1950s owing to detailed histological examination of the resected stomachs [74, 96–98, 104, 130], and the detection of many cases of EGC promoted these studies greatly [53, 100, 101, 105, 106, 112, 116, 117].

At present, intestinal metaplasia of the gastric mucosa is studied in several ways – electron microscopically [59, 95, 103, 109, 115, 134, 136], histochemically [56, 60, 61, 67, 75–77, 86–89a, 102, 107, 127, 128, 137, 145, 146], enzyme histochemically [58, 80, 91, 92, 110, 111, 121, 122, 132], biochemically [55, 78, 79, 114, 135], immuno-histochemically [66, 133, 138, 139] autoradiographically [63], and epidemiologically [48, 49–51, 72, 73, 84, 85, 93, 99, 113, 126, 142], and most papers focus on its possible role in the development of gastric cancer.

It is known from recent studies [71, 78, 79, 91, 92, 108, 120] that mature intestinal metaplasia is far from being a risk factor for gastric cancer, while immature types – so-called incomplete types – seem to be far more closely linked with development of gastric cancer. From these results it appears probable that a decreased ability of generative cells to differentiate into ordinary gastric glands is intimately connected with the development of gastric cancer.

Pernicious Anemia

The characteristic feature of pernicious anemia is atrophy of the mucosa of the corpus and/or fundus, leaving the flat mucosa of the antrum relatively intact, and there are geographic differences in frequency. Histologically, atrophy of the mucosa of corpus or fundus is due to marked atrophy of the fundic glands [149, 152, 155, 164, 167] composed of chief cells, parietal cells, and mucous neck cells, and these cells are responsible for the secretion of acidic gastric juice containing hydrochloric acid and pepsin. The clinical diagnosis of this disease, therefore, is based chiefly on roentgenological, endoscopic, and biochemical examination of the stomach for the functional disorder of marked hypoacidity of gastric juice in the patient. Intestinal metaplasia confined to the mucosa of corpus and/or fundus is generally quite rare in the ordinary gastric mucosa, but is not uncommon in this disease.

Many papers [150, 153–157, 160, 161, 163, 168] stress that the risk of developing gastric cancer is higher in patients suffering from pernicious anemia than in the general population. The cancerous lesions derived from this disease also have a predilection for the mucosa of the corpus or of the fundus [154, 159]. Since this disease is so rare in Japan, the author has had almost no experience with cases of gastric cancer which seemed to have been preceded by pernicious anemia.

On the basis of the findings reported, it is supposed that histogenesis of this type of gastric cancer is not essentially different from the cancer derived from the usual type of chronic atrophic gastritis, but from the viewpoints of pathogenesis and etiology it is characterized by a genetic background [162, 165, 166], unlike the other variants of gastric cancer, and an autoimmune nature of the disease is suspected by some investigators [151].

The formation of nitroso compounds from nitrates to nitrites and their chemical reaction with secondary amines owing to intrinsic changes in the stomach, such as achlorhydria and subsequent activation of the intragastric bacteria, are proposed as possible carcinogenetic mechanisms in the stomach in pernicious anemia [148, 158].

In summary, it can be said that pernicious anemia is definitely a significant precancerous condition of the stomach, but without atypical epithelial changes in the affected mucosa it cannot be cited as a precancerous change.

Gastric Remnant

A gastric remnant is the part of the stomach remaining after partial gastrectomy; in most cases resection is performed in the distal half of the stomach. The presence of a gastric remnant is easily recognized on X-ray and endoscopic examination of the stomach. In gastric remnants such changes as stomal ulcer, polypoid mucosal protrusion, or cancer can occur many years after gastrectomy, and these changes are most often found in the gastric mucosa adjacent to gastroduodenal or gastrojejunal anastomoses. Cancers that have developed in a gastric remnant are generally referred to as "stump carcinoma," but from the aspect of the histogenesis of gastric cancer it would be better if this term were confined to cancer developing in the gastric remnant after the resection of nonmalignant lesions, most of which are peptic ulcers. In fact, most investigators in Europe reporting on this subject have defined the term stump carcinoma in this way. Furthermore, to eliminate the possibility that the cancer already existed in the upper half of the stomach at the time of surgical operation but was overlooked, the interval between gastrectomy and the detection of cancer in the gastric remnant must be over 5 years. Since it is not unusual for stump carcinoma to develop many years after gastrectomy, gastric remnant has been cited as a precancerous condition of the stomach.

However, there are still differences of opinion as to whether patients with gastric remnants are more susceptible to the development of cancer than the general population. Most workers [169–178, 180, 181, 184, 186, 187, 190, 191, 195, 197]

support the view that they are, while others [182, 199] do not accept this opinion.
The frequency of stump carcinoma depends on the interval between surgical resection and the date of the examination. For this reason, it is necessary to carry
out a statistical comparison of results recorded at 15-, 20-, 25-, and 30-year intervals after partial gastrectomy.

Most papers reporting this problem, including our own, point out that the frequency is higher following the BILLROTH II resection procedure than after the
BILLROTH I technique (Table 29), and the cancers were most often seen in the gastric mucosa adjacent to the anastomosis. It is also mentioned by all authors that
the interval between gastrectomy and the detection of carcinoma in the gastric
remnant can be more than 15 years.

Table 29. Frequency of stump carcinoma more than 18 years after partial gastrectomy

Procedure for partial gastrectomy	No. of patients subjected to gastrectomy	No. of cases with subsequent carcinoma	Frequency (%) of stump carcinoma
Billroth I	2535	2	0.08
Billroth II	1828	6	0.33
Total	4363	8	0.18

These results have brought about general acceptance of the opinion that long-
standing refluxed bile flow from the duodenum to the gastric remnant plays an
essential role in development of the cancer, especially at the site of anastomoses.

Similar results were also deduced from our own examination of stump carcinoma [184a]. There were 27 cancerous lesions in the 25 patients, the primary diseases being gastric ulcer in 13, duodenal ulcer in 11, and other in 1 cases; 8 lesions
were found in stomachs in which the Billroth I resection procedure was done,
while the other 19 lesions were found in the stomachs treated by the BILLROTH II
method. Carcinoma at the site of anastomosis accounted for 12 cases (63.2%) following the latter procedure, but for none after the former (Table 30).

More than half the cancers were sited in the gastric mucosa adjacent to the
anastomosis and did not appear until more than 15 years after surgery (Fig. 130

Table 30. Methods of initial surgery and sites of cancer in stomach remnant

Method of surgery \ Site of cancer	Anastomosis	Cardia	Other	Total numbers of lesions
Billroth II (17 cases)	12	1	6	19
Billroth I (8 cases)	0	5	3	8
Total	12	6	9	27

and 131). Protruded lesions with the histology of poorly differentiated medullary adenocarcinoma were relatively frequent (Table 31 and Fig. 132).

Intestinal metaplasia around the cancer was seen in a few cases. Some protruding and sessile mucosal lesions close to the anastomosis showed characteristic histological features similar to "gastritis cystica polyposa" or "gastric stomal polypoid hyperplasia" [183, 183a]. The changes seem to be specific for the anastomotic area of gastric remnants. These characteristic histological features were also recognized in and around protruding cancerous lesions with poorly differentiated and medullary histology in two cases. These findings strongly suggest the precancerous nature of gastritis cystica polyposa as a factor in the development of stump carcinoma (Figs. 133 and 134).

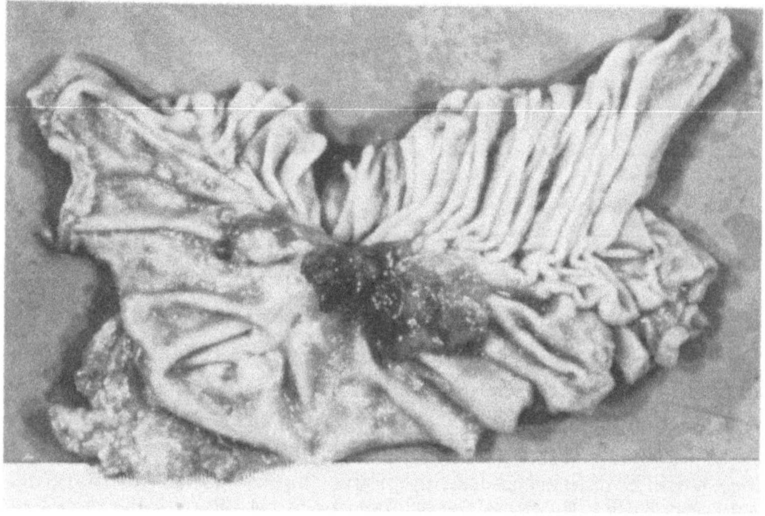

Fig. 130. Polypoid carcinoma developed 20 years after gastrectomy for duodenal ulcer by Billroth II procedure. Besides the polypoid and advanced cancer, smaller mucosal protrusion is visible along the line of gastrojejunal anastomosis. (Pt no. 15 103, 53 years, m)

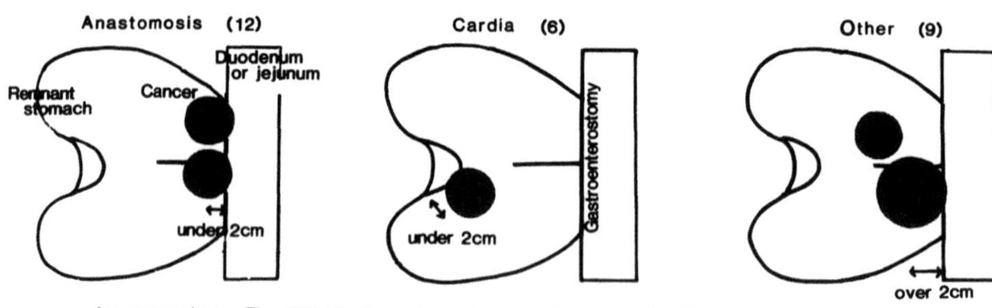

Fig. 131. Sites of cancer in gastric remnants

Table 31. Sites and histological types of remnant cancers

Histological type	Anastomosis	Cardia	Other	Total numbers of lesions
tub$_1$	0	3	0	3
tub$_2$	2	2	0	4
muc	0	0	1	1
por	9 med 6 sci 1	0	6 med 2 sci 1	15 med 8 sci 2
sig	1	1	2	4
Total	12	6	9	27

Tub$_1$: well differentiated adenocarcinoma
Tub$_2$: moderately differentiated adenocarcinoma

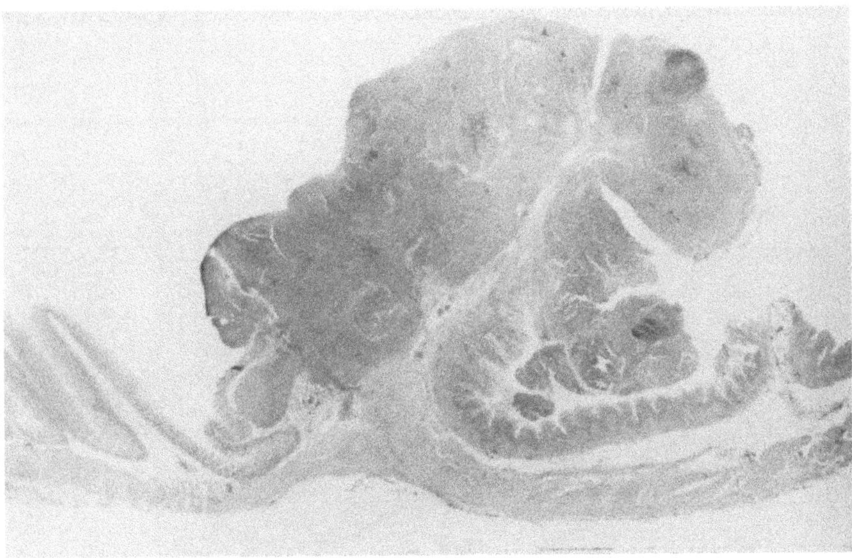

Fig. 132. Large, polypoid mass developed in the gastric mucosa adjacent to gastrojejunal anastomosis shows poorly differentiated adenocarcinoma with medullary stroma. Jejunal mucosa is seen to *left* of the figure. (Pt no. 14 253, ×7)

123

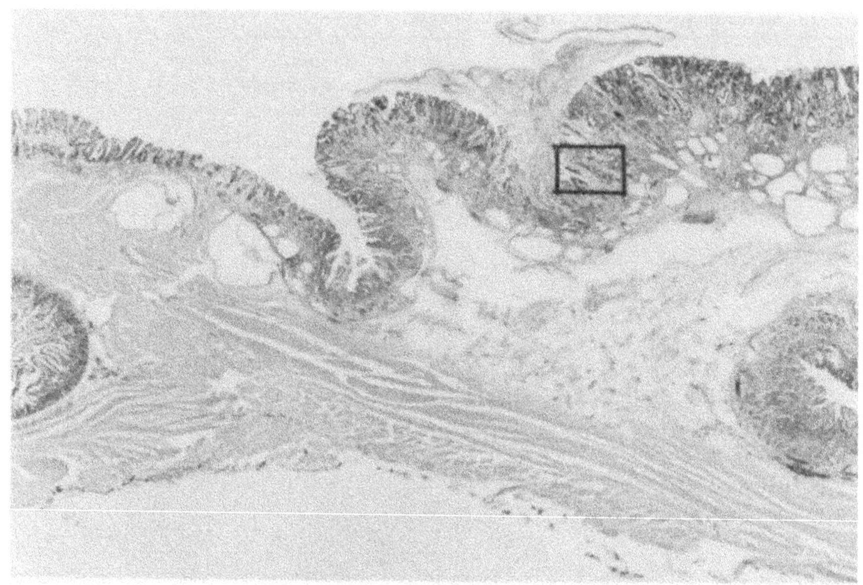

Fig. 133. Low-power view of the samller protrusion seen in Fig. 130. The elevated mucosa shows histologically severe dysplasia with many glandular cysts in its lower half. (Pt no. 15 103, × 20)

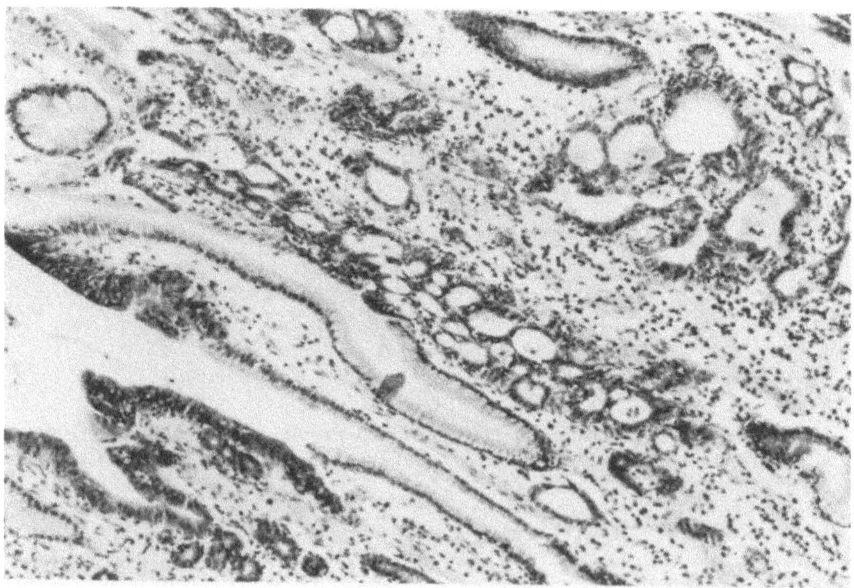

Fig. 134. Higher magnification of a part (rectangle) of the specimen shown in Fig. 133. Small cancerous glands composed of cuboidal epithelial cells are seen among the elongated foveolar tubules. (Pt no. 15 103, × 40)

124

The results obtained from animal experiments on this subject strongly support the hypothesis of bile reflux as a cause of stump carcinoma [170, 171, 174, 184a, 185, 187, 188, 194, 198, 202].

Followup examination of the patients with gastric remnants by means of endoscopy and biopsy is quite important, especially for those who have undergone gastric surgery more than 15 years before, and followup reports [176, 177, 179, 183, 189, 191–193, 196, 200, 201] have increased in frequency in recent years.

Menetrier's Disease and Aberrant Pancreas

Gastric cancer can occur on the basis of Menetrier's disease. The characteristic features of this condition are giant hypertrophy of the mucosal folds, looking like gyri of the brain in an area of the corpus and fundus with hypoproteinemia. A few cases of cancerization of this disease have been reported [203–208]. We ourselves have also experienced such a case (Fig. 135).

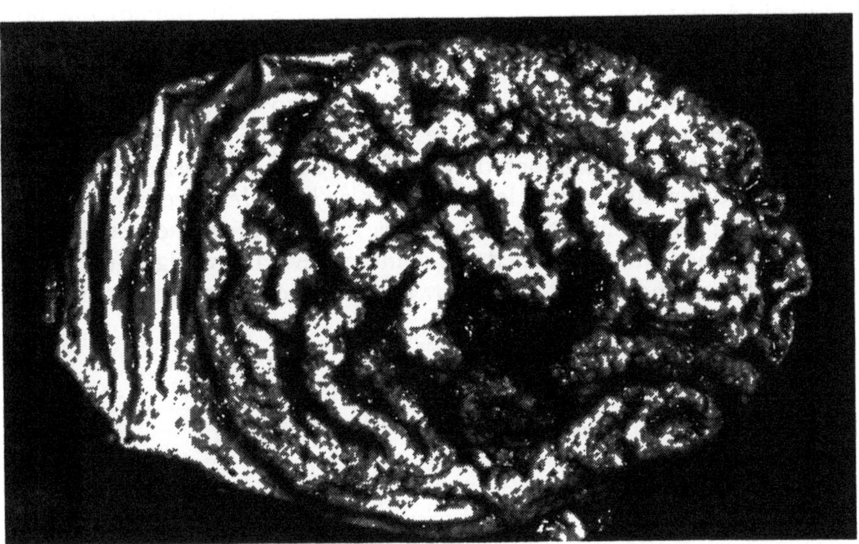

Fig. 135. Giant hypertrophy of the mucosal folds in the corpus and fundus (Menetrier's disease), accompanied by crater-forming and well-defined cancer in central part of the hyperplastic mucosa. The carcinoma showed the histology of tubular adenocarcinoma. Antral mucosa remained unaffected. (Pt no. 15 544, 52 years, m)

Aberrant pancreas is by no means uncommon in the stomach, having the macroscopical appearance of a focal submucosal tumor, but cases with histological evidence of malignant transformation from these aberrant tissues are exceptional [209–211].

125

Gastric Dysplasia Including Borderline Lesion

In the field of pathological histology, the term dysplasia has been used mainly for mucosal changes covered by squamous epithelium, for example in the esophagus, uterine cervix, and bronchus, and grading of the dysplasia is of the utmost importance for the prognosis of the lesion. This term has scarcely been used for the glandular mucosa, however.

During histological examination of the resected stomachs broad-based and flat elevations of the mucosa showing growth of metaplastic and atypical foveolar epithelium but lacking histological evidence of malignancy in the upper half of the elevated lesions were quite often encountered, and I [233] tentatively named these as "borderline lesions", because of their adenoma-like nature intermediate between benign and malignant change. It was noted during the studies that atypical foveolar epithelial cells were almost always accompanied by cystic dilatation of the glands in the lower half, and these two changes combined to form the elevated lesion. The higher the grade of cellular atypia of the foveolae, the more irregular is the form of the cystically dilated gland, while lower grades of epithelial atypia are accompanied by lessening degrees of deformity of the glandular cysts.

These findings, together with an analysis of the distribution pattern of the mitotic cells within the elevated lesions [223 a], led me to the opinion that borderline lesions with cellular and structural atypia are different from adenoma or simple maturation-arrested epithelial hyperplasia and are better classified as a type of abnormal cell growth. Most of these lesions seems to have a neoplastic nature, and when the lesions are severe in grade they cannot be distinguished clearly from carcinoma in situ. Even though they are fewer in number, lesions having the same nature as borderline elevated lesions have also been detected in focally depressed mucosa. But the definition of and criteria for the borderline lesion were not yet fully established when I reached this opinion. Several investigators have also used different terms and criteria of their own for these quite atypical epithelial changes (Table 32).

Table 32. Comparison of different grading systems for gastric dysplasia

Nagayo (1971)	No atypia	Slight atypia	Borderline	Probable cancer	Cancer
Grundman (1979)	Inflammatory	Mild dysplasia	Moderate dysplasia	Severe dysplasia	
Oehlert (1979)		Grade I	Grade II	Grade III	
Ming (1979)	Grade 1	Grade 2	Grade 3	Grade 4	
Cuello (1979)	Hyperplastic mild	Dysplasia severe	Adenomatous mild	Dysplasia severe	
Morson (1980)	Inflammatory regenerative	Mild dysplasia	Moderate dysplasia	Severe dysplasia	
Isggc[a] (1982)	——— Hyperplasia ———		——— Dysplasia ———		
	Simple	Atypical		Possible carcinoma	

[a] International study group of gastric cancer

This was the background to the World Health Organization Workshop on Histological Criteria of Precancerous Change of the Stomach (London 1978), at which the participants, including myself, agreed to use the term dysplasia, which includes the following three histological changes:

1) Cellular atypia
2) Abnormal differentiation
3) Disorganized mucosal architecture

The dysplasia was graded into (a) mild, (b) moderate, and (c) severe, according to the severity of the atypical changes of the lesions as a whole. Proceedings of this workshop have been published in detail [232] and in a summarized version [248].

Mild dysplasia is seen in several kinds of mucosal changes, from regenerative but maturation-arrested mucosa following deep erosion to hyperplastic lesions with slight structural derangement. In general, the lesion that can be diagnosed as mild dysplasia shows no histological changes that are likely to become malignant, and some of them can regress so that the normal state is regained. This grade of dysplasia is seen in both elevated and depressed mucosa, but the histological features of the lesions suggest that reversibility to nondysplastic mucosa is more frequent in depressed than in elevated mucosa (Figs. 136–138).

The borderline lesion with broad-based and flat mucosal elevation is a typical example of moderate dysplasia (Figs. 139–142). The prominent disorganized mucosal structure, especially with many large glandular cysts, and irregular increase of the mitotic cell zone in the atypical epithelia [223a] mean that reversibility of the lesion to nondysplastic mucosa can hardly be expected. The possibility that the lesion will progress to a severe grade of dysplasia or transform directly into

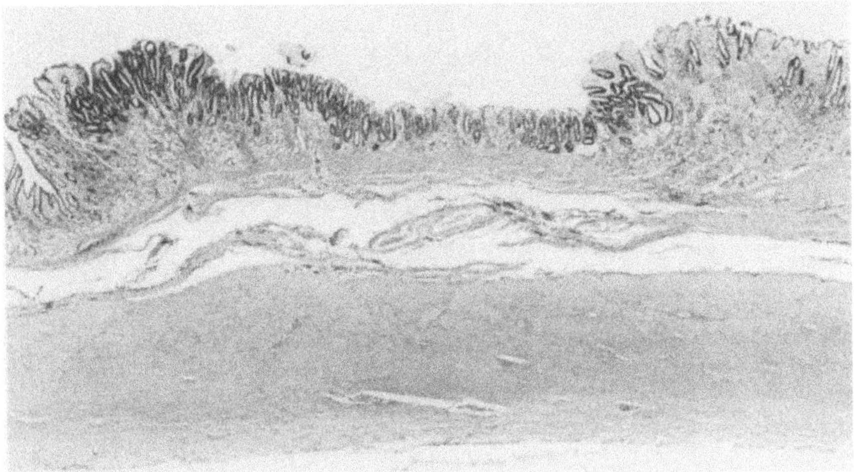

Fig. 136. Mild dysplasia of the depressed mucosa. Upper half of the depressed lesion is occupied by metaplastic foveolar tubules lacking in goblet cells, but no apparent cellular and structural abnormality is visible. (Pt no. 12398, × 40)

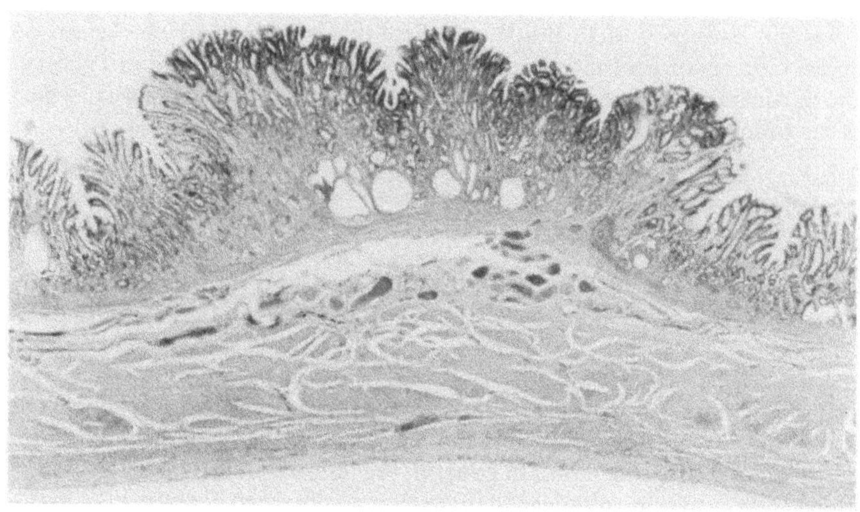

Fig. 137. Mild dysplasia of elevated mucosa. Darkly stained foveolar tubules are seen in upper half of the elevated mucosa only, and its lower half is composed of hyperplastic and non-metaplastic gastric mucosa with a few glandular cysts. (Pt no. 8909, × 7)

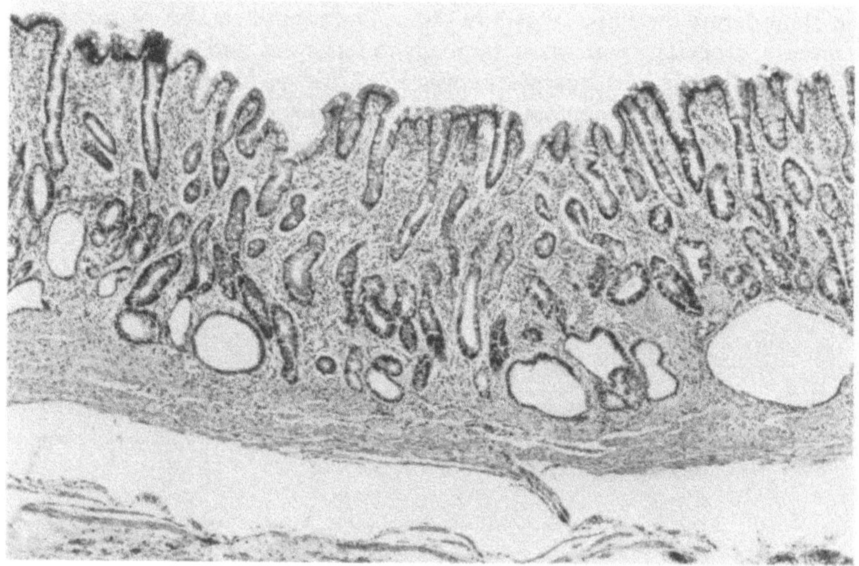

Fig. 138. Mild dysplasia of flat mucosa. The mucosa shows diffuse intestinal metaplasia without any proper gastric glands. In lower half of the metaplastic mucosa, oval cystically dilated glands are visible. Goblet cells are sparse and no Paneth's cells are visible. (Pt no. 10069, × 40)

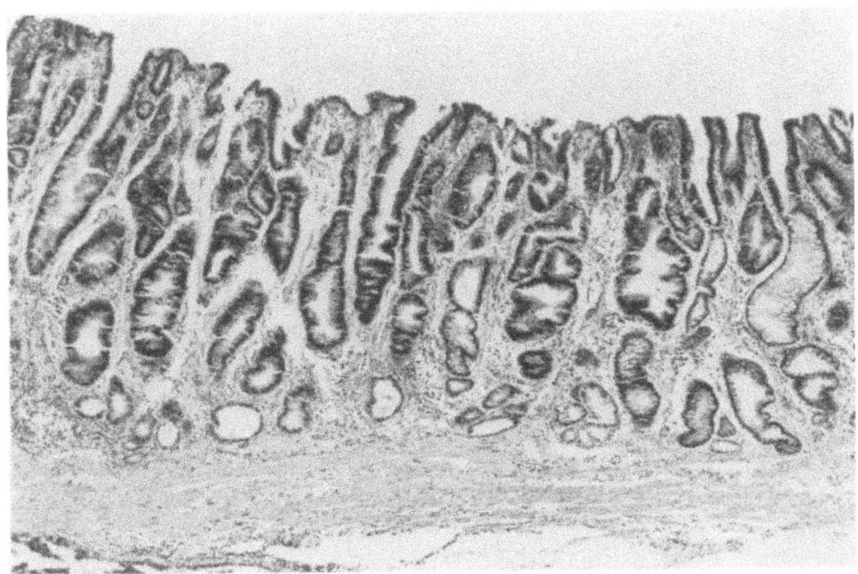

Fig. 139. Moderate dyplasia of slightly atrophic mucosa. The mucosa is composed of elongated, twisted foveolar tubules with densely arranged hyperchromatic nuclei and is lacking in goblet cells. Proper gastric glands have almost disappeared. (Pt no. 11 321, × 60)

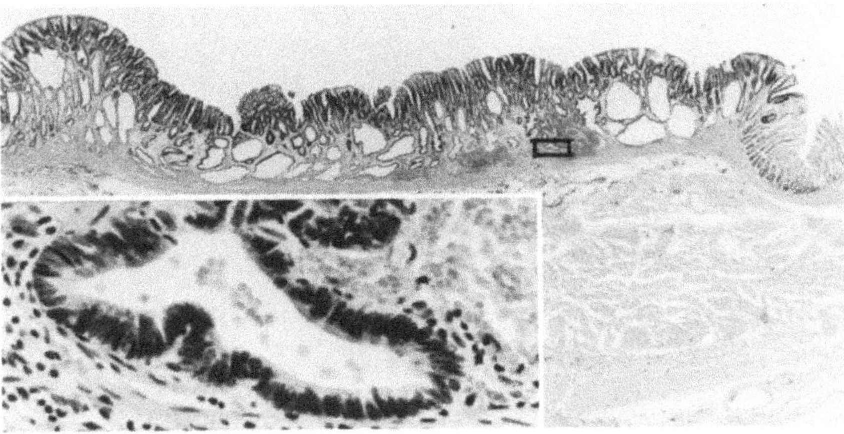

Fig. 140. Moderate dysplasia of broad-based, flatly elevated mucosa. Entire layer of the mucosa is made up of dark-stained, partly papillate foveolar tubules with cystic dilatation of the glands. In *central* part of figure, downward growth of the tubules reaching to the deepest layer of the mucosa is visible, but still no invasive growth of it is noted. (Pt no. 11 149, × 40)

carcinoma in situ cannot be entirely ruled out, but the condition of the atypical epithelium is mostly stationary, as indicated by the results of followup of these lesions recorded over many years in several institutions (Fig. 143).

In contrast to mild and moderate dysplasia, severe dysplasia (Figs. 144–148) is very close to the state of carcinoma in situ or adenocarcinoma without prominent

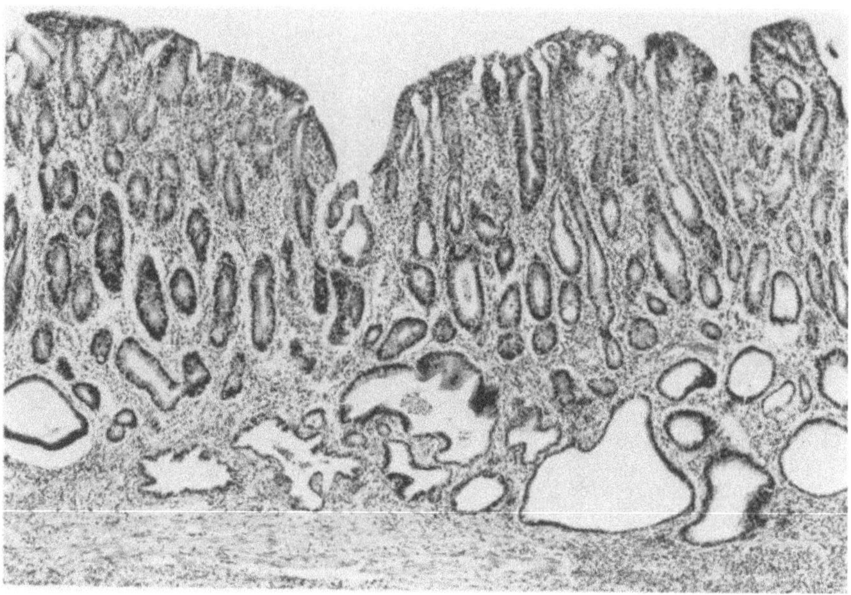

Fig. 141. Moderate dysplasia of flat mucosa. The mucosa shows diffuse intestinal metaplasia lacking in goblet cells and Paneth's cells. In basal zone of the mucosa, irregularly dilated glands composed of small cuboidal epithelial cells with a high nucleus-to-cytoplasm ratio are visible. (Pt no. 6321, × 40)

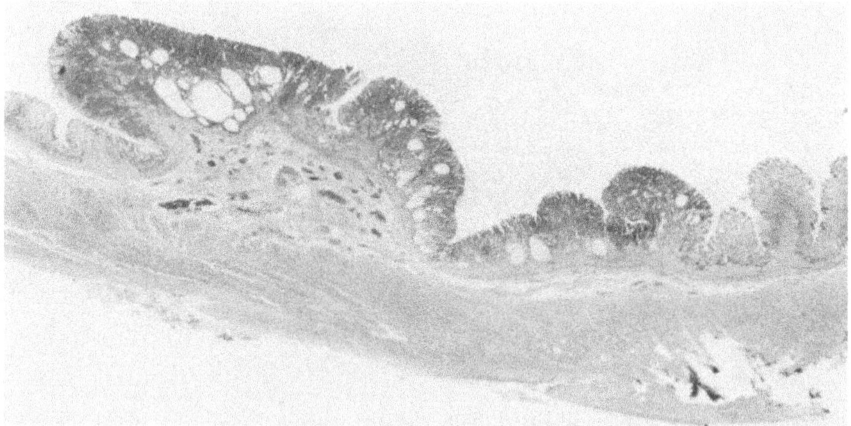

Fig. 142. General view of borderline elevated lesion (moderate dysplasia). The elevation is made up of aggregation of the areae gastricae and has a relatively flat surface. The upper half of the elevated mucosa is composed of densely arranged and dark-stained atypical foveolar tubules accompanied by many glandular cysts in the lower half. (Pt no. 16825, × 4)

130

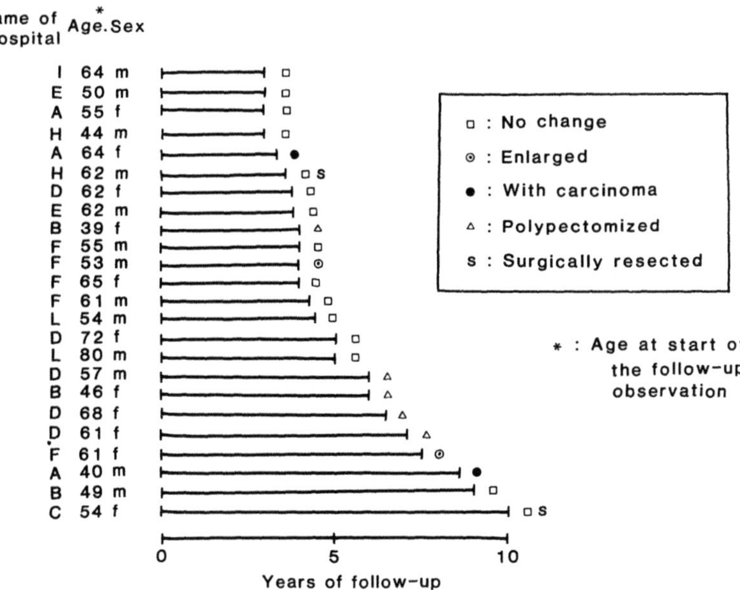

Fig. 143. Followup data on patients treated for borderline elevated lesion of the stomach

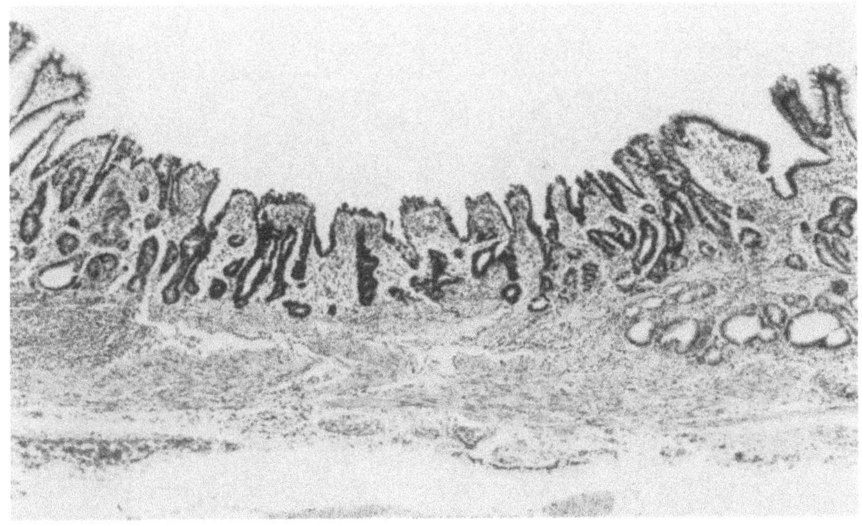

Fig. 144. Severe dysplasia of depressed mucosa. The depressed lesion is composed of distorted and dark-stained foveolar tubules, some of them disoriented and fused together. These findings strongly suggest that the lesion is in an incipient phase of malignancy. (Pt no. 12084, × 20)

invasive growth (Figs. 149–157), and in fact it is often very difficult to discriminate clearly between the two changes.

Since the cellular atypia, abnormal differentiation, and disorganization of the mucosal architecture are similar in degree in most cases, the diagnosis of severe dysplasia is made on the basis of the changes as a whole, but there are some cases

131

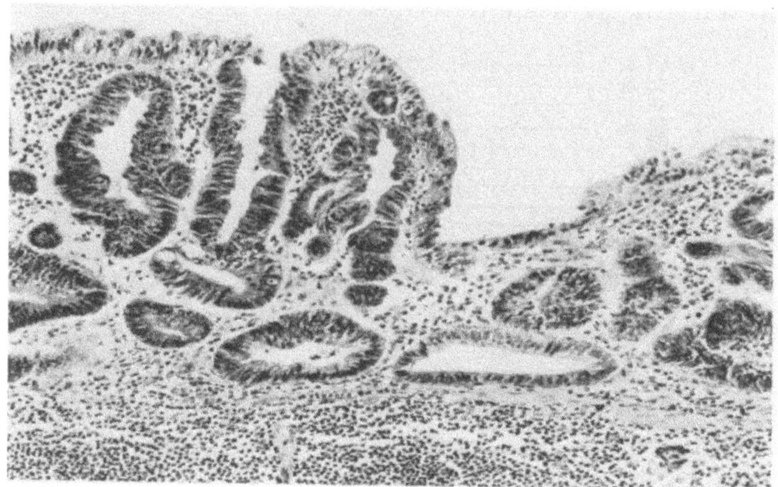

Fig. 145. Severe dysplasia of depressed mucosa. Foveolar tubules forming the depressed lesion are composed of tall columnar epithelial cells with slender, elongated, hyperchromatic and densely distributed nuclei, but neither invasion nor pleomorphy of the nuclei is recognizable. (Pt no. 10346, ×100)

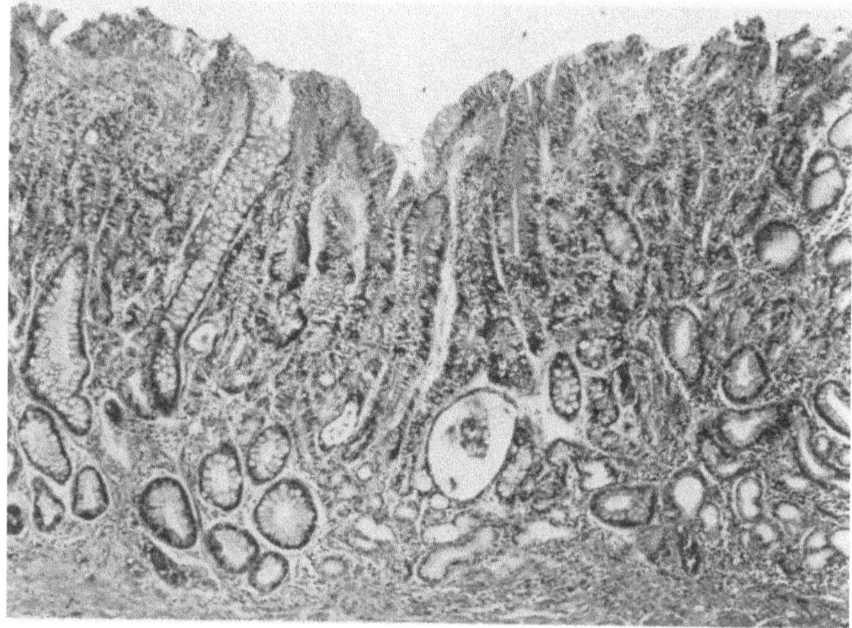

Fig. 146. Severe dysplasia of flat mucosa. The mucosa shows severe intestinal metaplasia; the metaplastic tubules containing mature goblet cells are sporadic and are intermingled with tubules containing very few goblet cells. (Pt no. 3527, ×40)

132

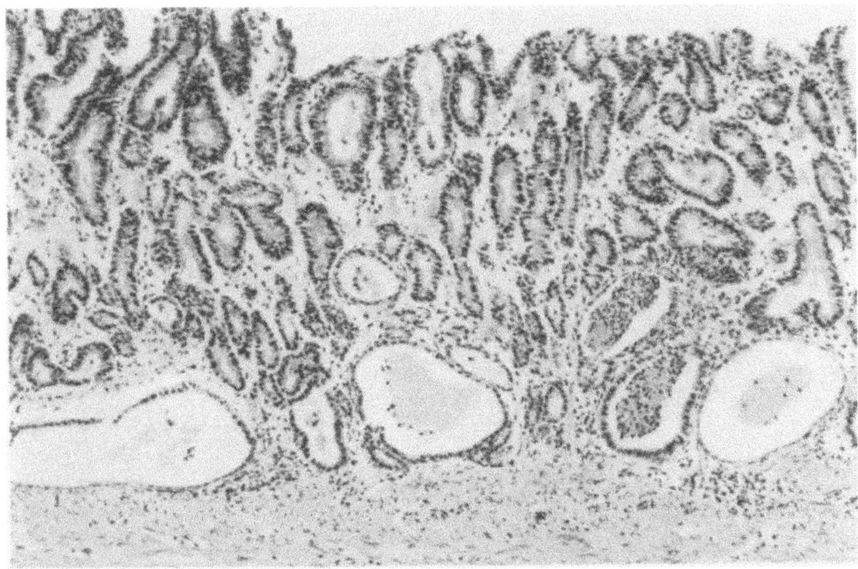

Fig. 147. Severe dysplasia of flat mucosa. Structural abnormality of the foveolar tubules is not prominent, but the whole mucosa is composed of slender tubules of cuboidal epithelial cells with a high nucleus-to-cytoplasm ratio suggestive of malignancy. (Pt no. 15 146, × 40)

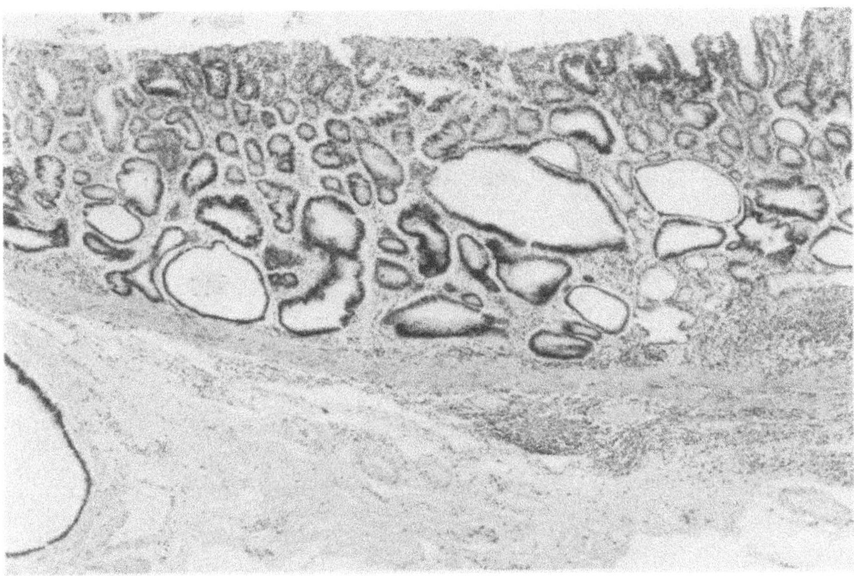

Fig. 148. Severe dysplasia of atrophic mucosa. Original structure of the atrophic mucosa is greatly disturbed, and irregularly arranged tubules and glands composed of cuboidal epithelial cells are seen diffusely. Cellular atypia is more intense in upper layer than in lower layer. (Pt no. 16 983, × 40)

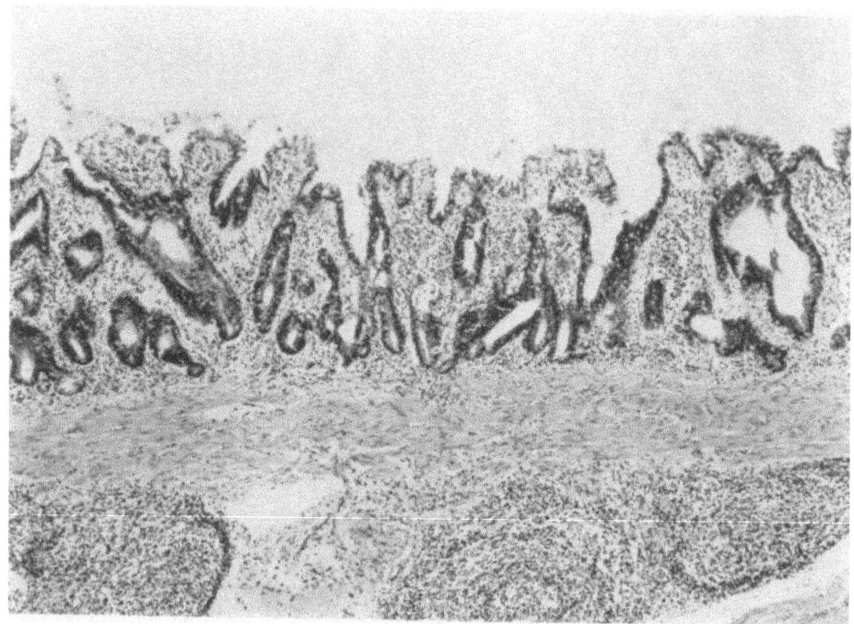

Fig. 149. Severe dysplasia of atrophic mucosa. The mucosa is composed widely of irregularly arranged, cleft-like foveolar tubules of metaplastic and atypical nature. Fusion of the neighboring tubules is also noted. (Pt no. 13 320, × 30)

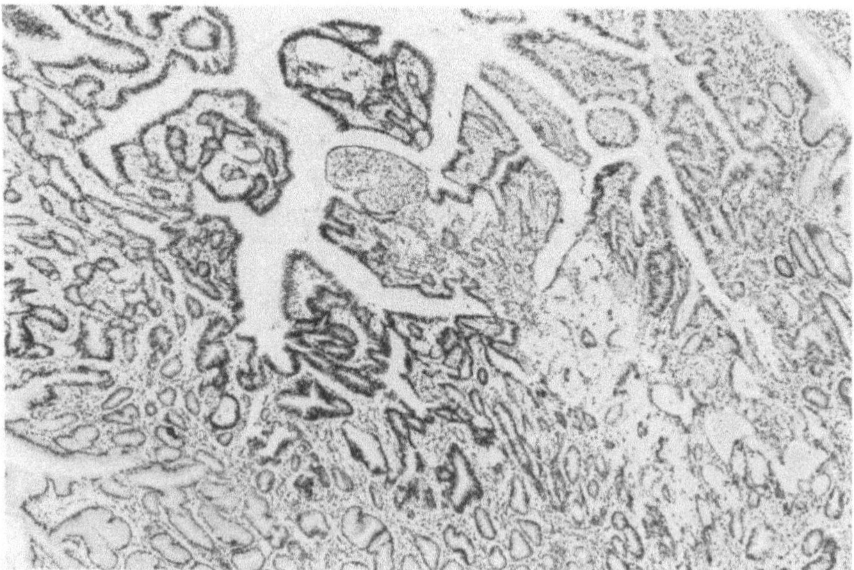

Fig. 150. Intramucosal cancer of proliferated mucosa. The hyperplastic and proliferated mucosa is composed mainly of slender adenocarcinomatous tissue forming a reticular structure. The tubules are made up of small cuboidal epithelial cells with densely arranged, round nuclei, and part of the lesion is infiltrative with mucinous degeneration. (Pt no. 11 109, × 40)

134

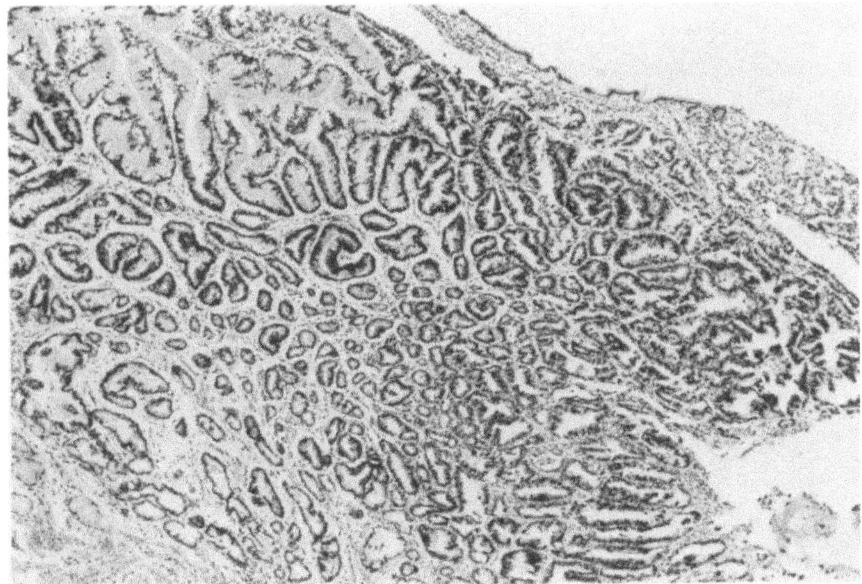

Fig. 151. Intramucosal cancer of hyperplastic mucosa. The mucosa is made up of tubular adenocarcinoma with a few connective tissue stroma and cystic/papillary structure of the tubules indicative of a malignant nature in several parts of the lesion. (Pt no. 12 468, × 40)

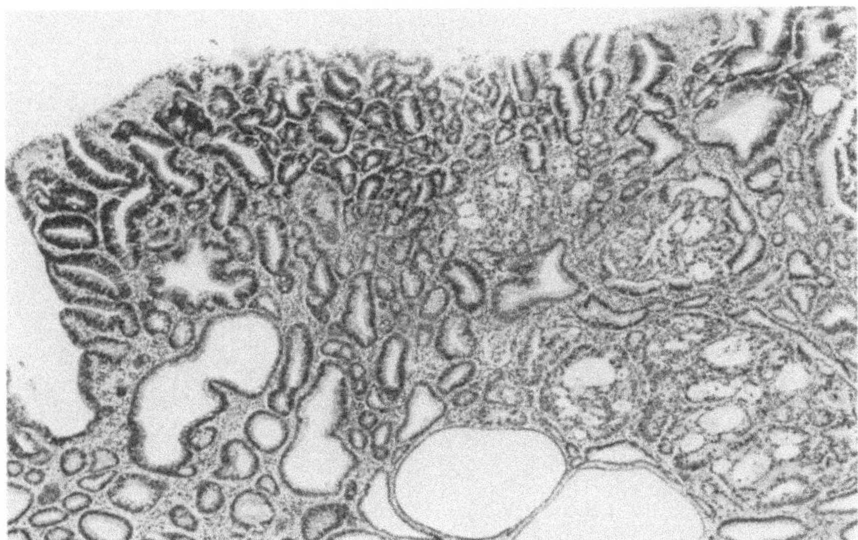

Fig. 152. Intramucosal cancer of elevated mucosa. In the elevated mucosa composed mainly of severe dysplasia, tiny cancerous foci composed of small cuboidal epithelial cells forming an acinar structure are visible in the *right half* of the figure. (Pt no. 12 468, × 40)

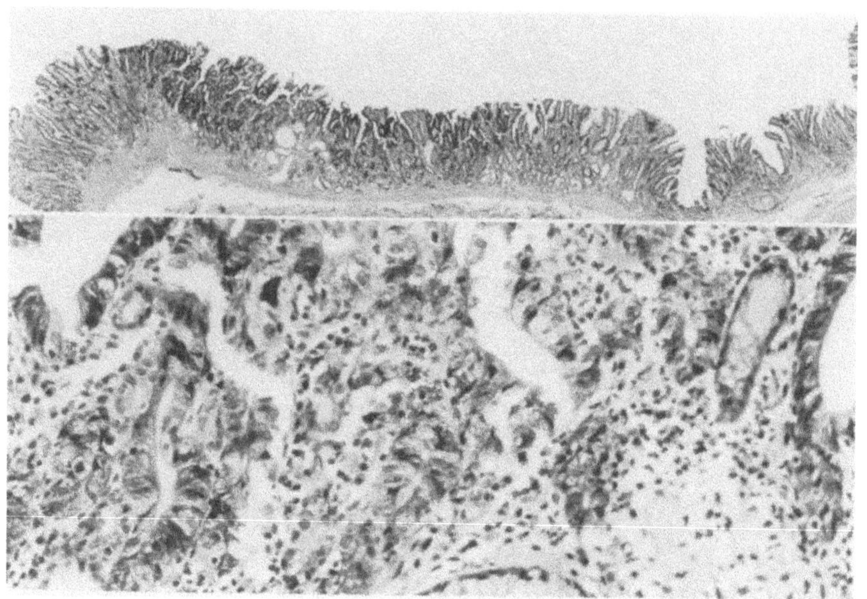

Fig. 153. Intramucosal cancer of flatly elevated mucosa. The mucosa as a whole shows severe dysplasia of intestinal metaplastic nature. In the central part of the elevated lesion cancerous tissues made up of cuboidal epithelial cells are detected in the zone below the surface, as shown by the *lower enlarged photograph.* (Pt no. 11725, × 6 and × 100)

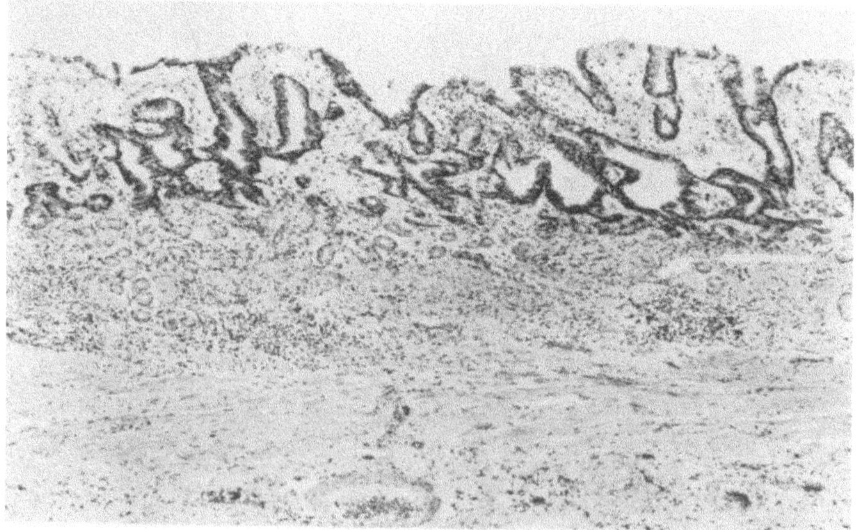

Fig. 154. Intramucosal cancer of atrophic mucosa. Histological appearance is similar at first glance to that shown in Fig. 149 but disorganized foveolar tubules are composed of cuboidal epithelial cells containing small, densely arranged nuclei. Irregular fusion of neighboring tubules indicative of a malignant nature is seen diffusely. (Pt no. 14529, × 35)

136

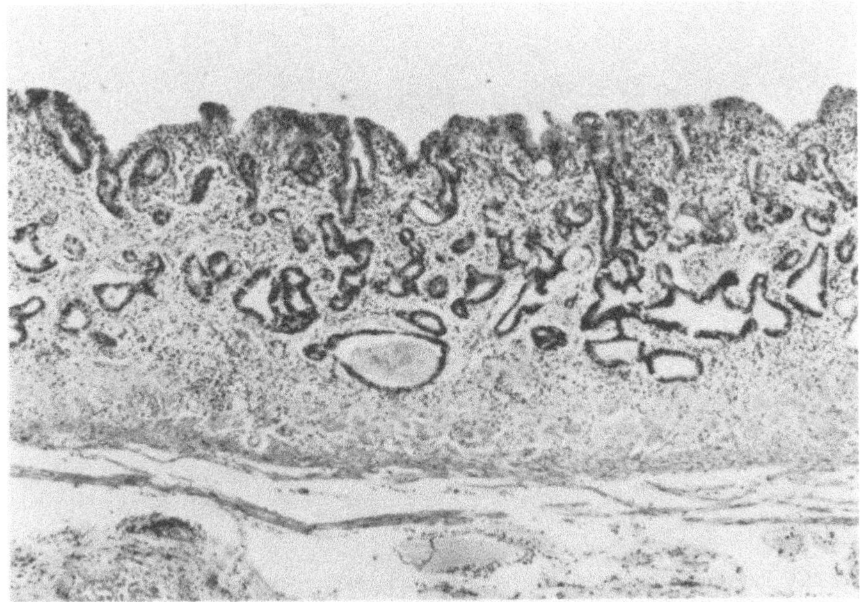

Fig. 155. Intramucosal cancer of atrophic mucosa. Original structure of the mucosa is severely disturbed, and irregularity of shape, structure, and distribution of the foveolar tubules is more marked than in Fig. 154. (Pt no. 8390, × 40)

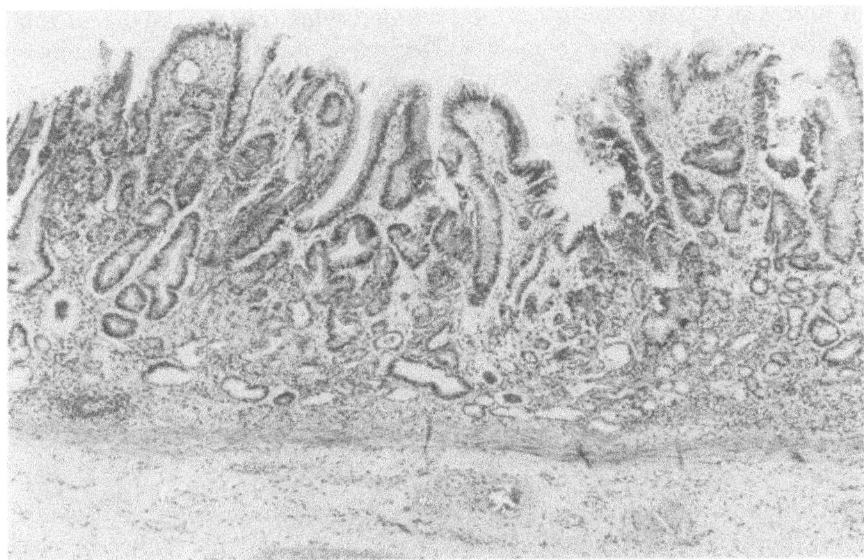

Fig. 156. Intramucosal cancer of flat mucosa. The mucosa shows mild dysplastic change with a few metaplastic foveolae, but close examination reveals downward budding growth of small cancerous glands composed of cuboidal epithelial cells at base of the foveolae. (Pt no. 3527, × 40)

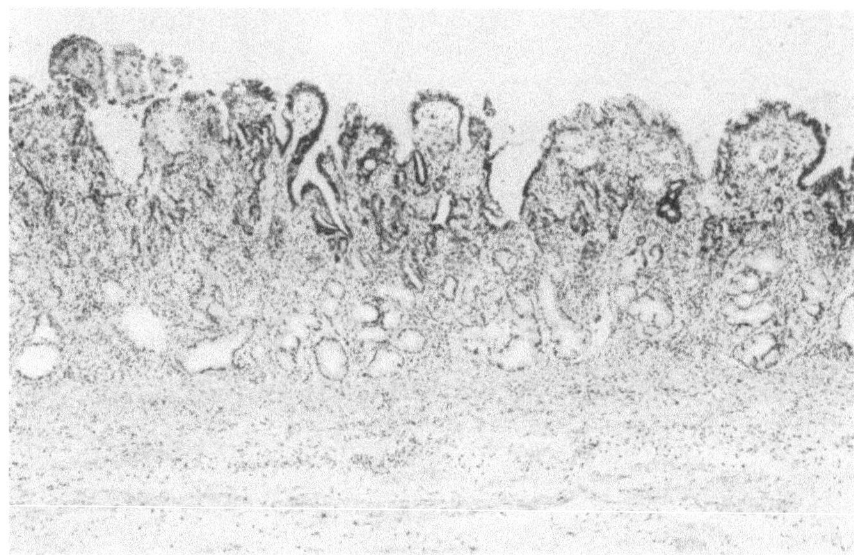

Fig. 157. Intramucosal cancer of flat mucosa. Slender cancerous tubules are seen widely in neck zone between foveolae and pyloric glands. No lateral invasion of the cancer is visible. (Pt no. 16 592, × 40)

in which the grade of cellular atypia is relatively slight compared with the degree of structural abnormality, while in other cases the grade of cellular atypia is really high enough to suggest malignancy even though structural changes are relatively slight. Nevertheless, it can be said that the essential change in severe dysplasia consists in cellular atypia and is not a structural one. In other words, a diagnosis of severe dysplasia should not be recorded when cellular atypia of tubules or glands is not clearly recognizable. Difference in the findings between intramucosal cancer and severe dysplasia of the stomach are listed (Table 33).

Table 33. Differences of the histology of intramucosal cancer from that of severe dysplasia

1. Pleomorphy and loss of polarity of the nuclei are noted
2. Nucleo-cytoplasmic ratio is more markedly increased
3. Loss of cellular differentiation is prominent
4. Abnormal course of the glandular tubulus is visible
5. Invasive growth of epithelia into the surrounding stroma is noticed
6. Small clusters of glands detaching from neck zone may be seen in non-metaplastic but atrophic mucosa
7. Epithelium-stroma relationship is disturbed
8. Surface of the affected mucosa loses smoothness and abnormal mitoses may be seen on the surface
9. Whole layers of the mucosa are often occupied by neoplastic tissues
10. Border of the lesion to the surrounding mucosa is serrated to varying degrees

It is important to note that in the resected stomachs severely dysplastic changes were found most frequently in or adjacent to the apparent cancerous lesions in the early and intermediate stages, but owing to the difficulties involved in reexamining all the surgically resected cancers histologically from this viewpoint, the number and frequency of cases are still not certain; the raw data show that there

138

were more than 300 cases. Isolated dysplastic lesions apart from the primary lesion of cancer or ulcer, mostly the former, were found in 115 cases. Owing to resectability of the stomach, the lesions with dysplastic changes alone accounted for only 40 cases, and most of these were elevated lesions (Table 34).

Table 34. Materials used in this study: specimens taken from 16 606 stomachs resected during the period 1953–1979

Dysplastic lesions	
In or adjacent to cancer	Many
Separate from cancer or ulcer	115 cases
Alone	40 cases
Elevated type	31 cases
Hollowed type (focal atrophy or erosion)	9 cases

From the viewpoint of general pathology, dysplasia of gastric mucosa is intermediate between hyperplasia and neoplasia, and some types of hyperplasia may change their nature gradually to dysplasia in the course of progressive change while some types of dysplasia may transform into carcinoma after many years in a latent growth state (Fig. 158).

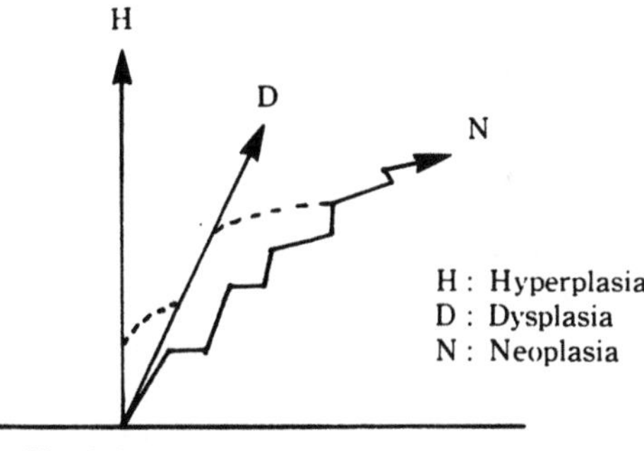

Fig. 158. Relationships between hyperplasia, neoplasia, and dysplasia

It is certain that dysplasia is a typical example of a precancerous lesion of the stomach, but the question as to whether or not all precancerous lesions have the histological features of dysplasia as defined in this chapter is still obscure.

The reports in which the term dysplasia of the stomach is used have been increasing in number recently, and many of them [212, 215, 216, 225, 228, 232a, 242–245, 250, 251] refer to the clinical significance of dypslasia when these change are visible in the biopsy specimens or resected stomachs. With reference to the possible precursor to the development of gastric cancer, Grundmann [217–222] classified dysplastic lesions into low-grade and high-grade and commented on the latter as "in full awareness of their fluent transition into the intestinal type of early gastric cancer." With studies on cell kinetics, karyometry, and histochemistry, OEHLERT [238–241] classified dysplasia into grades I, II, and III, and as characteristic findings in dysplasia grade III he specified "Umwandlung der kryptenartigen Foveolae gastricae" [transformation of the crypt-like foveolae gastricae], "mehrreihigen Epithel mit deutlicher Kernpolymorphie" [laminated epithelium with obvious nuclear polymorphism], and "vergrößerte Nukleolen und zytoplasmatische Basophilie mit völligem Verlust der Schleimbildung" [enlarged nucleoli and cytoplasmic basophilia with complete loss of mucus formation]. He also commented on the possible reversibility or persistence of the lesion without transition into early cancer. CUELLO [213, 214] classified dysplasia into hyperplastic and adenomatous types, and each type was subdivided into mild and severe grades. For severe grades of adenomatous dysplasia he noted the following characteristics:

a) elongated rod-shaped hyperchromatic nuclei of irregular size;
b) pseudostratification of the nuclei;
c) frequent mitosis;
d) increased nucleocytoplasmic ratio;
e) inconspicuous nucleoli;
    and
f) less abundant lamina propria.

MING [229, 230] denoted dysplasia of gastric epithelia as "deviation from the histological feature of the normal stomach, both structurally and cytologically" and classified it into four grades. Grades I and II are found in benign conditions, while grades III and IV are seen in severe atrophic gastritis, adenoma, or mucosa bordering on adenocarcinoma. In conclusion, he said: "grade IV dysplasia, exhibiting prominent cellular pleomorphism, is occasionally difficult to differentiate from carcinoma." SCHADE [247] also described a borderline lesion of the stomach and concluded that various histological findings, such as piled-up multinucleated epithelial cells with absence of goblet cells, are a good guide for the diagnosis of intraepithelial neoplasm. In his book entitled *Early Gastric Cancer. A Contribution to the Pathology and to Gastric Cancer Histogenesis*, JOHANSEN [226] described dysplasia as "malignant change without convincing evidence of invasion" and said that "there are some highly differentiated tumors," and "distinction of it from severe grades of dysplasia is very difficult."

Recently, MING et al [230a] reported on the definition, criteria, and histopathological classification of gastric dysplasia, which were discussed at the Workshop of the International Study Group on Gastric Cancer held at St. Miniato near Florence in 1982.

In Japan, papers using the term dysplasia of gastric mucosa are few, but papers using other, synonymous terms, such as "atypical epithelium," "atypical epithelial hyperplasia," or "borderline lesion," are not uncommon. SUGANO et al. [249] and NAKAMURA et al. [237] reported the atypical epithelial lesions of the stomach in full detail, with ample descriptions and photomicrographs. I myself have also reported the histological features of borderline lesions or gastric dysplasia, starting 10 years ago [234–236]. Besides treating on elevated atypical lesion, the report of Iwanaga et al. [224] seems to be noteworthy from the viewpoint of precancerous change of the stomach. These authors reported 12 cases of superficial gastric cancer, all of which were accompanied by diffuse and heterotopic glandular cysts in

140

the submucosa, and the distributions of the two changes were almost coincident. KATO et al. [227] and RUBIO et al. [246, 246 a] stressed the higher frequency of intramucosal glandular cysts in the stomach with cancer than without cancer.

At present, we still have no reliable indicator or marker for precancerous changes of the stomach, even though this subject has been discussed in some detail by HAMPERL [223]. Without analysis of the constituent cells of the dysplastic lesions from several aspects, this problem can hardly be touched upon.

Summary on Precancerous Changes in the Stomach

On the basis of findings described in Chap. 5 and in this chapter, precancerous lesions of the stomach can be divided into the following three sorts of changes:

a) adenoma,
b) dysplasia,
   and
c) atrophy of the gastric mucosa with severe cellular atypia.

A certain type of gastric cancer develops through a stage of severe dysplasia, but this is by no means mandatory, since most of the gastric mucosa in and around the minute cancers merely shows atrophy of the gastric glands proper with or without intestinal metaplasia and there are no recognizable dysplastic changes as defined in this chapter (Fig. 159). On the other hand, there are some

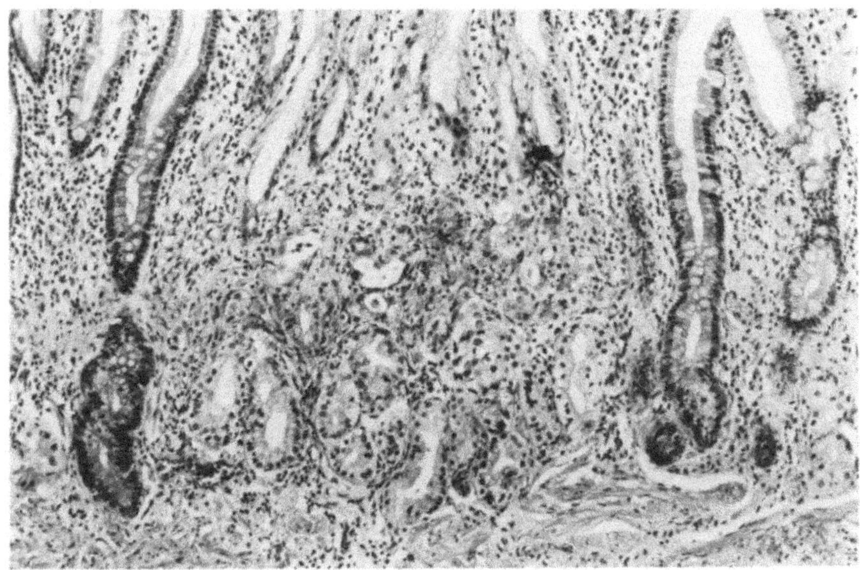

Fig. 159. Cancerous focus of microscopical size, composed of clustering of small cuboidal epithelial cells, is seen in deeper layer of the metaplastic mucosa. No cellular atypia and no disorganized mucosal structure are visible in the surrounding mucosa. (Pt no. 12956, × 100)

141

types of adenomatous polyp that coexist with carcinoma, in which the neoplastic proliferative lesion is made up of de novo-developed epithelium showing tubular, papillary, or villous structures and no disorganized mucosal architecture can be seen (Fig. 160).

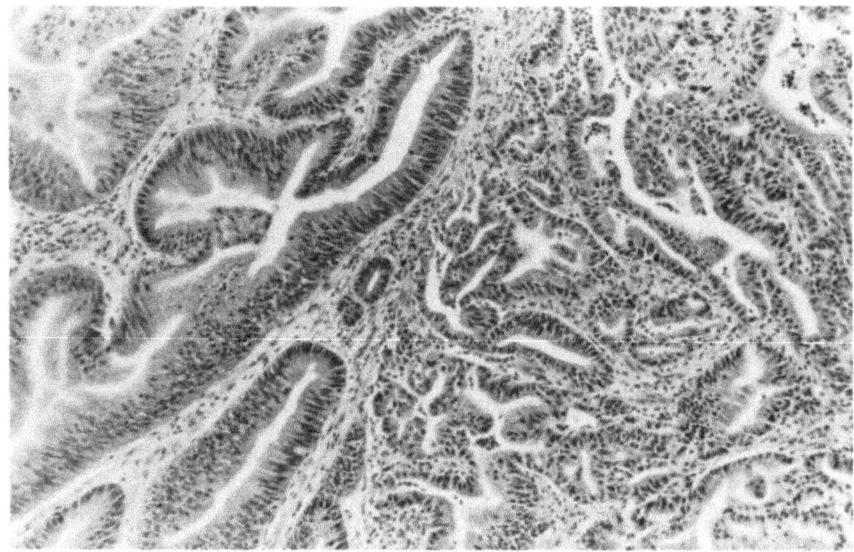

Fig. 160. Small, well-defined lesion composed of tubulopapillary adenocarcinoma *(right)* detected in the gastric polyp with the histology of tubular adenoma *(left)*. No dysplastic change recognizable in the adenomatous growth. (Pt no. 15 342, × 100)

However, it must also be mentioned here that atrophy and atrophic dysplastic mucosa, adenoma, and dysplastic lesion of the elevated or protruding type share some common histological features. According to these ideas, the histogenesis of gastric cancer can be summarized as in Fig. 161.

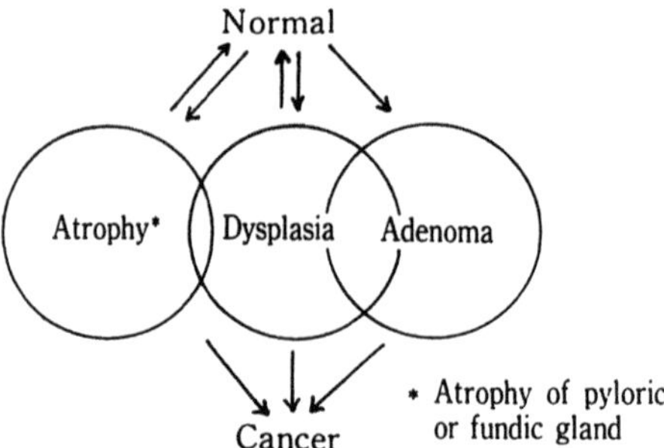

Fig. 161. Histogenesis of gastric cancer

References

Polyp

1. Berg JW (1958) Histological aspects of the relation between gastric adenomatous polyps and gastric cancer. Cancer 11: 1149–1155
2. Elster K (1976) Histological classification of gastric polyps. Curr Top Pathol 77–93
3. Elster K (1974) A new approach to the classification of gastric polyps. Endoscopy 6: 44–47
4. Goldman DS, Appelman HD (1972) Gastric mucosal polyps. Am J Clin Pathol 58: 434–444
5. Hay LJ (1953) Polyps and adenomas of the stomach. Surgery 33: 446–467
6. Hermanek P (1979) Gastric polyps and gastric cancer. In: Herfarth C, Schlag P (eds) Gastric cancer. Springer, Berlin Heidelberg New York, pp 147–148
7. Holmes EJ (1966) Morphogenesis of gastric adenomatous polyps. Transformation to invasive carcinoma of intestinal type. Cancer 19: 794–802
8. Johansen A (1983) Gastric polyps: Pathology and malignant potential. In: Sherlock P et al (eds) Precancerous lesions of the gastrointestinal tract. Raven, New York, pp 171–188
9. Kümmerle F, Schmitt-Köppler A (1971) Magenpolypen. Morphologie, Klinik und Therapie. Dtsch Med Wochenschr 38: 1485–1489
10. Laxen F, Sipponen P, Ihamaki T, Hakkiluoto A, Dortscheva Z (1982) Gastric polyps: The morphological and endoscopical characteristics and relation to gastric carcinoma. Acta Pathol Microbiol Immunol Scand [A] 60: 221–228
11. Majima S (1963) Histopathological study on gastric polyps and their malignant degeneration. Tohoku J Exp Med 80: 355–369
12. Marshak RH, Feldmann F (1965) Gastric polyps. Am J Dig Dis 10: 909–935
13. Ming SC (1984) Precancerous states of the oesophagus and stomach. In: Carter RL (ed) Precancerous states. Oxford University Press, London New York Toronto, p 185–229
14. Ming SC (1977) The classification and significance of gastric polyps. In: Yardley JH, et al (eds) The gastrointestinal tract. Williams and Wilkins, Baltimore, pp 149–175
14 a. Ming SC, Goldman H (1965) Gastric polyp: A histogenetic classification and its relation to carcinoma. Cancer 18: 721–726
15. Monaco AP, Roth ST, Castleman B, Welch CE (1962) Adenomatous polyps of the stomach: A clinical and pathological study of 153 cases. Cancer 15: 456–466
16. Morson BC (1955) Gastric polyps composed of intestinal epithelium. Br J Cancer 9: 550–557
17. Muto T, Oota K (1970) Polypogenesis of gastric mucosa. Gann 61: 435–442
18. Nakamura T (1970) Pathologische Einteilung der Magenpolypen mit spezifischer Betrachtung ihrer malignen Entartung. Chirurg 41: 122–130
19. Nakamura T (1965) Histopathological classification of gastric polyp and its malignant change. In: Badenach JB, et al (eds) Recent advances gastroenterology. I. Brooke JB, pp 477–480
20. Tomasulo J (1971) Gastric polyps. Histologic types and their relationship to gastric carcinoma. Ulcer Cancer 27: 1346–1355

Ulcer

21. Ackerman LV (1964) Carcinoma of the stomach. In: Surgical pathology, 3rd edn, Mosby, St Louis, pp 391–398
22. Bamforth J (1955) Early carcinomatous changes in the stomach. Br J Surg 43: 292–296
23. Becker T, Mayland J (1966) Das Ulcuskarzinom des Magens. Zentralbl Chir 91: 68–75
24. Boyd W (1956) Gastritis and carcinoma. Text-book of pathology. 16th edn Lea and Febiger, Philadelphia, p 460
25. Büchner F (1966) Die Histogenese des Karzinoms. In: Allgemeine Pathologie. Pathologie als Biologie und als Beitrag zur Lehre vom Menschen, Büchner F 5th edn. Urban and Schwarzenberg, Munich, pp 344–349
26. Davis BA, Moroney MJ (1952) "Ulcer-cancer" of the stomach. Br J Cancer 6: 215–229
27. Imai T, Kubo T (1968) Relationship between gastric ulcer and gastric cancer (in Japanese). Stomach Intestine 3: 677–679
28. Kubo T (1971) Histology of gastric ulcer with reference to criteria of "ulcer cancer". Gann 62: 1–11

29. Kuru M (1953) On cancers developed upon ulcerative lesions of the stomach. A study of the regeneration of the mucous membrane of the stomach with special reference to its malignant transformation. Gann 44: 47–54
30. Majima S, Yamaguchi I, Karube K (1965) On malignant change of gastric ulcer. Tohoku J Exp Med 86: 255–276
31. Marshall SF (1953) The relation of gastric ulcer to carcinoma of the stomach. Ann Surg 137: 891–903
32. Morgan AD, Lee ED (1954) The incidence of ulcer-cancer. Br J Surg 41: 595–598
33. Murakami T (1968) Significance of ulcers. Gann Monogr 3: 153–156
34. Nagayo T (1979) Early histogenesis of human gastric carcinoma. In: Pfeiffer CF (ed) Gastric cancer. Etiology and pathogenesis. Witzstrock, Baden-Baden, pp 128–138
35. Nagayo T, Yokoyama H (1974) Early phases and diagnostic features of gastric cancer. JAMA 228: 888–889
36. Nakamura K, Sugano H, Takagi K, Fuchigami A (1967) Histopathological study on early carcinoma of the stomach. Some considerations on the ulcer-cancer by analysis of 144 foci of the superficial spreading carcinoma. Gann 58: 377–387
37. Oehman U, Wetterfors J, Moberg A (1972) Ulcer-cancer of the stomach. Acta Chir Scand 138: 391–395
38. Olsson O, Endresen R (1956) Ulcer cancer of the stomach. Acta Chir Scand 111: 16–21
39. Oota K (1968) On the nature of the ulcerative changes in early carcinoma of the stomach. Gann Monogr 3: 141–151
40. Ostertag H, Georgi A (1974) Histology of early carcinoma of the stomach. Verh Dtsch Ges Pathol 58: 548
41. Paikova LV (1982) Cancer of the stomach arising from chronic ulcers (Histological and histogenetical problems). Arkh Patol 44: 13–19
42. Sano R (1971) Pathological analysis of 300 cases of early gastric cancer with special reference to cancer associated with ulcers. Gann Monogr Cancer Res 11: 81–89
43. Schenken J, Burns EL (1957) Ulcer-carcinoma of the stomach. Anderson WAD (ed) Pathology 3rd edn. Mosby, St Louis, p 753
44. Stout AP (1950) The relationship of gastric ulcer to gastric carcinoma. Cancer 3: 515–552
45. Sugano H, Nakamura K (1968) Frequency of the ulcer cancer in early gastric cancer. Gann Monogr 3: 133–137
46. Takagi K, Someya M (1959) Histopathological study of mucosal carcinoma of the stomach. Gastritis and intest. metapl. Gann 50: 147–148

Gastritis and intestinal metaplasia

47. Cheli R, Giacosa A (1983) Atrophic gastritis. In: Sherlock P et al (eds) Precancerous lesions of the gastrointestinal tract. Raven, New York, pp 155–169
48. Cheli R, Santi L, Ciancamerla G, Canciani G (1973) A clinical and statistical follow-up study of atrophic gastritis. Am J Dig Dis 18: 1061–1066
49. Correa P (1983) Chronic atrophic gastritis as a precursor of cancer. In: Sherlock P, et al (eds) Precancerous lesions of the gastrointestinal tract. Raven, New York, pp 145–153
50. Correa P, Cuello C, Haenszel W (1979) Epidemiologic pathology of precursor lesions and pathogenesis of gastric carcinoma in Colombia. In: Pfeiffer CJ (ed) Gastric cancer. Etiology and pathogenesis. Witzstrock, Baden-Baden, pp 112–127
51. Correa P, Cuello C, Duque E (1970) Carcinoma and intestinal metaplasia of the stomach. J Natl Cancer Inst 44: 297–306
52. Cox AJ (1949) Chronic atrophic gastritis: .dentifikakatation of different varieties. J Natl Cancer Inst 10: 523–532
53. Elster K, Reiss S, Heinkel K (1960) Histotopographische Untersuchungen über die intestinal Metaplasie in Karzinom- und Ulcusmägen. Z Inn Med 15: 1053–1058
54. Faber K (1927) Chronic gastritis, its relation to achylia and ulcer. Lancet 2: 901–907
55. Furihata C, Tatematsu M, Miki K et al (1984) Gastric- and intestinal type properties of human gastric cancers transplanted into nude mice. Cancer Res 44: 727–733
56. Gad A (1969) A histochemical study of human alimentary tract. Mucosubstances in health and disease. I. Normal and tumour. Br J Cancer 23: 52–63

57. Geissendörfer R (1928) Untersuchungen über Vorkommen, Lokalisation und Ausbreitungsweise der Umbaugastritis in Carcinommägen. Langenbecks Arch Klin Chir 153: 235–252
58. Glass GBJ, Pitchumoni CS (1975) Atrophic gastritis. Structural and ultrastructural alterations, exfoliative cytology and enzyme cytochemistry and histochemistry, proliferation kinetics, immunological derangements and other causes and clinical association and sequelae. Hum Pathol 6: 219–250
59. Goldman H, Ming SC (1968) Fine structure of intestinal metaplasia and adenocarcinoma of the human stomach. Lab Invest 18: 203–210
60. Goldman H, Ming SC (1968) Mucins in normal and neoplastic gastrointestinal epithelium. Arch Pathol 85: 580–586
61. Graham RI, Schade ROK (1965) The distribution of intestinal metaplasia in macroscopic specimen demonstrated by a histochemical method. Acta Pathol Microbiol Scand 65: 53–59
62. Guiss LW, Stewart FW (1943) Chronic atrophic gastritis and cancer of the stomach. Arch Surg 46: 823–843
63. Hattori T, Fujita S (1979) Tritiated thymidine autoradiographic study on histogenesis and spread of intestinal metaplasia in human stomach. Pathol Res Pract 164: 224–237
64. Hebbel R (1949) The topography of chronic gastritis in cancer-bearing stomachs. J Natl Cancer Inst 10: 505–522
65. Hebbel R (1949) The topography of chronic gastritis in otherwise normal stomach. Am J Pathol 25: 125–142
66. Häkkinen I, Järvi O, Grönroos J (1968) Sulphoglycoprotein antigens in the human alimentary canal and gastric cancer. An immunohistological study. Int J Cancer 3: 572–581
67. Heilmann KL, Reipker WW (1979) Loss of differentiation in intestinal metaplasia in cancerous stomachs. A comparative morphologic study. Pathol Res Pract 164: 249–258
68. Hillenbrand K (1930) Histotopographische und histologische Untersuchungen über die sogenannte chronische Gastritis. Beitr Pathol Anat 85: 1–32
69. Hitchcock CR, MacLean LD, Sullivan WA (1957) The secretory and clinical aspects of achlorhydria and gastric atrophy as precursors of gastric cancer. J Natl Cancer Inst 18: 795–811
70. Hurst AF (1929) Precursors of carcinoma of the stomach. Lancet 2: 1023–1028
71. Iida F, Kusama J (1982) Gastric carcinoma and intestinal metaplasia: Significance of types of intestinal metaplasia upon development of gastric carcinoma. Cancer 10: 2854–2858
72. Imai T, Murayama H (1983) Time trend in the prevalence of intestinal metaplasia in Japan. Cancer 52: 353–361
73. Imai T, Kubo T, Watanabe H (1971) Chronic gastritis in Japanese with reference to high incidence of gastric carcinoma. J Natl Cancer Inst 47: 179–195
74. Järvi O, Laurén P (1951) On the role of heterotopias of the intestinal epithelium in the pathogenesis of gastric cancer. Acta Pathol Microbiol Scand 29: 26–44
75. Jass JR (1980) Role of intestinal metaplasia in the histogenesis of gastric carcinoma. J Clin Pathol 33: 801–810
76. Jass JR, Filipe MI (1980) Sulphomucins and precancerous lesions of the human stomach. Histopathology 4: 271–279
77. Jass JR, Filipe MI (1979) A variant of intestinal metaplasia associated with gastric carcinoma: A histochemical study. Histopathology 3: 191–199
78. Kawachi T, Kurisu M, Numanyu N et al (1976) Precancerous changes in the stomach. Cancer Res 36: 2673–2677
79. Kawachi T, Kagure K, Tanaka N et al (1974) Studies of intestinal metaplasia in the gastric mucosa by detection of disaccharidases with "Tes-tape". J Natl Cancer Inst 53: 19–30
80. Kobori O, Oota K (1974) Mucous substance and enzyme histochemistry of non-neoplastic and neoplastic gastric epithelium in man. Acta Pathol Jpn 24: 119–130
81. Konjetzny GE (1943) Die Beziehungen zwischen Gastritis und Magenkrebsentwicklung. Langenbecks Arch Klin Chir 204: 4–63
82. Konjetzny GE (1913) Über die Beziehung der chronischen Gastritis mit ihren Folgeerscheinungen und des chronischen Magenulkus zur Entwicklung des Magenkrebses. Bruns Beitr Klin Chir 85: 455–519
83. Konturek SJ, Urban A (1969) The correlation between gastric acid secretion and histology of fundic and antral gland area. Scand J Gastroenterol 4: 463–468

84. Kubo T, Imai T (1971) Intestinal metaplasia of gastric mucosa in autopsy materials in Hiroshima and Yamaguchi districts. Gann 62: 49–54
85. Lambert R (1972) Chronic gastritis. A critical study of the progressive atrophy of the gastric mucosa. Digestion 7: 83–126
86. Laurén P (1967) Histochemical study on enzyme distribution in diffuse and intestinal type of gastric carcinoma. Acta Pathol Microbiol Scand [Suppl] 187: 62
87. Lei DN, Yu JV (1984) Types of mucosal metaplasia in relation to the histogenesis of gastric carcinoma. Arch Pathol Lab Med 108: 220–224
88. Lev R, Siegel HL, Glass GBJ (1969) The enzyme histochemistry of gastric carcinoma in man. Cancer 23: 1086–1093
89. Lev R (1965) The mucin histochemistry of normal and neoplastic gastric mucosa. Lab Invest 14: 2080–2100
89a. Ma J, DeBoer GRM, Nayman J (1982) Intestinal mucinous substances in gastric intestinal metaplasia and carcinoma studied by immunofluorescence. Cancer 49: 1664–1667
90. Magnus HA (1937) Observations on the presence of intestinal epithelium in the gastric mucosa. J Pathol Bacteriol 44: 389–398
91. Matsukura N, Kinebuchi M, Kawachi T, Sato S, Sugimura T (1979) Quantitative measurement of intestinal marker enzymes in intestinal metaplasia from human stomach with cancer. Gann 70: 509–513
92. Matsukura H, Yamamoto T, Sekine I, Ochi Y, Otake M (1980) Distribution of marker enzymes and mucin in intestinal metaplasia in human stomach and relation of complete type of intestinal metaplasia to minute gastric carcinomas. J Natl Cancer Inst 65: 231–240
93. Matsuura H, Yamamoto T, Sekine I, Ochi Y, Otake M (1983) Pathological and epidemiological study of gastric cancer in atomic bomb survivors, Hiroshima and Nagasaki, 1950–1977. 12: 1–22 RERF TR (Radiation Effects Research Foundation Technical Report)
94. McManus JFA (1946) Histological demonstration of mucin after periodic acid. Nature 158: 202
95. Ming SC, Goldman H, Freiman DG (1967) Intestinal metaplasia and histogenesis of carcinoma in human stomach. Light and electron microscopic study. Cancer 20: 1418–1429
96. Morson BC (1956) Intestinal metaplasia of the gastric mucosa. Gastroenterologia 85: 181–191
97. Morson BC (1955) Carcinoma arising from areas of intestinal metaplasia. Br J Cancer 9: 377–385
98. Morson BC (1955) Intestinal metaplasia of the gastric mucosa. Br J Cancer 9: 365–376
99. Muñoz N, Connelly P (1971) Time trends in intestinal and diffuse types of gastric cancer in the United States. Int J Cancer 8: 158–164
100. Murakami T, Nakamura S, Suzuki I (1955) A histological study on the mechanism of intestinal epithelial metaplasia in gastric mucous membrane. Gann 46: 9–14
101. Nagayo T, Komagoe T (1961) Histological studies of gastric mucosal cancer with special reference to relationship of histological pictures between the mucosal cancer and the cancer-bearing gastric mucosa. Gann 52: 109–119
102. Nakahara K (1978) Special features of intestinal metaplasia and its relation to early gastric carcinoma in man. Observation by a method in which leucine aminopeptidase activity is used. J Natl Cancer Inst 61: 693–702
103. Nevaleinen T, Järvi O (1977) Ultrastructures of intestinal and diffuse type gastric carcinoma. J Pathol 122: 129–136
104. Oohara T, Tohma A, Aono G et al. (1983) Intestinal metaplasia of the regenerative epithelia in 549 gastric ulcers. Hum Pathol 14: 1066–1071
105. Oota K, Tanaka N (1952) On the mechanism of regeneration of the gastric mucosa, especially of reparation of the metaplastic epithelium. Gann 43: 365–367
106. Oota K (1950) On metaplastic gastritis. Some consideration on its histogenesis. Gann 41: 72–75
107. Pagnini CA, Bozzola L (1981) Precancerous significance of colonic type intestinal metaplasia. Tumori 67: 113–116
108. Pagnini CA, Rugge W (1983) Gastric cancer: Problems in histogenesis. Histopathology 7: 699–706
109. Pfeiffer CJ (1970) Surface topology of the stomach in man and the laboratory ferret. J Ultrastruct Res 33: 252–262

146

110. Planteydt HT, Willighagen RGJ (1963) Enzyme histochemistry of gastric carcinoma. J Pathol Bacteriol 90: 393–398
111. Planteydt HT, Willighagen RGT (1960) Enzyme histochemistry of human stomach with special reference to intestinal metaplasia. J Pathol Bacteriol 80: 317–323
112. Ringertz N (1961) The pathology of gastric cancer and its relationship to gastritis , polyp and ulcer. Acta Unio Int Contra Cancrum 17: 289–295
113. Rösch W, Demling L, Elster K (1975) Is chronic gastritis a reversible process? Follow-up study of gastritis by stepwise biopsy. Acta Hepatogastroenterol (Stuttg) 22: 252–255
114. Ruddell WS (1979) Gastric juice nitrite and thiocyanate as etiological factors in human gastric cancer. In: Pfeiffer CJ (ed) Gastric cancer. Etiology and pathogenesis. Witzstrock, Baden-Baden, pp 139–151
115. Sasano N, Nakamura K, Arai M, Akazaki K (1969) Ultrastructural cell patterns in human gastric carcinoma compared with non-neoplastic gastric mucosa. Histogenetic analysis of carcinoma by mucin histochemistry. J Natl Cancer Inst 43: 783–802
116. Schade ROK (1962) Pathologisch-anatomische Frühdiagnose des Magenkarzinoms. Chirurg 33: 193–197
117. Schade ROK (1960) Chronic gastritis, a precancerous condition. Acta Unio Int Contra Cancrum 16: 1402–1406
118. Schindler R (1965) Gastric carcinoma and gastritis. With reference to coexistences of carcinoma and chronic hypertrophic glandular gastritis. Am J Dig Dis 10: 607–624
119. Segal HL, Samloff IM (1973) Gastric cancer: Increased frequency in patients with achlorhydria. Am J Dig Dis 18: 295–299
120. Segura DI, Montero C (1983) Histochemical characterization of different types of intestinal metaplasia in gastric mucosa. Cancer 52: 498–503
121. Sipponen P, Kekki M, Siurala M (1983) Atrophic chronic gastritis and intestinal metaplasia. Comparison with a representative population sample. Cancer 52: 1062–1068
122. Sipponen P, Sepälä K, Varis K et al (1980) Intestinal metaplasia with colonic type sulphomucins in the gastric mucosa; its association with gastric carcinoma. Acta Pathol Microbiol Immunol Scand [A] 88: 217–224
123. Siurala M, Villako T, Ihamäki T et al (1977) Atrophic gastritis: Its genetic and dynamic behavior and its relation to gastric carcinoma and pernicious anemia. In: Farber E, et al (eds) Pathophysiology of carcinogenesis in Digestive organs. University of Tokyo Press, Tokyo, pp 135–148
124. Siurala M, Varis K, Wiljasulo M (1966) Studies on patients with atrophic gastritis – a 10–15 years follow-up. Scand Gastroenterol 1: 40–48
125. Siurala M, Seppala K (1960) Atrophic gastritis as a possible precursor of gastric carcinoma and pernicious anemia. Results of follow-up examinations. Acta Med Scand 166: 455–461
126. Stemmermann GN, Hayashi T (1968) Intestinal metaplasia of the gastric mucosa. A gross and microscopic study of its distribution in various disease state. J Natl Cancer Inst 41: 627–634
127. Stemmermann GN (1967 Comparative study of histochemical patterns in non-neoplastic and neoplastic gastric epithelium. A study of Japanese in Hawaii. J Natl Cancer Inst 39: 375–383
128. Stemmermann H, Ishidate T, Samlott M, Masuda H, Walsh JH (1978) Intestinal metaplasia of the stomach in Hawaii and Japan. A study of its relation to serum pepsinogen I, gastric and parietal cell antibodies. Am J Dig Dis 23: 815–820
129. Stewart MJ (1931) Precancerous lesions of the alimentary tract. Lancet 2: 617–622
130. Stout AP (1953) Gastritis. Atlas of tumor pathology, sect 6, fasc 21. AFIP, Washington
131. Strickland RG, MacKay IR (1973) A reappraisal of the nature and significance of chronic atrophic gastritis. Am J Dig Dis 18: 426–440
132. Sugimura T, Matsukura N, Sato S (1982) Intestinal metaplasia of the stomach as a precancerous stage. IARC Sci Publ 32: 515–530
133. Sumiyoshi H, Taniyama K, Ito H et al (1984) Secretory component and immunoglobulin in human gastric carcinoma: An immunohistochemical study. Gann 75: 166–176
134. Takebayashi S, Takagi T, Shiraishi M (1979) Scanning electronmicroscopy of human gastric cancer and intestinal metaplasia. In: Pfeiffer CJ (ed) Gastric cancer. Etiology and pathogenesis. Witzstrock, Baden-Baden, pp 209–227
135. Tannenbaum SR, Sinsky AJ, Weisman M, Bishop W (1974) Nitrite in human saliva, its possible relationship to nitrosamine formation. J Natl Cancer Inst 53: 79–84

136. Tarpila S, Telkkä A, Siurala M (1969) Ultrastructure of various metaplasia of the stomach. Acta Pathol Microbiol Scand 77: 187–195
137. Teglbjärg PS, Nielson HO (1978) "Small intestinal type" and "Colonic type" intestinal metaplasia of the human stomach. Acta Pathol Microbiol Scand 86: 351–355
138. Tsutsumi Y, Nagura H, Watanabe K (1984) Immune aspects of intestinal metaplasia of the stomach: an immunohistochemical study. Virchows Arch [A] 403: 345–359
139. Twomey JJ (1978) Immunological dysfunction with atrophic gastritis and gastric malignancy. In: Lipkin M et al (eds) Gastrointestinal tract cancer. Plenum, New York, pp 93–111
140. Usland O (1935) Über die Bedeutung der chronischen Gastritis für die Entwicklung des Magenkrebses. Acta Chir Scand 76: 485–500
141. Varis K (1971) A family study of chronic gastritis. Scand J Gastroenterol [Suppl] 6
142. Walker IR, Strickland RG, Ungar B, Mackay IR (1971) Simple atrophic gastritis and gastric carcinoma. Gut 12: 906–911
143. Warren S, Meissner WA (1944) Chronic gastritis and carcinoma of the stomach. Gastroenterology 3: 251–256
144. Watanabe T (1981) Chronic gastritis observed from a standpoint of chronic organ inflammation. Acta Pathol Jpn 31: 717–732
145. Wattenberg LW (1959) Histochemical study of aminopeptidase in metaplasia and carcinoma of the stomach. AMA Arch Pathol 67: 281–286
146. Wolff G (1970) Über einige morphologische Strukturen der Magenschleimhaut bei verschiedenen Formen der chronischen Gastritis und ihre Beeinflussung durch die Verdauung. Z Gastroenterol 8: 168–175
147. Wolff G (1968) Chronische Gastritis und Magenkrebs. Arch Geschwulstforsch 31: 184–199

Pernicious anemia

148. Bartholomew BA, Hill MJ, Hudson MJ, Ruddell WS, Walters CL (1980) Gastric bacteria, nitrate, nitrite and nitrosamines in patients with pernicious anemia and in patients treated with cimetidine. IARC Sci Publ 31: 595–608
149. Cox AJ (1943) The stomach in pernicious anemia. Am J Pathol 19: 491–501
150. Elsborg L, Mosbeck J (1979) Pernicious anemia as a risk factor in gastric cancer. Acta Med Scand 206: 315–318
151. Irvine WJ, Cullen DR, Mawhinney H (1974) Natural history of autoimmune achlorhydric atrophic gastritis. Lancet 2: 482–485
152. Johansen AA, Rödbro P (1968) The histology of the gastric mucosa in pernicious anemia. Acta Pathol Microbiol Scand 73: 145–155
153. Magnus HA (1958) A reassessment of gastric lesions in pernicious anemia. J Clin Pathol 2: 289–294
154. Magnus HA, Ungley CC (1938) The gastric lesion in pernicious anemia. Lancet 1: 420–421
155. Mosbech J (1954) Pernicious anemia and cancer of the stomach. Acta Med Scand 148: 305–315
156. Mosbech J, Videbaek A (1950) Mortality from and risk of gastric carcinoma among patients with pernicious anemia. Br Med J 2: 390–394
157. Rigler RG, Kaplan HS (1945) Pernicious anemia and the early diagnosis of tumor of the stomach. JAMA 128: 426–432
158. Ruddell WSJ, Bone ES, Hill MJ, Walters CL (1978) Pathogenesis of gastric cancer in pernicious anemia. Lancet 1: 521–523
159. Schell R, Dockerty MB (1954) Carcinoma of the stomach associated with pernicious anemia. A clinical and pathologic study. Surg Gynecol Obstet 98: 710–720
160. Siurala M, Villako K, Ihamäki T et al (1977) Atrophic gastritis. Its genetic and dynamic behaviors and its relation to gastric carcinoma and pernicious anemia. In: Farber E et al (eds) Pathophysiology of carcinogenesis in digestive organs. University of Tokyo Press, Tokyo, pp 135–148
161. Siurala M, Varis K, Wiljasuh M (1966) Studies on patients with atrophic gastritis – a 10-, 15 years follow-up. Scand Gastroenterol 1: 40–48
162. Siurala M, Seppata K (1960) Atrophic gastritis as a possible precursor of gastric carcinoma and pernicious anemia. Results of follow-up examination. Acta Med Scand 166: 451–461

148

163. Stockbrugger W, Menon GG, Beilby JO, Mason RR, Cotton PB (1983) Gastroscopic screening in 80 patients with pernicious anemia. Gut 24: 1141–1147
164. Torgersen J (1944) Localization of gastritis and gastric cancer, especially in cases of pernicious anemia. Acta Radiol (Stockh) 25: 845–855
165. Varis K (1983) Surveillance of pernicious anemia. In: Sherlock P et al (eds) Precancerous lesions of the gastrointestinal tract. Raven, New York, pp 189–194
166. Varis K, Stenman UH, Lehtola J, Siurala M (1978) Gastric lesion and pernicious anemia: a family study. Acta Hepatogastroenterol (Stuttg) 25: 62–67
167. Wood JJ (1951) The value of gastric biopsy in the study of chronic gastritis and pernicious anemia. Br Med J 2: 823–825
168. Zancheck N (1955) Occurrence of gastric cancer among patients with pernicious anemia at Boston City Hospital. N Engl J Med 252: 1103–1110

Gastric remnant

169. Clémençon G (1979) Risk of carcinoma of the gastric remnant after gastric resection for benign conditions. In: Herfarth Ch, Schlag P (eds) Gastric cancer. Springer, Berlin Heidelberg New York, pp 129–136
170. Dahm K, Werner B, Eichen R, Mitschke H (1979) Experimental cancer of the gastric stump. In: Herfarth Ch, Schlag P (eds) Gastric cancer. Springer, Berlin Heidelberg New York, pp 44–59
171. Dahm K, Werner B (1973) Experimentelles Anastomosencarcinom. Ein Beitrag zur Pathogenese des Magenstumpfcarcinoms. Langenbecks Arch Chir 333: 211–236
172. Domellöf L, Reddy BS, Weisburger JH (1980) Microflora and deconjugation of bile acids in alkaline reflux after partial gastrectomy. Am J Surg 140: 291–295
173. Domellöf L, Eriksson S, Janunger KG (1977) Carcinoma and possible precancerous changes of the gastric stump after Billroth II resection. Gastroenterology 73: 462–468
174. Domellöf L, Eriksson S, Janunger KG (1975) Late occurence of precancerous changes and carcinoma of the gastric stump after Billroth II resection. Acta Chir Scand 141: 292–297
175. Dougherty SH, Foster CA, Eisenberg MM (1982) Stomach cancer following gastric surgery for benign disease. Arch Surg 117: 294–297
176. Fischer AB, Graen N, Jensen ON (1983) Risk of gastric cancer after Billroth II resection for duodenal ulcer. Br J Surg 70: 552–554
177. Graem N, Fischer AB, Hastrup N, Poulsen CO (1981) Mucosal changes of the Billroth II resected stomach. A follow-up study of patients resected for duodenal ulcer, with special reference to gastritis, atypia and cancer. Acta Pathol Microbiol Immunol Scand [A] 89: 227–234
178. Griesser G, Schmidt H (1964) Statistische Erhebung über die Häufigkeit des Karzinoms nach Magenoperation wegen eines Geschwürleidens. Med Welt 35: 1836–1840
179. Hammer E (1976) The localization of precancerous change and carcinoma after previous gastric operation for benign conditions. Acta Path Microbiol Immunol Scand [A] 84: 495–507
180. Helsingen N, Hillestad L (1956) Cancer development in the gastric stump after partial gastrectomy for ulcer. Ann Surg 143: 173–179
181. Hilbe G, Salzer GM, Hassel H (1968) Die Carcinomgefährdung des Resektionsmagens. Langenbecks Arch Klin Chir 323: 142–153
182. Inokuchi K, Tokudome S, Ikada M et al (1984) Mortality from carcinoma after partial gastrectomy. Gann 75: 588–594
183. Jablokow VR, Aranba GY, Reyes CV (1982) Gastric stomal polypoid hyperplasia: Report of four cases. J Surg Oncol 19: 106–108
184. Krause U (1957) Late prognosis after partial gastrectomy for ulcer. Acta Chir Scand 114: 341–354
184a. Kondo K, Suzuki H, Nagayo T (1982) Pathology of stump carcinoma. Gan No Rinsho (in Japanese) 28: 1615–1625
185. Kondo K, Suzuki H, Nagayo T (1984) The influence of gastrojejunal anastomosis on gastric carcinogenesis in rats. Gann 75: 362–369
186. Kühlmayer R, Rokitansky O (1954) Das Magenstumpfkarzinom als Spätproblem der Ulcuschirurgie. Langenbecks Arch Klin Chir 278: 361–375

187. Lawson HH (1979) Duodenal reflux and epithelial lesions. In: Herfarth Ch, Schlag P (eds) Gastric cancer. Springer, Berlin Heidelberg New York, pp 112–119
188. Meister H, Schlag P (1979) Epithelium at the gastroenteral borderline – Comparison of animal experiment and clinical-pathological investigations. In: Herfarth Ch, Schlag P (eds) Gastric cancer. Springer, Berlin Heidelberg New York, pp 32–43
189. Myren J (1983) Markers of cancer risk and surveillance of the gastric stump. In: Sherlock P et al (eds) Precancerous lesions of gastrointestinal tract. Raven, New York, pp 195–203
190. Peitsch W (1979) Remarks of frequency and pathogenesis of primary gastric stump cancer. In: Herfarth Ch, Schlag P (eds) Gastric cancer. Springer, Berlin Heidelberg New York, pp 137–144
191. Rösch W (1979) Prospective studies in patients with resected stomach and stump carcinoma. In: Herfarth Ch, Schlag P (eds) Gastric Cancer. Springer, Berlin Heidelberg New York, pp 145–146
192. Salvadori G (1983) Endoscopic and histologic appearances of the gastric mucosa more than 10 years after partial gastrectomy. Acta Endosc 13: 301–307
193. Savage A, Jones S (1979) Histological appearances of the gastric mucosa 15–27 years after partial gastrectomy. J Clin Pathol 32: 179–186
194. Schlag P, Böckler R, Meyer H, Beloklavek D (1979) Nitrite and N-nitrosocompounds in the operated stomach. In: Herfarth Ch, Schlag P (eds) Gastric Cancer. Springer, Berlin Heidelberg New York, pp 120–128
195. Schrumpf E, Serck-Hanssen A, Stadaas J et al (1977) Mucosal changes in the gastric stump 20–25 years after partial gastrectomy. Lancet 2: 467–469
196. Serck-Hansen A et al (1977) Mucosal changes in the gastric stump 20–25 years after resections for ulcer. A follow-up study. In: International Conference of Gastrointestinal Cancer. Karger, Basel, p 273
197. Stalsberg H, Taksdal S (1971) Stomach cancer following gastric surgery for benign conditions. Lancet 2: 1175–1177
198. Sturniolo G, Carditello A, Bonavita CT, Bartolatta M, Saitta E (1983) Risk factors for development of primary cancer in the gastric stump. Intragastric nitrites and nitrosocompounds after surgery for duodenal ulcer. Acta Chir Scand 149: 591–596
199. Tokudome S, Kono S, Ikeda M et al (1984) A prospective study on primary gastric stump cancer following partial gastrectomy for benign gastroduodenal diseases. Cancer Res 44: 2208–2212
200. Totten J, Burns HJ, Kay AW (1983) Time of onset of carcinoma of the stomach following surgical treatment of duodenal ulcer. Surg Gynecol Obstet 157: 431–433
201. Welvaart K, Warsiuck HM (1982) The incidence of carcinoma of the gastric remnant. J Surg Oncol 21: 104–106
202. Wolter FH, Heinrich P, Dittrich S, Theuring F (1982) Experimental study on the pathogenesis of gastric stump neoplasms. Exp Chir 15: 167–171

Menetrier's disease and aberrant pancreas

203. Benichou J, Ohana S, Testas P, Monod-Broca P (1980) Menetrier's disease and gastric tumors. J Chir (Paris) 117: 161–163
204. Chusid EL (1964) Spectrum of hypertrophic gastropathy, giant rugal folds, polyposis and carcinoma of the stomach. Case report and review of the literatures. Arch Intern Med 114: 621–628
205. Dirschmid K (1980) Early gastric carcinoma in Menetrier's disease. Med Klin 75: 448–450
206. Rubin RG, Fuik H (1967) Giant hypertrophy of the gastric mucosa associated with carcinoma of the stomach. Am J Gastroenterol 47: 379–388
207. Texter EC, Legerton CW, Reeves RJ, Smith AG, Ruffin JM (1953) Coexistent carcinoma of the stomach and hypertrophic gastritis. Gastroenterology 24: 579–586
208. Woods MG (1983) Intramucosal carcinoma of the gastric antrum complicating Menetrier's disease. J Clin Pathol 36: 1071–1075
209. Goldfarb WB, Bennett D, Monafo W (1963) Carcinoma in heterotopic gastric pancreas. Ann Surg 158: 56–58
210. Hickman DM, Frey CF, Carson JW (1981) Adenocarcinoma arising in gastric heterotopic pancreas. West J Med 135: 57–62
211. Tanimura A, Yamamoto H, Shibata H, Sano E (1979) Carcinoma in heterotopic gastric pancreas. Acta Pathol Jpn 29: 251–257

Dysplasia

212. Barwick KW (1982) Gastric epithelial dysplasia: How reliable can it be recognized and what does it mean? J Clin Gastroenterol 4: 493–496
213. Cuello C, Correa P (1979) Dysplastic changes in intestinal metaplasia of the gastric mucosa. In: Herfarth C, Schlag P (eds) Gastric cancer. Springer, Berlin Heidelberg New York, pp 83–90
214. Cuello C, L'opez L, Correa P et al. (1979) Histopathology of gastric dysplasias: Correlations with gastric juice chemistry. Am J Surg Pathol 3: 491–500
215. Farini R, Pagnini CA, Mario F Di et al (1983) Is mild gastric epithelial dysplasia an indication for follow up? J Clin Gastroenterol 5: 307–310
216. Gedigk P, Bechtelsheimer H, Müller-Wallraf R (1979) Premalignant lesions of the stomach. J Med Sci 15: 405–409
217. Grundmann E (1973) Die Bedeutung der Präcancerösen Zell- und Gewebsveränderungen in Experiment und Klinik. Arch Klin Exp Ohren Nasen Kehlkopfheilkd 205: 55–67
218. Grundmann E (1983) Classification and clinical consequences of precancerous lesions in the digestive and respiratory tract. Acta Pathol Jpn 33: 195–217
219. Grundmann E, Schlake W (1979) Histology of possible precancerous stages in the stomach. In: Herfarth C, Schlag P (eds) Gastric cancer. Springer, Berlin Heidelberg New York, pp 72–82
220. Grundmann E (1978) Early gastric cancer today. Pathol Res Pract 162: 347–360
221. Grundmann E (1976) Precancer. Histology, trends and prospects. Z Krebsforsch 85: 1–11
222. Grundmann E (1975) Histologic types and possible initial stages in early gastric carcinoma. Beitr Pathol 154: 256–280
223. Hamperl H (1974) Praecancerosen der von Zylinderepithel bekleideten Schleimhäute. b. Magen. In: Grundmann E (ed) Geschwülste/Tumors I. Springer, Berlin Heidelberg New York, pp 383–387 (Handbuch der allgemeinen Pathologie, vol 6/5)
223 a. Hanawa K, Kubota K, Suzuki H, Nagayo T (1980) Proliferative activities of epithelia in atypical and cancerous elevated lesion of the stomach. From the viewpoint of distribution and frequency of the mitotic cells (in Japanese). Gan No Rinsho 26: 429–436
224. Iwanaga T, Koyasha H, Takahashi Y, Taniguchi H, Wada A (1975) Diffuse submucosal cysts and carcinoma of the stomach. Cancer 36: 606–614
225. Jass JR (1983) A classification of gastric dysplasia. Histopathology 7: 181–193
226. Johansen A (1981) Border-line lesion of the stomach. In: Early gastric cancer. A contribution to the pathology and to gastric cancer histogenesis. By Johansen A. Bispebjorg Hospital, Copenhagen, pp 48–50
227. Kato Y, Sugano H, Rubio CA (1983) Classification of intramucosal cysts of the stomach. Histopathology 7: 931–938
228. Meister H, Holubarsh Ch, Haferkamp O, Schlag P, Herfarth Ch (1979) Significance and location of atrophic gastritis and of glandular dysplasia in benign and malignant gastric disease. In: Herfarth Ch, Schlag P (eds) Gastric Cancer. Springer, Berlin Heidelberg New York, pp 105–107
229. Ming SC (1979) Dysplasia of gastric epithelium. Front Gastrointest Res 4: 164–172
230. Ming SC (1974) Histogenesis and premalignant lesions. JAMA 228: 886–888
230 a. Ming SC, Bajtai A, Conea P et al (1984) Gastric dysplasia. Cancer 54: 1794–1801
231. Morson BC, Sobin LH, Grundmann E et al (1980) Precancerous condition and epithelial dysplasia. J Clin Pathol 33: 711–721
232. Morson BC (1962) Precancerous lesions of upper gastrointestinal tract. JAMA 179: 311–315
232 a. Morson BC, Jass JR (1985) Precancerous lesions of the gastric intestinal tract. In: Stomach. Bailliere Tindall, London, pp 52–96
233. Nagayo T (1981) Dysplasia of the gastric mucosa and its relation to the precancerous state. Gann 72: 813–823
234. Nagayo T (1980) Dysplastic changes of the digestive tract related to cancer. Acta Endosc 10: 69–80
235. Nagayo T (1977) Precursors of human gastric cancer: Their frequencies and histological characteristics. In: Farber E et al (eds) Pathophysiology of carcinogenesis of digestive organs. University of Tokyo Press, Tokyo, pp 151–160
236. Nagayo T (1971) Histological diagnosis of biopsied gastric mucosa with special reference to that of borderline lesions. Gann Monogr 11: 245–256

237. Nakamura K, Sugano H, Takagi K, Fuchigami A (1966) Histopathological study on early carcinoma of the stomach: Criteria for diagnosis of atypical epithelium. Gann 57: 613–620
238. Oehlert W (1983) Präkanzerosen des Ösophagus und des Magen-Darm-Traktes. MMW 125: 242–247
239. Oehlert W (1979) Biological significance of dysplasia of the epithelium and of atrophic gastritis. In: Herfarth C, Schlag P (eds) Gastric cancer. Springer, Berlin Heidelberg New York, pp 91–104
240. Oehlert W, Keller P, Henke M, Strauch M (1979) Gastric mucosal dysplasia: What is its clinical significance. Front Gastrointest Res 4: 173–182
241. Oehlert W, Keller P, Henke M, Strauch M (1975) Die Dysplasien der Magenschleimhaut. Das Problem ihrer klinischen Bedeutung. Dtsch Med Wochenschr 100: 1950–1956
242. Pilotti S, Rilke F (1977) Atypical epithelium of the protuberant lesions in the stomach. Acta Cytol (Baltimore) 21: 1–2
243. Potet F, Camilleri JP (1982) High risk populations and precancerous dysplasia in the stomach: Definition and management. Gastroenterol Clin Biol 6: 454–461
244. Riemann JF, Schmidt H, Hermanek P (1983) Comparative morphologica and morphometric analysis of the borderline lesion of the antral mucosa of the stomach. In: Sherlock P et al (eds) Precancerous lesions of the gastrointestinal tract. Raven, New York, pp 137–144
245. Riemann JF, Schmidt H, Hermanek P (1983) On the ultrastructure of the gastric "borderline lesion". J Cancer Res Clin Oncol 105: 285–291
246. Rubio CA, Kato Y, Sugano H (1983) The intramucosal cysts of the stomach in Japanese subjects having focal (elevated) dysplasia. Gann 74: 391–397
246a. Rubio CA, Kato Y, Sugano H (1984) The intramucosal cysts of the stomach VI. Their quantitative and qualitative characteristics in focal (elevated) neoplastic lesions. Path Res Pract 179: 105–109
247. Schade ROK (1974) The borderline between benign and malignant lesions in the stomach. In: Grundmann E et al (eds) Early gastric cancer. Springer, Berlin Heidelberg New York, pp 45–53
248. Serck-Hansen A (1979) Precancerous lesions of the stomach. Scand J Gastroenterol [Suppl] 54: 104–105
249. Sugano H, Nakamura K, Takagi K (1971) An atypical epithelium of the stomach. A clinico-pathological entity. Gann Monogr Cancer Res 11: 257–269
250. Thomas C, Oehlert W (1983) Dysplasias of the gastric mucosa. Med Welt 34: 20–21
251. Zhdanov US, Kodrian AA (1982) Dysplasia of the epithelium of the gastric mucosa. Arkh Patol 44: 86–90

7. Chronologic Development and Prognosis of Early Gastric Cancer

Development and Growth

As described in Chap. 6, gastric cancer does not develop suddenly in a healthy stomach but develops through latent periods of chronic disorder. From the viewpoint of chronology, the best example of a precancerous condition is the presence of a gastric remnant after partial gastrectomy for a nonmalignant disease, most commonly peptic ulcer. The average interval from resection of the stomach to the development of the cancers in the remnant is reported by several investigators as around 20 years, and the same tendency has also been confirmed by our own experience.

Gastric cancers having histological evidence of the ulcer-cancer sequence are seen only in the mucosa around chronic or callotic peptic ulcers and never in the mucosa around subacute or subchronic ulcers. Unlike the cases of gastric remnant, the development of peptic ulcer cannot be precisely dated, but from the symptoms and from histological features of the lesions, such as dense collagenous or sometimes callous connective tissues occupying the base of the ulcer, most of the chronic gastric ulcers that underwent malignant change later on in the surrounding mucosa are thought to have at least preexisted for more than 5 years. It is also certain from its characteristic histological features and from followup data that the protruding or elevated type of EGC has had protracted and gradually progressing precancerous periods before development of the cancer. The frequency of intestinal metaplasia of gastric mucosa, the most important histological marker of chronic atrophic gastritis, becomes proportionally higher with advancing age, and it is reasonable to consider that the metaplasia has been developing for many years before it becomes apparent. Thus, gastric cancer, and especially that with intestinal-type histology, is thought to have a long latent period before it develops.

On the basis of the data available, it is generally accepted that often more than 5 years pass between the stages of EGC and AGC. This means that superficial or minute cancers that develop in the gastric mucosa do not grow so rapidly as once supposed, probably owing to the immune response of the host tissue. This opinion is derived from (a) statistics on the average ages of patients with EGC and AGC; (b) retrospective studies on recurrent EGC; and (c) followup observations in EGC.

As suggested by Figs. 18 and 27, the average age of 510 patients with intramucosal EGC (51.3 years) was 3.0 years lower than that of 3567 with AGC

(54.3 years), and the highest frequency of AGC was in the 7th decade, while it fell in the 6th decade in cases of EGC, even though the age and sex distribution patterns were quite similar in the two groups.

Comparison of the ages of patients in the same series with the same macroscopical and histological types but different grades of cancerous growth revealed that the average age was a few years lower in EGC than in AGC in the case of ill-defined morphology, but to our surprise, in cases of well-demarkated morphology no such significant difference was observed (Table 35).

Table 35. Average age of patients with EGC and AGC

	Well-demarkated type			Ill-defined type	
EGC (*n*=1192)	I 61.4	IIa 58.6	IIc' 56.5	IIc'' 48.7	III 50.8
AGC (*n*=3771)	I 59.0		II 56.3	III 51.3	IV 52.4

As will be described later in more detail, the prognosis of EGC after gastrectomy is quite hopeful, especially in the case of mucosal cancer. However, in four cases of mucosal cancer (0.7%) and in seven cases of submucosal cancer (1.2%), the cancer did recur in the gastric remnants, and most of these cancers were in an advanced stage. Retrospective studies of the resected stomachs revealed that in all these cases moderately to poorly differentiated cancer cells had infiltrated microscopically to the proximal cut end on the stomach (ow +), and in all of them recurrence of the cancer in the gastric remnant was recognized more than 5 years after the resection, the longest interval being 19 years (Table 36; Figs. 162 and 163).

Table 36. Cases of EGC with recurrence (ow + cases alone)

	No.	Serial no.	Age	Sex	Macro. type	Size (mm)	Site	Histol. type	Survival (years)	Form of recurrence
Mucosal (m) cancer	1	1249	33	f	IIc+III	33×30	M	por	13.3	Peritoneal Ca
	2	3120	48	m	IIc+III	45×40	M	tub	13.9	Peritoneal Ca
	3	4876	52	f	IIc+III	90×80	M	tub	6.8	Esophageal Ca
	4	6044	49	f	IIc+III	77×80	M	por	6.3	Stump Ca
Submucosal (sm) cancer	1	275	47	m	IIc+III	40×30	M	por	19.0	Stump Ca
	2	2288	44	f	IIc+III	55×45	M	por	12.10	Peritoneal Ca
	3	2930	47	m	IIc	90×90	M	por	6.3	Stump Ca
	4	5347	58	f	IIc	90×95	M	por	11.4	Stump Ca
	5	8804	43	f	IIc	100×90	M	por	6.0	Stump Ca
	6	9319	43	f	IIc	100×70	M	por	5.4	Stump Ca
	7	12470	43	m	IIc+III	70×50	M	tub	6.2	Stump Ca

M: Middle part of the stomach

154

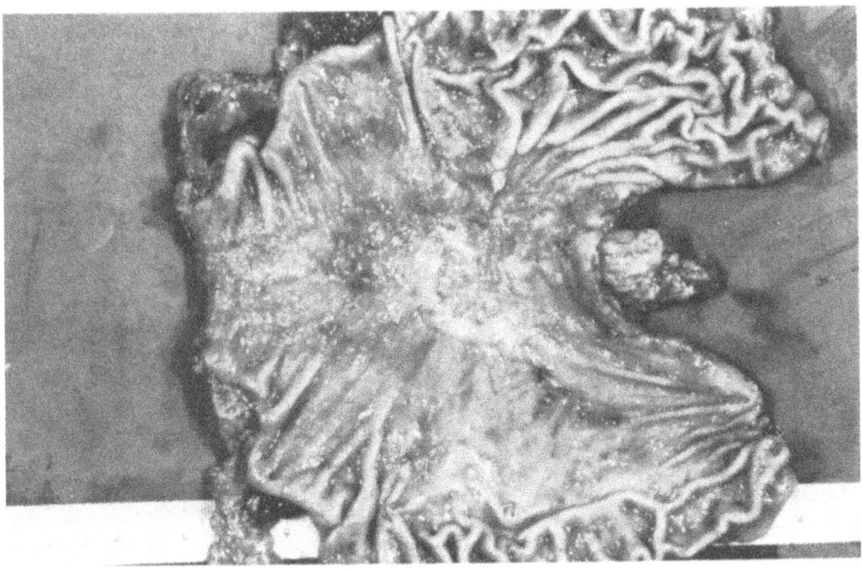

Fig. 162. Large cancerous erosion with central shallow ulceration developed in the angulus. Periphery of the eroded lesion can be followed to proximal (oral) cut end of the resected stomach. (Pt no. 15 995, 43 years, m)

Fig. 163. Schematic of the lesion shown in Fig. 162. Cancerous change of the eroded mucosa, with infiltrating poorly differentiated adenocarcinoma containing signet-ring cancer cells was confirmed by histological examination extending to the proximal cut end of the stomach

These unexpected observations indicate that tiny cancerous foci remaining in a gastric remnant grow to clinically detectable cancer only over a long period of time.

The cases in which EGC has been diagnosed by biopsy but has not been subjected to surgical treatment, owing to refusal by the patients or for some other reason, include some of the patients who visited the same or another hospital after many years, when the cancerous lesion had become larger and was already at a more advanced stage. There are other cases of EGC for which the chronological growth can be estimated. For example, slight cancerous lesions overlooked at the time of initial X-ray or endoscopic examination can be recognized later on as

an earlier stage of the cancer on retrospective scrutiny of the films. Even though
these cases are few in number, the data on them are highly significant for chronological plotting of the growth of gastric cancer within the stomach, and such cases
have been reported by some investigators [27, 37, 39].

From the data obtained it is concluded that it takes many years for the precancerous state to develop into microscopically recognizable cancer, many years
from this state to clinically detectable EGC, and some years again for EGC to
progress to AGC. A crude growth curve for gastric cancer can be illustrated as the
figure (Fig. 164).

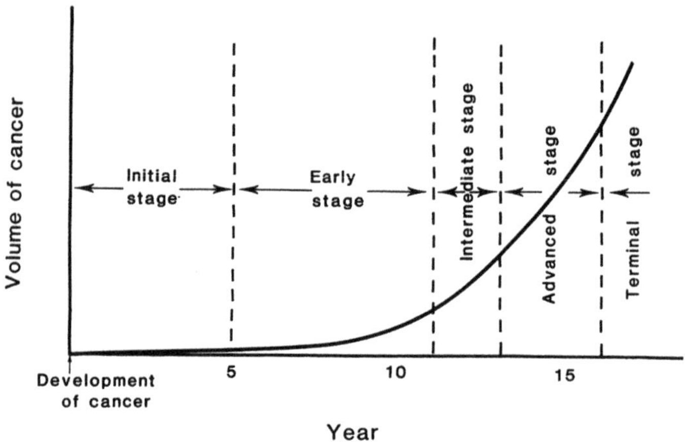

Fig. 164. Natural history of gastric cancer

Prognosis

As is well known, the survival rate after surgical resection for gastric cancer is far
higher in EGC than in AGC. For 1007 patients who underwent partial gastrectomy at Yokoyama Hospital during the 27 years from 1953 to 1979 and for whom a
final diagnosis of EGC was made on the basis of histological examination, enqui-
ries as to the present status were sent out by letter, and answers were received
from 992 patients or their families. The response rate therefore was 98.5%.
Among these 992 cases, the patients who had died from diseases other than cancer were excluded from the statistics and those whose present status was un-
known were classed with those who had died of cancer. Survival rates for the patients were calculated from the data with these adjustments.

Survival rates of the patients with mucosal cancer (m) and submucosal cancer
(sm) were 97.6% and 91.8%, respectively, at 5 years after surgery; 91.2% (m) and
82.7% (sm) at 10 years after; and 87.3% (m) and 75.0% (sm) at 15 years after.
These results demonstrate that the survival rates are always higher in (m) than
(sm) cancer and the difference in the rate between (m) and (sm) becomes wider
with increasing time after surgery (Fig. 165).

156

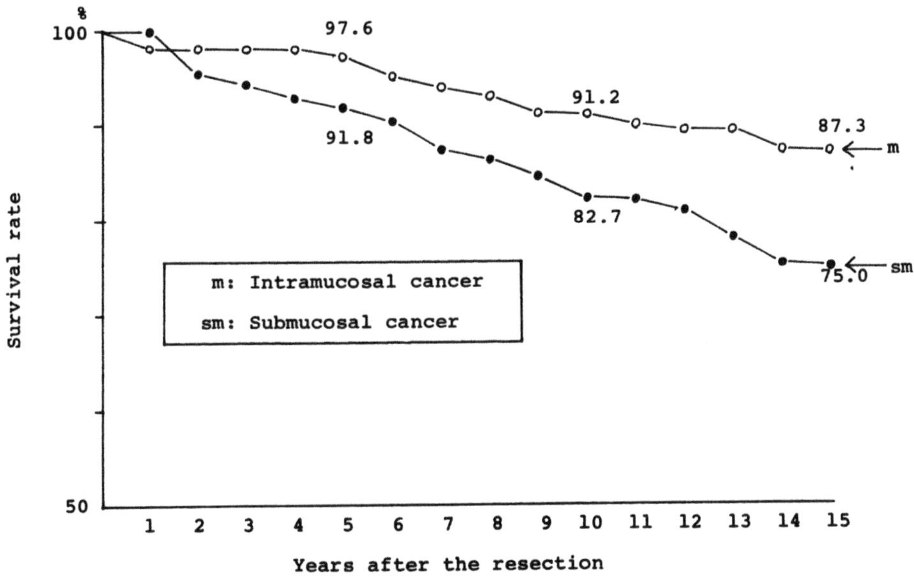

Fig. 165. Survival rate after surgical resection the lesion in EGC (Yokoyama Hospital, 1953–1979)

A similar result on the survival rate was obtained in 1209 cases of surgical resection performed for gastric cancer at Aichi Cancer Center Hospital from 1965 to 1975: the 335 cases of EGC without lymphnode metastasis·n (−) had a higher survival rate than the 33 cases of EGC with metastasis·n (+) (Fig. 166).

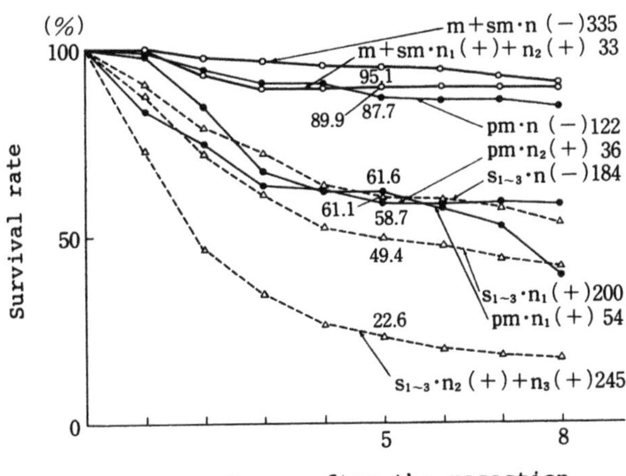

Fig. 166. Survival rate after resection of the stomach. (Aichi Cancer Center Hospital, 1965–1975)

On analysis of a few recurrent cases of EGC, it became apparent that except in the case of heterochronous double primaries cancer never recurred in cases of (m) less than 5 years after the surgical operation, while it was not uncommon in the cases of (sm), owing to lymphatic or hematogenous metastasis. As mentioned above, all the recurrent cases of (m) more than 5 years after surgery were due to an inadequate length of the proximal cut end of the stomach [ow(+) in Fig. 167].

157

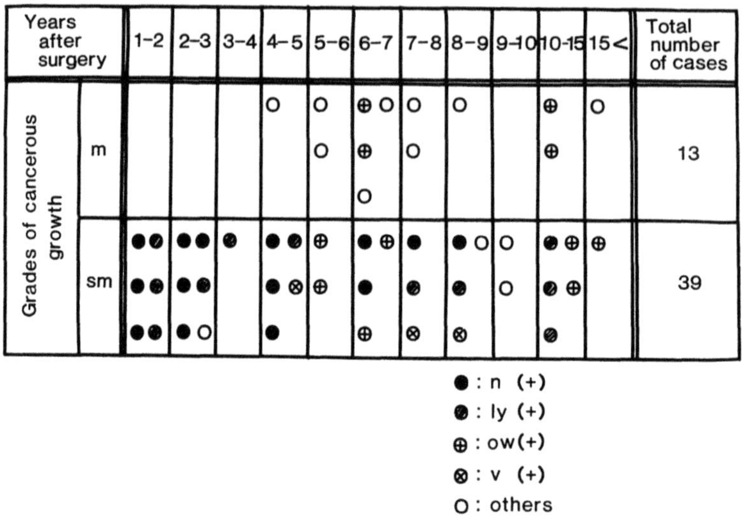

Years after surgery	1–2	2–3	3–4	4–5	5–6	6–7	7–8	8–9	9–10	10–15	15<	Total number of cases
m				○	○ ○	⊕ ○ ⊕ ○	○ ○	○		⊕ ⊕	○	13
sm	● ◍ ● ● ● ● ◍	● ● ◍ ● ● ● ○	◍	● ● ◍ ● ⊗ ●	⊕ ⊕	● ⊕ ● ⊕	● ◍ ⊗	● ○ ◍ ⊗	○ ○	● ◍ ⊕ ◍ ⊕ ◍	⊕	39

(*Grades of cancerous growth*)

● : n (+)
◍ : ly (+)
⊕ : ow(+)
⊗ : v (+)
○ : others

Fig. 167. Deaths from EGC following surgery by grade of cancerous growth

As shown in Table 36, most of these cases have fairly large cancerous erosions, often more than 5 cm^2 in area, with the center located in the angulus or lower half of the corpus and showing diffuse infiltration of cancer cells with an ill-defined boundary especially at its proximal cut ends (Fig. 167).

The prognosis of EGC, however, is less hopeful when cancer cells are seen in the venules of the resected stomach. These changes have been observed with a relatively high frequency in (sm) gastric cancer with the intestinal type of histology, and hematogenous spread of the adenocarcinoma cells into the liver and other remote organs was the main cause of early death in such cases.

The frequency of metastasis to the regional lymph nodes was compared in 3567 cases of resected gastric cancer by the grade (depth) of cancerous invasion within the stomach wall. It became obvious from the examination that the frequency of lymph node metastasis was lowest (1.8%) in (m) cancer, and it became far higher in proportion to increasing grade of cancerous invasion (Table 37) [24 a].

Table 37. Frequency of lymph node metastasis by grade of cancerous invasion. (Yokoyama Hospital 1965–1982)

Deepest layer of cancerous growth	Number of cases	No. with LN metastasis	Frequency (%) of metastasis
m	502 (14.1%)	9	1.8
sm	488 (13.7%)	91	18.6
pm	375 (10.5%)	166	44.3
ss and s	2202 (61.7%)	1611	73.2
Total	3567 (100.0%)	1877	52.6

m, mucosa; sm, submucosa, pm, muscularis propria; ss, subserosa; s, serosa

A similar but better result on the rate of lymph node metastasis was obtained in 1253 cases at the Aichi Cancer Center Hospital (Table 38).

Table 38. Frequency (%) of lymph node metastasis by grade (depth) of cancerous invasion within the stomach. (Aichi Cancer Center Hospital 1965~1975)

Grade	No. of cases	$n_{(-)}$	$n_1 (+)$	$\geqq n_2 (+)$
m	132	99.2	0.8	0
sm	241	86.3	10.4	3.3
pm	215	57.2	25.1	17.7
ss	24	58.3	20.8	20.8
$s_1 \sim s_3$	641	29.3	31.4	39.3

It must be noted here that lymph node metastasis of (m) cancer was seen only in cases with cancerous erosion (type IIc″), and when the frequency of metastasis was confined to this type it was 4.6%. In contrast, in the cases with (sm) cancer the frequency of lymph node metastasis was significantly higher than average in the protruding (I) and elevated (IIa) types (18.6%) (Table 39).

Table 39. Rate of lymph node metastasis from EGC

Macroscopical type / Grade of cancerous growth		Lymph node metastasis			
		Mucosa (m)		Submucosa (sm)	
		No.	%	No.	%
Protruding	I	0/24	0	11/30	36.7
Elevated	IIa	0/51	0	11/40	27.5
Flat	IIb	0/16	0		
Depressed	IIc′	0/98	0	29/148	19.6
Eroded	IIc″	9/194	4.6	28/177	15.8
Ulcerated	III	0/119	0	12/93	12.9
Total		9/502	1.8	91/488	18.6

The present status of nine cases of (m) cancer with lymph node metastasis (Figs. 168 and 169) was checked by inquiries directed to the patients' families, and this approach revealed that the general condition of all the patients was good (Table 40).

From the results described above, it is apparent that the difference in survival rates between (m) and (sm) cancer after surgery is due mainly to the presence or absence of lymph node metastasis, to the grade of its extension, and to the presence or absence of cancer cell invasion into the venules at the time of surgery.

Over the past 40 years or so, many papers have reported survival rates of gastric cancer after partial or total gastrectomy [2, 5, 6–8, 12, 21, 29, 30, 38, 40, 41],

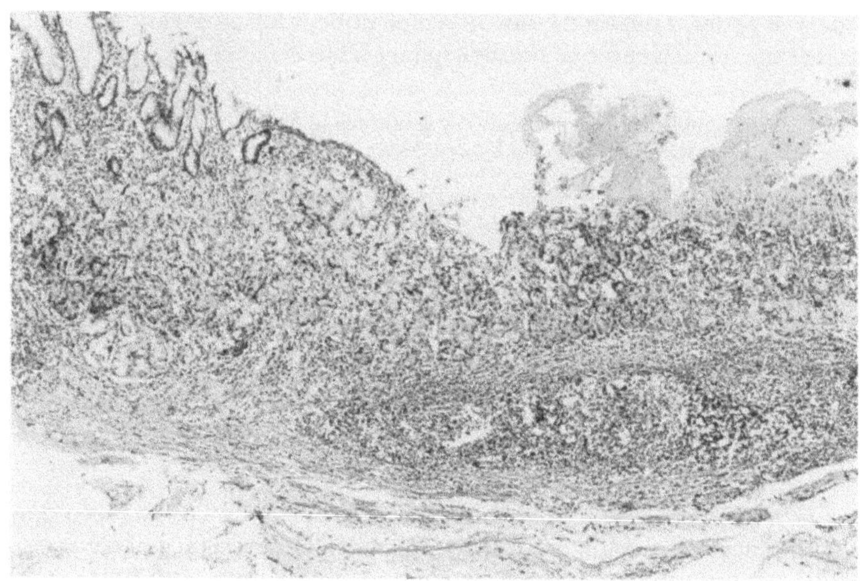

Fig. 168. Histology of peripheral part of cancerous erosion with central ulceration (type II c″ + III) developed in the angulus. The eroded lesion is diffusely infiltrated by poorly differentiated cancer cells, but no submucosal infiltration was visible in this case. (Pt no. 6634, 42 years, m, × 15)

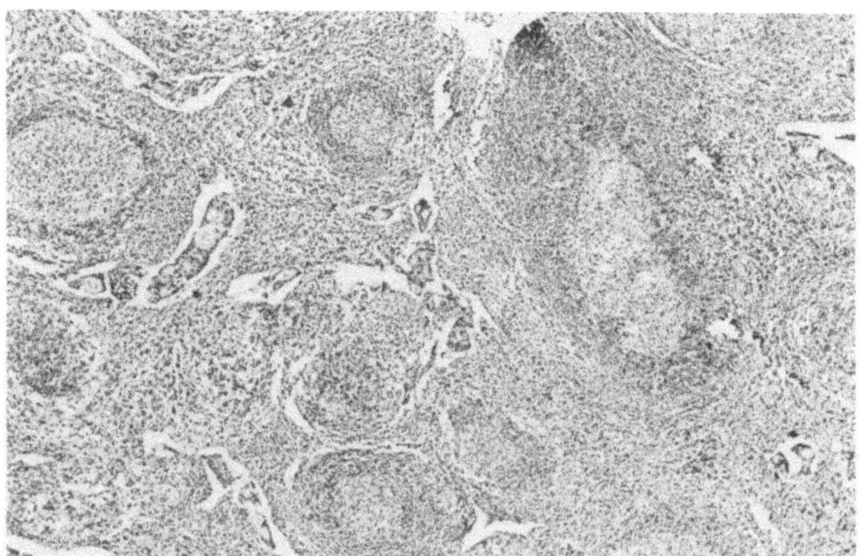

Fig. 169. Histology of the regional lymph node corresponding to the lesion shown in Fig. 168. Cancerous glands composed of small cuboidal cells are visible in the sinus of the node. Cancerous infiltration into the parenchyma of the node was not detected, however. The patient is in good condition 14 years after surgery. (Pt no. 6634, × 15)

160

Table 40. Cases of intramucosal cancer with lymph node metastasis

No.	Series no.	Age	Sex	Macroscopical type	Size (mm)	Site	Histological type	Prognosis (years)
1	6 634	42	m	II c″ + ul	32 × 27	Angulus	C	Alive (14.1)
2	9 039	46	m	″	45 × 23	″	B	″ (11.4)
3	9 301	34	m	″	42 × 40	″	B	″ (14.6)
4	13 645	58	f	″	30 × 20	Antrum	C	″ (5.11)
5	14 578	41	f	″	60 × 40	Angulus	C	″ (5.3)
6	15 645	52	f	″	60 × 35	Corpus	C	″ (8.0)
7	15 672	28	m	″	50 × 25	Angulus	B	″ (5.3)
8	16 142	52	f	″	50 × 60	Corpus	C	″ (5.3)
9	16 729	35	f	″	35 × 30	Angulus	C	″ (5.6)

B, moderately differential adenocarcinoma; C, poorly differentiated adenocarcinoma

And in all the reports the conclusion is reached that the more advanced the stage of the cancerous growth at the time of surgery the lower the survival rate of the patients. This applies to both (m) and (sm) cancers (Table 41).

Table 41. Published work on survival rates after gastrectomy for EGC

Authors	Years of exam.	Year of publ.	No. of cases		5-year survival (%)		10-year survival (%)		Published in
			m	sm	m	sm	m	sm	
Inokuchi et al.	1951–1972	1976	83	81	94.1	88.3	79.2	69.2	Gann no Rinsho 13: 1017
Takasugi et al.	1962–1976	1977	376	356	100.0	95.3	99.5	93.1	I to Cho 12: 933
Kishimoto et al.	1948–1971	1977	90	115	92.3	86.1	80.6	62.5	Gann no Rinsho 23: 957
Kohzaki et al.	1961–1975	1978	292	302	100.0	98.3	100.0	96.6	Geka Chiryo 39: 674
Yamada et al.	1965–1976	1979	156	262	94.1	95.2	91.0	84.6	Geka 41: 346
Furusawa et al.	1964–1979	1982	161	179	99.5	97.0	96.2	87.8	Shokaki Geka 16: 32

Pessimism about the prognosis of gastric cancer even after radical gastrectomy faded with the introduction of new diagnostic methods such as double-contrast roentgenography, fibergastroscopy, and biopsy to the field of gastroenterology, since these allow the detection of gastric cancer at earlier stages of growth with no great technical difficulties.

Owing to the great progress made in clinical diagnosis, 5-year survival rates for EGC after surgery have risen to 90% or more, as shown in Figs. 165 and 166. The administration of adjuvant chemotherapy after gastrectomy will raise the survival rate for EGC still further.

The prognosis of EGC after gastrectomy is analyzed by many investigators – mostly surgeons – from several viewpoints, e. g., grade of cancerous invasion [5, 5 a, 9 a, 16, 18, 20, 22, 42], extent of lymph node metastasis [4, 9, 10, 23, 38], curative or noncurative operation [3, 11, 17, 26 a, 41 a], histological type according to Lauren's classification [13, 21, 26, 31, 33, 36, 37], growth pattern of the cancer [14, 19], and stromal reaction [1, 15, 32, 34, 35, 40], and most authors point out the importance of summation of multiple factors [24, 25, 28] in evaluation of the prognosis.

The most reliable data on the survival rate of gastric cancer after surgery have been reported recently by the group of MIWA [23 a], who is in charge of the statistics for cases of surgically resected gastric cancer in Japan. They analyzed the survival rates of the 15 589 cases registered with the National Cancer Center · WHO CC in Tokyo by collaborators in 56 institutions throughout the country from several aspects. This statistical analysis confirmed that the survival rates correlate best with staging according to the TNM classification devised by the World Health Organization, modified by pathological examination of the resected stomachs (p. TNM).

References

1. Black MM, Freeman C, Mork T, Harvei S, Cutler SJ (1971) Prognostic significance of microscopic structure of gastric carcinoma and their regional lymphnodes. Cancer 27: 703–711
2. Blalock J, Ochsner A (1957) Carcinoma of the stomach: A study of 18 five-year survivors. Ann Surg 145: 726–737
3. Bonnichon PH, Lacaine F, Fatnassy B, Hay JM (1983) Postoperatic follow-up surveillance of patients with gastric cancer. J Chir (Paris) 120: 229–231
4. Cantreu EG (1971) The importance of lymph nodes in the assessment of gastric carcinoma at operation. Br J Surg 58: 384–386
5. Dochat GR, Gray HK (1943) Carcinoma of the stomach: prognosis based on a combination of Duke's and Broder's methods of grading. Am J Clin Pathol 13: 441–449
5 a. Douglass HO (1982) Potentially curable cancer of the stomach. Cancer 50: 2582–2589
6. Ederer F, Cutler SJ, Eisenberg H, Keogh JR (1960) Survival of patients with cancer of the stomach, Connecticut 1953–54. J Natl Cancer Inst 25: 1005–1021
7. Ferguson LK, Nusbaum M (1963) Survival after surgical treatment of carcinoma of the stomach. Ann Surg 158: 51–55
8. Fielding JWL, Fellis PJ, Jones BG et al. (1980) Natural history of "early gastric cancer". Results of a 10-year regional survey. Br Med J 281: 965–967
9. Georgi A, Ostertag H (1982) Pathology and survival times in early gastric cancer. Clin Oncol 1: 571–585
9 a. Green PHR, O'toole KM, Weinberg LM, Goldfarb JP (1981) Early gastric cancer. Gastroenterology 81: 247–256
10. Hamley PR, Westenhoby P, Morson BC (1970) Pathology and prognosis of carcinoma of the stomach. Br J Surg 57: 877–883
11. Hermanek P (1973) Frühdiagnose und Frühbehandlung des Magenkrebses. Aus der Sicht der chirurgischen Pathologie. MMW 115: 1509–1512
12. Hoerr SO (1965) Malignant lesions of the stomach. Analysis fifty-four five year survivors. Am J Surg 109: 14–20

13. Inberg MV, Lauren P, Vuori J, Viikari SJ (1973) Prognosis of intestinal type and diffuse gastric carcinoma with special reference to the effect of the stromal reaction. Acta Chir Scand 139: 273–278

14. Inokuchi K, Inutsuka S, Furusawa M, Soejima K, Ikeda T (1967) Stromal reaction around tumor and metastases and prognosis after curative gastrectomy for carcinoma of the stomach. Cancer 20: 1924–1929

15. Inokuchi K, Inutsuka S, Furusawa M, Soejima K, Ikeda T (1966) Development of superficial carcinoma of the stomach: Report of late recurrence. Ann Surg 164: 145–151

16. Kajitani T (1976) Surgical treatment for gastric cancer. Their contribution to improvement in the five-year survival rate. Asian Med J 19: 915–935

17. Kato K, Kato T, Nakazato H, Miyaishi S, Yamada E (1975) Gastric cancer: Survival rates with special reference to "early gastric cancer". Nagoya J Med 38: 35–42

18. Kidokoro T (1971) Frequency of resection, metastasis and five-year survival rate of early gastric carcinoma in a surgical clinic. Gann Monogr Cancer Res 11: 45–49

19. Kodama Y, Inokuchi K, Soejima K et al. (1983) Growth patterns and prognosis in early gastric carcinoma. Superficially spreading and penetrating growth types. Cancer 51: 320–326

20. Kuhlencordt F (1959) Das carcinoma in situ des Magens und der kleine Magenkrebs. Katamnestische Untersuchungen von 42 Fällen. Dtsch Med Wochenschr 84: 2111–2115

21. Laurén P, Vikari S, Hytinen A, Autio V (1962) Pathological features of gastric cancer affecting survival after curative resections. Ann Chir Gynecol 51: 342–350

22. Maruta K, Shida H 1968) Some factors which influence prognosis after surgery for advanced gastric cancer. Ann Surg 167: 313–318

23. Matsusaka T, Kodama Y, Soejima K et al. (1980) Recurrence in early gastric cancer: A pathologic evaluation. Cancer 46: 168–172

23 a. Miwa K (1984) Evaluation of the TNM classification of stomach cancer and proposal for its rational stage-grouping. Jpn J Clin Oncol 14: 385–410

24. Monafo WW, Krause GL, Medina JG (1962) Carcinoma of the stomach. Morphological characteristics affecting survival. Arch Surg 85: 754–763

24 a. Nagayo T, Yokoyama H, Yokoyama Y (1984) Lymphnode metastasis of intramucosal cancer of the stomach. Verh Dtsch Ges Path 68: 276–283

25. Nakazato H, Kato K, Goto M, Matsubara M (1979) A statistical trial on evaluation for prognosis of gastric cancer. Herfarth C, Schlag P (eds) Gastric cancer. Springer, Berlin Heidelberg New York, pp 187–192

26. Noda S, Soejima K, Inokuchi K (1980) Clinicopathological analysis of the intestinal type and diffuse type of gastric carcinoma. Jpn J Surg 10: 277–283

26 a. Ohman U, Emas S, Rubio C (1980) Relation between early and advanced gastric cancer. Am J Surg 140: 351–355

27. Okabe H (1971) Growth of early gastric cancer. Clinical study of growth and invasion pattern of early gastric cancer: its position in the natural history of gastric cancer. Gann Monogr Cancer Res 11: 67–80

28. Okada M, Kojima S, Murakami M et al. (1983) Human gastric carcinoma: Prognosis in relation to macroscopic and microscopic features of the primary tumor. J Natl Cancer Inst 71: 275–279

29. Remine WH, Gomes MMR, Dockerty MB (1969) Long-term survival (10 to 56 years) after surgery for carcinoma of the stomach. Am J Surg 117: 177–184

30. Remine WH, Dockerty MB, Priestly JT (1953) Some factors which influence prognosis in surgical treatment of gastric carcinoma. Ann Surg 138: 311–319

31. Ribeiro MM, Salmento JA, Simões S, Bastos J (1981) Prognostic significance of Laurén and Ming classification and other pathologic parameters in gastric carcinoma. Cancer 47: 780–784

32. Schachenmayer W, Haferkamp O (1979) Prognostic significance of stromal reaction in gastric carcinoma. In: Herfarth C, Schlag P (eds) Gastric cancer. Springer, Berlin Heidelberg New York, pp 182–186

33. Schmidt C (1983) Intestinal and diffuse type of gastric carcinoma: A survival study. Int J Gastroenterol 15: 6–9

34. Schmitz-Moormann P, Heider HA, Thomas C (1979) Cancer of the stomach – Prognosis, independent of therapy. In: Herfarth C, Schlag P (eds) Gastric cancer. Springer, Berlin Heidelberg New York, pp 172–181

35. Steiner PE, Maimon SN, Palmer WL, Kirsner JB (1948) Gastric cancer: Morphologic factors in five-year survival after gastrectomy. Am J Pathol 24: 947–969
36. Stemmermann GN, Brown C (1974) A survival study of intestinal and diffuse types of gastric carcinoma. Cancer 33: 1190–1195
37. Sugano H, Nakamura K, Kato Y (1982) Pathological studies of human gastric cancer. Acta Pathol Jpn [Suppl 2] 32: 329–347
38. Thomas WD, Waugh JM, Dockerty MB (1951) Prognosis of gastric carcinoma. Arch Surg 62: 847–855
39. Tsukuma H, Mishima T, Oshima A (1983) Prospective study of "early" gastric cancer. Int J Cancer 31: 421–426
40. Urban CH, McNeer G (1959) The relation of the morphology of gastric carcinoma to long and short term survival. Cancer 12: 1158–1162
41. Walters W, Berkson J (1953) An improvement of 180 per cent in the five-year-survival rate of patients with carcinoma of the stomach. Ann Surg 137: 884–891
41 a. Weed TE, Nuessle W, Ochsner A (1981) Carcinoma of the stomach. Why are we failing to improve survival? Ann Surg 193: 407–413
42. Yamada E, Nakazato H, Koike A, Suzuki K, Kato K (1974) Surgical results for early gastric cancer. Int Surg 59: 7–14

8. Histological Diagnosis of Early Gastric Cancer
   by Biopsy Examination

EGC can be detected clinically by double-contrast X-ray examination and/or endoscopic examination with a fibergastroscope, but a definite diagnosis cannot be obtained without histological examination of biopsies taken from lesions suspected of being malignant. In earlier periods of our studies it was not possible to confirm the diagnosis of EGC before surgical resection of the stomach, but the possibility of taking biopsies under direct vision with the aid of endoscopy later allowed clear evidence of EGC to be obtained before surgery.

To ensure a high level of reliability in the clinical diagnosis of EGC, the following conditions must be met when the biopsy is taken.

1) Biopsy material should be taken from an adequate site. If a biopsy is taken from an inadequate site misdiagnosis is possible even if malignant change is present in the stomach. To avoid this risk, the endoscopist must be fully aware of the macroscopical and microscopical features of EGC.

2) Histological specimens should be prepared in an adequate manner. Even if material is taken from an adequate site, the diagnosis will be less reliable if the histological specimens are prepared inadequately or wrongly handled because of technical errors. Since many tiny specimens need to be processed within a limited time, it would also be easy for the tissues to be lost from the histological slides or labeled with wrong numbers. Therefore, preparation of the histological specimens requires great care on the part of the technicians.

3) Information on the lesion seen in the endoscope should be given to the pathologist. Without such information, the pathologists responsible for histological examination of the biopsied specimens cannot have any idea of the gross appearance of the lesion. It is important for the pathologist to know whether the specimens were taken from an elevated, flat, or eroded lesion or from the mucosa around an ulcer, etc. A schematic of the lesion seen in the endoscope with a simple explanation is adequate for this purpose. On the other hand, pathologists should have a wide knowledge of the various histological changes occasioned by gastric lesions.

4) Pathologists responsible for the examination must not overestimate or underestimate the lesion. There is no question that the utmost care must be taken to avoid such mistakes as far as possible, but in fact there really are cases in which only one of several specimens contains slight cancerous changes and these are microscopical in size. This might be overlooked on routine examinations, especially when many specimens have to be examined in a limited time or infiltrating cancer cells are of the pale-staining signet-ring cell type. To avoid this risk, specimens stained with both PAS and H & E are recommended.

In any case, mutual communication among endoscopist, surgeon, pathologist, and technician is of the utmost importance, especially when questions arise as to the diagnosis.

Even if the conditions described above are satisfied, there are some cases in which the lesion, whether or not it is malignant, cannot be assessed unequivocally, owing to a completely atypical and dysplastic nature. Furthermore, pathologists not infrequently encounter cases in which a malignant nature of the lesion is quite possible but cannot be confirmed owing to a lack of evidence fulfilling the histological criteria of malignancy.

In these circumstances, the hope was expressed by clinicians that standardized criteria for histological classification of biopsies for the diagnosis of gastric cancer would be set up. In response to this hope, a Committee composed of experienced pathologists was set up in 1969 within the Japanese Research Society for Gastric Cancer. In the first part of the meeting all the histological findings observed in biopsy specimens were temporarily classified into three categories,

a) normal mucosa and mucosa affected by a benign condition such as superficial gastritis, simple regeneration, or simple hyperplasia;
b) doubtful cases with varying grades of cellular and structural abnormality; and
c) obvious carcinoma

After repeated discussions on the cases in the second category with reference to many macroscopical and histological slides, and after consideration of the practical usefulness of the classification for routine clinical examinations, the members agreed to subdivide this category into three groups, and thus the following five groups were finally settled on.

The criteria for and definition of the different groups were as follows:

Group I: Normal mucosa or benign lesion without atypia
Group II: Benign lesion with slight atypia
Group III: Borderline lesion
Group IV: Probable carcinoma
Group V: Obvious carcinoma

In this paper, no detailed explanation of each group will be given, as this has already been published elsewhere by the author [31]. It should be mentioned here that the term borderline lesion was then used mainly for atypical foveolar epithelia with the nature of intestinal metaplasia in the upper half of the elevated mucosa. Several studies conducted since have shown that there are borderline lesions that are nonmetaplastic in nature. In these circumstances, a minor revision of the classification was made recently by the new Committee.

The results of routine histological examination of gastric biopsy specimens in a General Hospital near Nagoya, where I have been in charge of the examination for the last 10 years, are shown (Table 42). Most (76.4%) of the 4845 cases examined were allocated to group I, followed by group V (17.4%) and group II (3.5%). The cases allocated to group III (1.4%) (Figs. 170 and 171) and group IV (1.3%) (Figs. 172–175) were relatively few in number. Among the cases allocated to group I, most lesions were taken from the mucosa around peptic ulcers, the scars of peptic ulcers, or from mucosa affected by superficial gastritis.

166

Table 42. Histological diagnoses of biopsied gastric specimens by criteria of Group Classification. (Okazaki City Hospital, 1974–1983)

Histological diagnosis	No. of cases	Frequency (%)
Group I	3701	76.4
Group II	171	3.5
Group III	66	1.4
Group IV	62	1.3
Group V	845	17.4
Total	4845	100.0

It should be added that the main purpose of the Group Classification of biopsy specimens is to discriminate malignant from nonmalignant lesions. This is why each piece of the biopsied specimen must be numbered for the examination. However, in both malignant and nonmalignant cases it is impossible to express the nature of the lesion by this numbering method alone. To overcome such over-simplification, it is recommended that brief comments be appended to the histological specimens, such as "superficial gastritis," "regenerative epithelium," "hyperplastic mucosa," "intestinal metaplasia" etc in the case of benign lesions, and "well-demarcated tubular adenocarcinoma," "mucoid adenocarcinoma," or "infiltrating signet-ring cell carcinoma" etc in the case of malignant lesions.

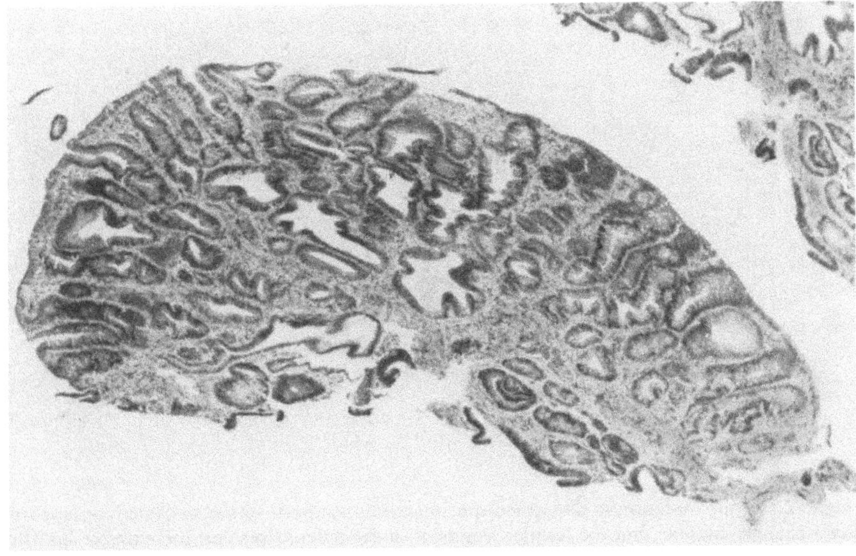

Fig. 170. Group III (borderline) lesion in a biopsied specimen taken from flatly elevated mucosa. Upper half of the mucosa is occupied diffusely by elongated, slightly twisted, foveolar tubules, some dilated and darkly stained. (Pt no. 3873, × 15)

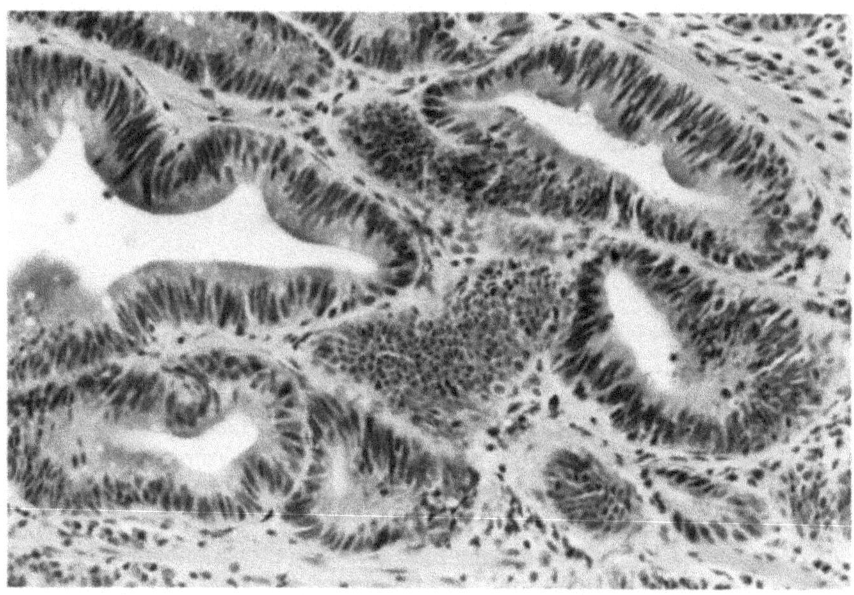

Fig. 171. High-power view of upper part of the specimen shown in Fig. 170. The elongated tubules are composed of tall columnar epithelial cells with slender and uniform nuclei in their lower half. No change suggestive of cancer is visible. (Pt no. 3873, × 85)

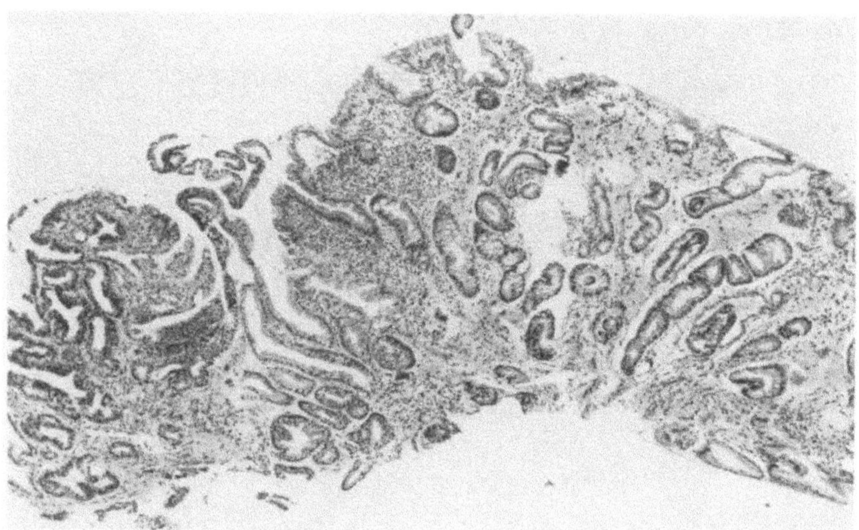

Fig. 172. Group IV lesion in a biopsied specimen. In most parts of the specimen, no apparent malignant change is visible, but the smaller fragment of the mucosa seen on the *extreme left* of the figure shows a tubular arrangement with an abnormal structure. (Pt no. 35974, × 15)

168

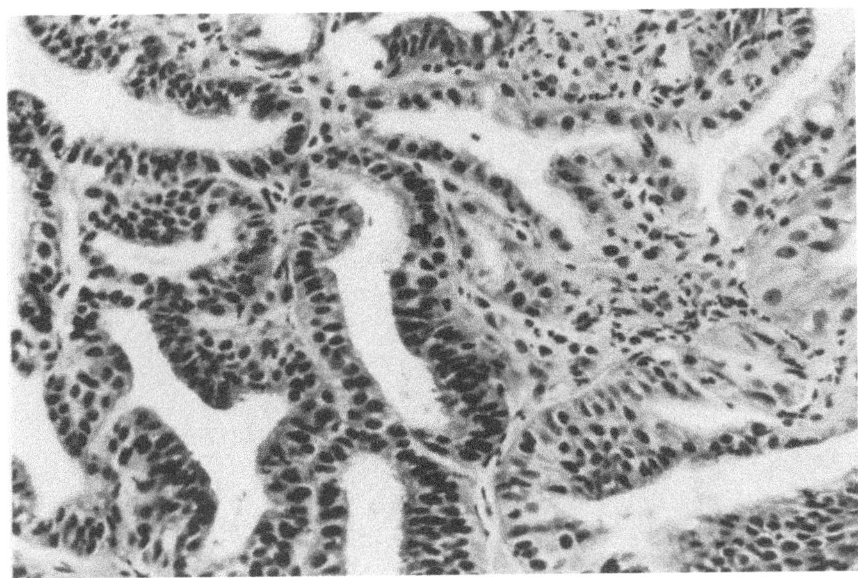

Fig. 173. Higher magnification of the specimen shown in Fig. 172 revealed that the tubules composed of cuboidal epithelial cells contained small, oval, and slightly piled-up nuclei with a high nucleus-to-cytoplasm ratio quite suggestive of incipient cancerization (group IV). EGC (type II a + II c, sm) was found in the resected stomach. (Pt no. 35974, × 75)

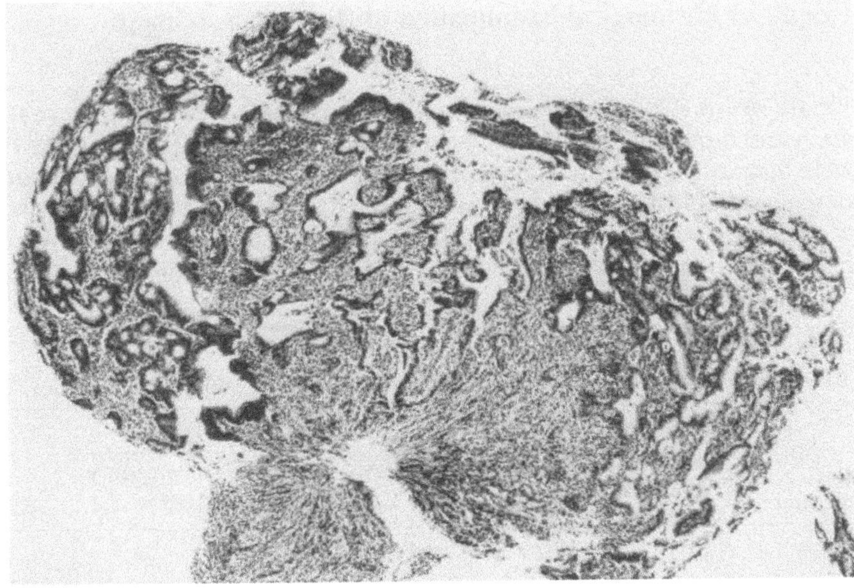

Fig. 174. Group V change (probably cancerous) in a biopsied specimen taken from a protruding lesion in a gastric remnant. The biopsied specimen shows various forms of adenocarcinoma. (Pt no. 38513, × 15)

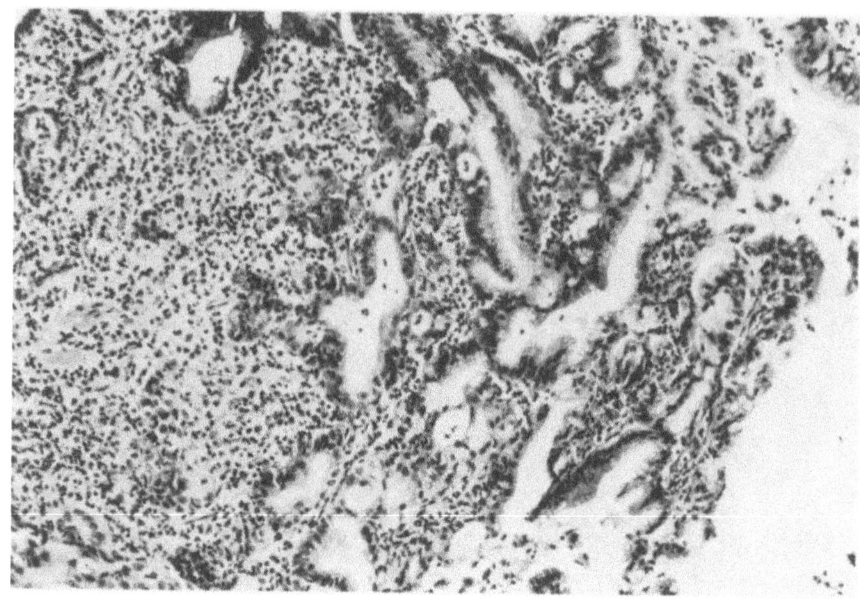

Fig. 175. Diagnosis of adenocarcinoma becomes more obvious on higher magnification of the biopsied mucosa shown in Fig. 174. (Pt no. 38 974, × 35)

Results of Histological Examination of Biopsied Specimens

From 1968 to 1979, histological examination of stomach biopsies from 6408 cases was carried out at Yokoyama Hospital. These included 6351 cases (99.1%) that were diagnosed correctly as benign or malignant, but in 57 cases (0.9%) the result of the histological examination of the resected stomach did not coincide with that of the biopsy and the frequency of false-positive cases (26, or 2.3%) was a little higher than that of false-negative cases (31, or 0.6%) (Table 43).

Table 43. Results of histological diagnoses of biopsied specimens. (April 1968 to March 1979)

Final diagnosis	Diagnosis in biopsy	Benign		Malignant		Total no. of cases
		No. of cases	Frequency (%)	No. of cases	Frequency (%)	
Benign		5243	99.4	26	2.3	5269
Malignant		31	0.6	1108[a]	97.7	1139
Total		5274	100.0	1134	100.0	6408

[a] Including 274 cases not subjected to surgery

170

It was known from retrospective studies that immature atypical regenerative glands or granulation tissue rich in capillaries with swollen endothelial cells overestimated or mistook as moderately or poorly differentiated adenocarcinoma were the most frequent cases (19/26: 73.1%) of false-positive findings (Figs. 176–179), while selection of inadequate biopsy sites was the most frequent reason (23/31: 74.2%) for false negatives, but failure to note slight infiltrations of signet-ring cell (Figs. 180 and 181) (two cases) and underestimation of well-differentiated tubular adenocarcinoma (Figs. 182 and 183) (four cases) also led to mistaken assessments (Table 44).

Table 44. Retrospective analysis of false-negative and false-positive cases

Type of incorrect diagnosis	Analysis	No. of cases	
False negative	Oversight or underestimation of cancerous change	6	
	Inadequacy of biopsy site	23	31
	Technical reason	2	
False positive	Atypical regenerative glands	19	
	Granulation tissue	2	26
	Borderline lesion	5	

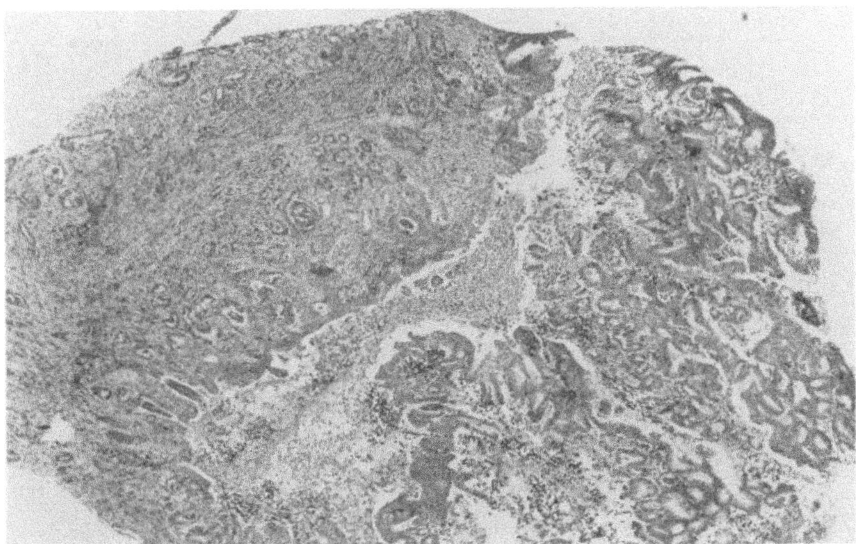

Fig. 176. False-positive case among the biopsy examinations. The biopsy specimen is composed of two parts. The *right half* in the figure is hyperplastic mucosa made up of fine glandular tubules and the *left half* is base of the ulcer with a few glands. (Pt no. 13586, × 15)

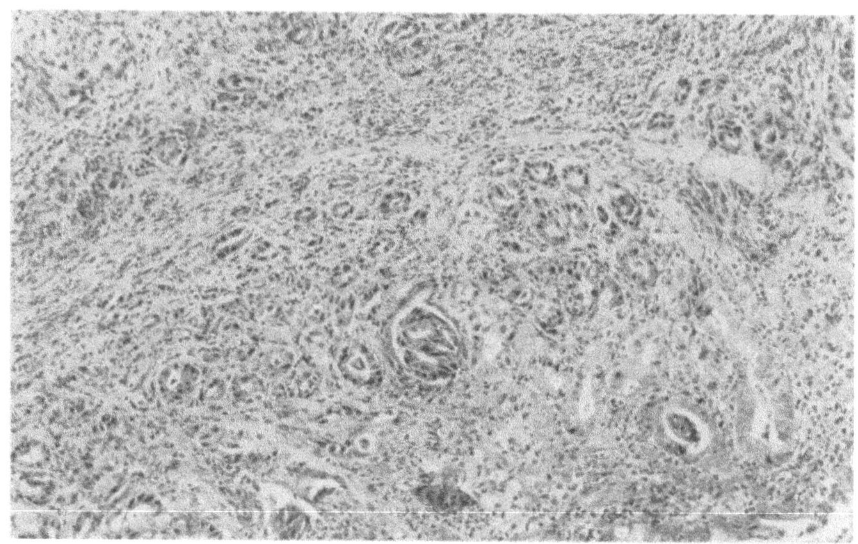

Fig. 177. High-power view of tissue from the base of the ulcer seen in Fig. 176. Small and immature regenerating glands are visible in the fibrotic tissue. These glands were mistaken for moderately differentiated adenocarcinoma. (Pt no. 13 586, × 35)

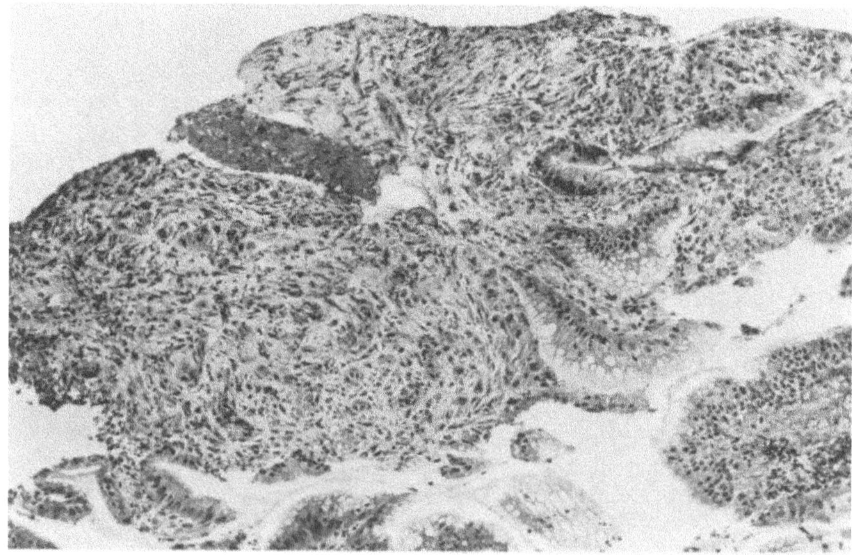

Fig. 178. False-positive case among the biopsy examinations. The biopsied mucosa is composed mainly of immature granulation tissue covered by surface epithelial cells. (Pt no. 13 636, × 15)

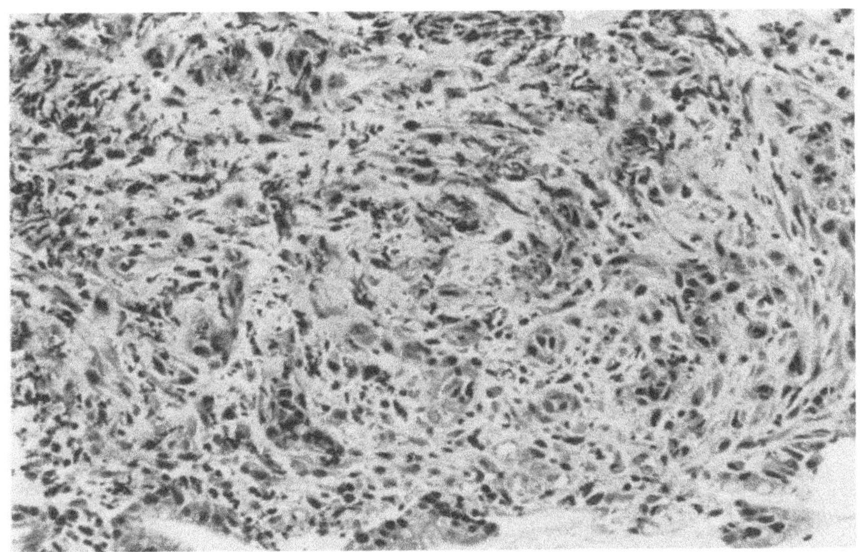

Fig. 179. Higher magnification of the granulation tissue shown in Fig. 178. Swollen and immature capillary endothelial cells were mistaken for poorly differentiated adenocarcinoma. (Pt no. 13636, ×70)

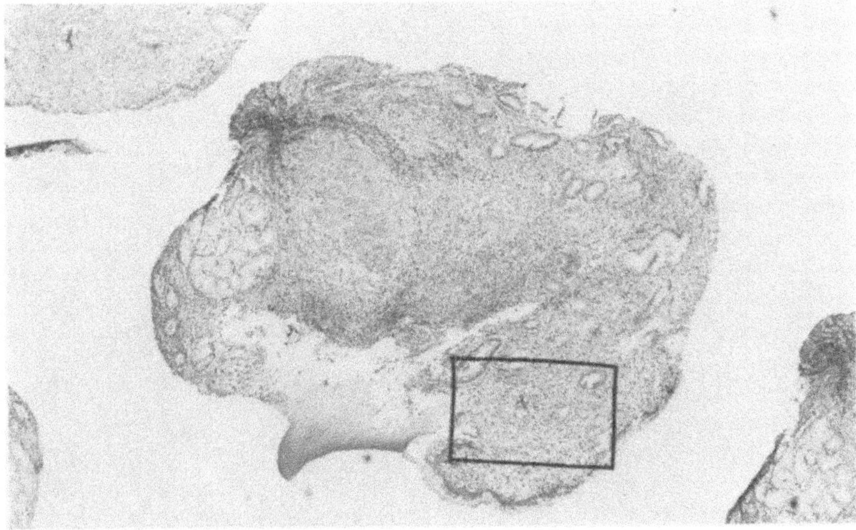

Fig. 180. False-negative case among the biopsy examinations. The biopsied mucosa was diagnosed merely as nonmetaplastic mucosa with inflammatory cell infiltration. (Pt no. 687, × 15)

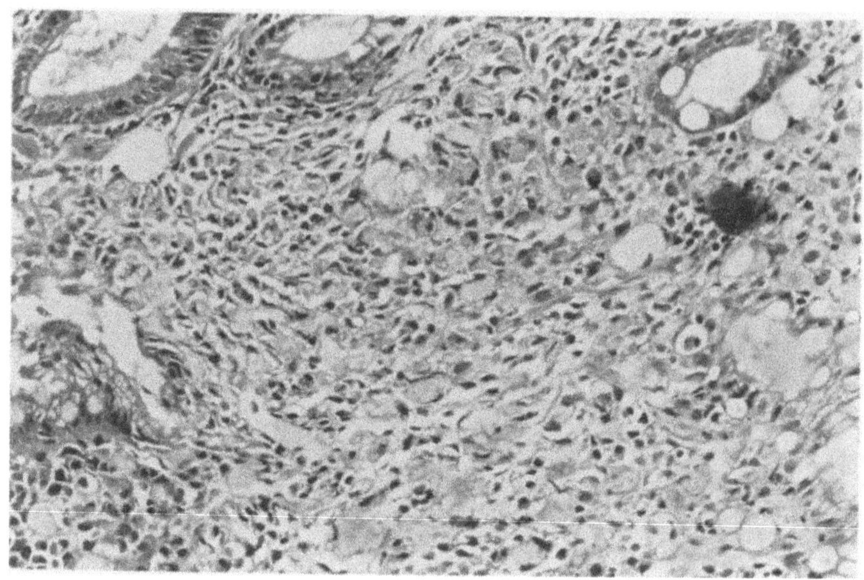

Fig. 181. Same biopsy specimen as in Fig. 180. Tiny cancerous focus composed of signet-ring cells outlined at *lower right* in Fig. 180 had been overlooked. (Pt no. 687, × 70)

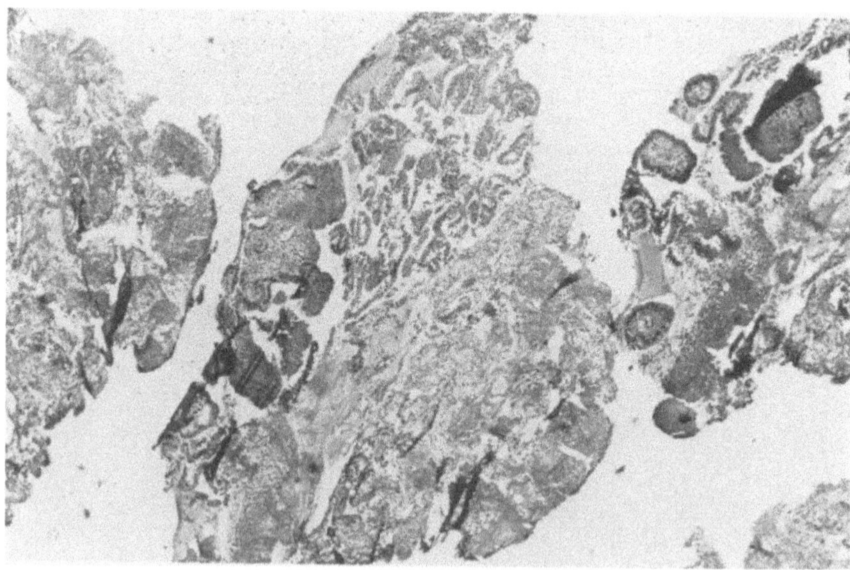

Fig. 182. False-negative case among the biopsy examinations. The biopsied mucosa was interpreted merely as nonmetaplastic and hyperplastic mucosa with inflammatory exudation and degeneration. (Pt no. 1335, × 15)

174

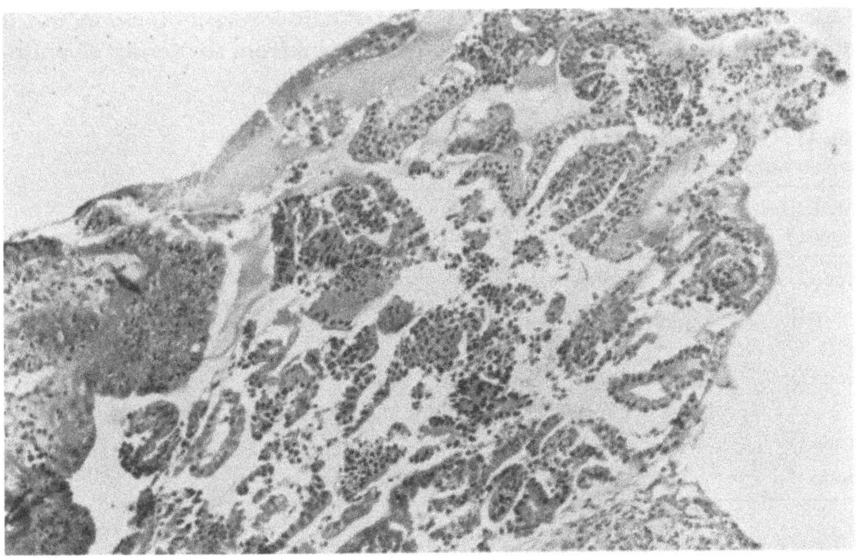

Fig. 183. High-power view of the epithelial part of the specimen shown in Fig. 182. The exfoliated and papillary tubules are composed of cuboidal epithelial cells with irregularly arranged small round nuclei with a high nucleus-to-cytoplasm ratio, which were underestimated as hyperplastic and regenerating epithelial cells. (Pt no. 1335, ×35)

Clinical Implications of Biopsy Findings

The histological diagnosis obtained from biopsies yields information that has important implications for the treatment of the patients. Indeed, at present, EGC and some other gastric diseases, such as malignant lymphoma, cannot decisively be diagnosed before surgery without biopsy.

When the biopsies show the changes classed in group I no active treatment is necessary for the patients. In group II cases reexamination after a long interval (6 to 12 month) is sufficient owing to the benign but slightly atypical epithelial changes. In the case of group III lesions, an interval of between 3 and 6 months is desirable, as it is known from followup examinations that almost all borderline lesions of the elevated type do not change their macroscopical and histological features for quite a long time, often more than 5 years. The interval should be shorter in cases with depressed lesions, however, owing to the more unstable condition of this lesion than of the elevated one. In contrast, close and careful scrutiny is immediately essential for lesions that fall in group IV, because there is a high probability that they are malignant. The best way to achieve this is by reexamination of the lesion as soon as possible by endoscopic biopsy. If the second examination gives a similar result, or if the circumstances do not allow reexamination, surgical treatment of the patients might be permissible, owing to the irreversible and high-risk nature of the lesions. Any group V lesions should of course

be surgically resected soon after detection, but before surgery the resection line of
the stomach has to be determined for the surgeon from the results of endoscopy
and of biopsy (Table 45).

Table 45. Clinical implications of the diagnoses
made in biopsied specimens

Histological diagnosis	Further procedure indicated
Group I	No active treatment
Group II	Followup examination (6- to 12-month interval)
Group III	Followup examination (3- to 6-month interval)
Group IV	Reexamination
Group V	Surgical treatment

In Chap. 6, dysplastic changes of the gastric mucosa were described. In my
opinion, the term "dysplasia" should better be applied to the resected stomachs
only and not to biopsies, because the tiny histological specimens taken for biopsy
often cannot yield information on the nature of the entire gastric mucosa, in addition to which probable carcinoma in the sense of the Group Classification and
severe dysplasia seen in the resected stomachs are not entirely synonymous.
Nevertheless, the standard criteria of both classifications are almost parallel. For
instance, mild dysplasia seen in the resected stomachs can be classified as group II
in the biopsied cases, while moderate dysplasia corresponds to group III. Cases of
severe dysplasia, the most important change with reference to the diagnosis, is almost always allocated to group IV.

The indispensable role of endoscopic biopsy in the diagnosis of EGC and other
gastric diseases owes its origin to the pioneering works of several investigators [2,
5, 14, 23, 32, 38, 44, 50], and especially of HIRSHOWITZ et al. [15], who enabled us
to bring biopsy of gastric lesions into routine practice by development of the flexible fibergastroscope. After his device became available several improvements
were made to the instrument, mostly by endoscopists [19–22, 37, 41, 42, 45] col-
laborating with technicians. These improvements opened the way in the early
1960s for reliable detection and diagnosis of gastric cancer even in its early stages.

The usefulness of biopsy in routine laboratory investigations has been stressed
by several investigators [1, 6–9 a, 17 a, 18, 24, 26–28, 30 a, 35, 36, 39, 43, 47, 48].
However, as described previously, endoscopic biopsying and histological examination of biopsies cannot play their essential role unless certain conditions are satisfied before, during, and after the biopsy is taken. It is known from several
studies that false-negative or false-positive results are possible in biopsies, but
their frequency has decreased significantly in recent years. Analysis of the cases of
incorrect diagnosis reported by several investigators [16, 17, 34, 40, 46] is of the
utmost importance for improved reliability of this method. It should be added
here that many European investigators [3, 4, 10–13, 25, 29, 30, 33, 49, 51] stress
the advantage of a combination of cytology and histology for this purpose.

176

References

1. Bearzi J, Ranaldi R (1982) Early gastric cancer: A morphologic study of 41 cases. Tumori 68: 223–233
2. Benedict EB (1948) An operating gastroscope. Gastroenterology 11: 281
3. Bertazzo S, Pesce G, Valmachino VG et al. (1981) Early gastric cancer: A retrospective study of our cases (1974–1979). Chir Ital 33: 213–214
4. Classen M, Rösch W (1974) Gastroscopy, biopsy and cytology in early detection of stomach cancer. In: Grundmann E, et al. (eds) Early gastric cancer. Current status of diagnosis. Springer, Berlin Heidelberg New York, pp 113–117
5. Debray C, Housset P (1962) A new direct vision biopsy gastroscope. Gut 3: 273–276
6. Demling L, Ottenjann R, Elster K (1982) Endoscopy and biopsy of the esophagus and stomach, 2nd edn. Saunders, Philadelphia
7. Elster K, Kudlich W (1972) Die diagnostische Effektivität der Gastrobiopsie. Endoscopy 4: 162–163
8. Elster K (1971) Die gastroskopische Biopsie in der Diagnostik umschriebener Prozesse. Leber Magen Darm 24: 24–27
9. Farini R, Leandro G, Di Mario F et al. (1981) Epithelial dysplasia in endoscopic gastric mucosal biopsies. Tumori 67: 589–598
9a. Fevre DI, Green PHR, Barrat PJ, Nagy GS (1976) Review of five cases of early gastric cancer. Gut 17: 41–47
10. Georgi A, Ostertag H, Atay Z, Seifert E (1974) Advantages of combined cytological-histological examinations in guided biopsies of the stomach. In: Grundmann E, et al. (eds) Early gastric cancer, Current status of diagnosis. Springer, Berlin Heidelberg New York, pp 127–130
11. Graham DV (1982) Prospective evaluation of biopsy number in the diagnosis of esophageal and gastric carcinoma. Gastroenterology 82: 228–231
12. Gupta RK, Rogers KE (1983) Endoscopic cytology and biopsy in the diagnosis of gastroesophageal malignancy. Acta Cytol (Baltimore) 27: 17–22
13. Gupta JP, Jain AK, Agrawal BK, Gupta S (1983) Gastroscopic cytology and biopsies in diagnosis of gastric malignancies. J Surg Oncol 22: 62–64
14. Hawksley JC, Cooray GH (1948) Observations on fragments of gastric mucous membrane found in aspirated resting gastric juice. J Pathol Bacteriol 60: 333–336
15. Hirschowitz BI, Curtis LE, Peter CW, Pollard HM (1958) Demonstration of a new gastroscope, the "fiberscope". Gastroenterology 35: 50–53
16. Isaacson P (1982) Biopsy appearance easily mistaken for malignancy in gastrointestinal endoscopy. Histopathology 6: 377–389
17. Itabashi M, Hirota T, Unakami M et al. (1984) The role of the biopsy in diagnosis of early gastric cancer. Jpn J Clin Oncol 14: 253–270
17a. Ito Y, Blackstone MO, Riddel RH, Kironer J (1979) The endoscopic diagnosis of early gastric cancer. Gastrointest. Endoscopy 25: 96–100
18. Joske RA, Finckle ES, Wood IJ (1955) Gastric biopsy. A study of 1,000 consecutive successful gastric biopsies. Q J Med 95: 269–294
19. Kasugai T (1982) Endoscopy of the stomach. In: Kasugai T (ed) Endoscopic diagnosis in gastroenterology. Igaku Shoin, Tokyo, pp 49–141
20. Kasugai T, Kobayashi S (1974) Evaluation of biopsy and cytology in the diagnosis of gastric cancer. Am J Gastroenterol 62: 199–203
21. Kawai K (1979) Early diagnosis of gastric cancer in Japan. In: Advances in medical oncology, research and education, vol 9. Pergamon, Oxford, p 211
22. Kawai K (1970) Gastrofiberscopic biopsy on early gastric cancer. Endoscopy 2: 82–87
23. Kenamore B (1940) A biopsy forceps for the flexible gastroscope. Am J Dig Dis Nutr 7: 539
24. Kobayashi S, Yoshii Y, Kasugai T (1976) Biopsy and cytology in the diagnosis of early gastric cancer. 10 year experience with direct vision techniques at a Japanese institution. Endoscopy 8: 53–58
25. Kobayashi S, Sugiura H, Kasugai T (1972) Reliability of endoscopic observation in diagnosis of early carcinoma of the stomach. Endoscopy 4: 61–65

26. Kurihara M, Shirakabe H, Izumi T et al. (1980) X-ray and endoscopy in the diagnosis of small early gastric cancer. In: Friedman M, et al. (eds) Diagnosis and treatment of upper gastrointestinal tumors. Excerpta Medica, Amsterdam, pp 15–24
27. Lusink C, Sali A, Chou ST (1983) Diagnostic accuracy of flexible endoscopic biopsy in carcinoma of the esophagus and cardia. Aust NZ J Surg 53: 545–549
28. MacDonald WC, Rublin CE (1967) Gastric biopsy. A critical evaluation. Gastroenterology 53: 143–170
29. Martinez CR, Bravo TA (1981) Diagnostic accuracy of biopsy and endoscopic cytology in cancer of the esophagus and stomach. Experience and analysis of error factors. Gastroenterol Mex 46: 59–62
30. Miller G, Kaufmann M (1975) Das Magenfrühkarzinom in Europa. Dtsch Med Wochenschr 100: 1946–1949
30a. Monissey JF (1976) The diagnosis of early gastric cancer. A survey of experience in the United State. Gastrointest Endosc 23: 13–15
31. Nagayo T (1971) Histological diagnosis of biopsied gastric mucosa with special reference to that of borderline lesions. Gann Monogr Cancer Res 11: 243–249
32. Ottenjann R (1955) Endoscopic snare biopsy with diathermy snare. In: Seifert E (ed) Results and clinical importance in surgical endoscopy. Witzstrock, Brussels
33. Prolla JC (1974) Gastroscopy, biopsy and cytology in early detection of stomach cancer. In: Grundmann E et al. (eds) Early gastric cancer. Current status of diagnosis. Springer, Berlin Heidelberg New York, pp 133–136
34. Reitzig P, Gutz HJ (1980) Errors in endoscopic diagnosis of early stomach cancer. Dtsch Z Verdau Stoffwechselkr 40: 165–168
35. Rösch W (1979) Early stomach cancer: New diagnostic and therapeutic aspects. Acta Med Austriaca [Suppl] 6: 291–295
36. Rösch W, Kock H (1976) Magenfrühkarzinom: Makroskopie und Biopsie. Erfahrungen bei 50 Fällen. Aktuel Gastrol 5: 239–246
37. Sakita T, Yoshimori M (1976) Early diagnosis of gastric cancer. Gann Monogr Cancer Res 18: 85–98
38. Schindler R (1955) On the comparison between gastric suction biopsies and gastroscopy. Am J Dig Dis 22: 336–337
39. Seifert E, Ostertag H, Otto P (1974) Incidence, localization and accuracy of endoscopy and guided biopsy. In: Grundmann E, et al. (eds) Early gastric cancer. Current status of diagnosis. Springer, Berlin Heidelberg New York, pp 54–57
40. Takeda T, Yamada S, Amakasu H et al. (1981) Histologic and cytologic studies on atypical epithelial growth of the stomach. Gastroenterol Jpn 16: 232–235
41. Takemoto T, Okita K (1981) Advance of endoscopy. Cancer Detect Prev 4: 385–399
42. Takemoto T, Ichioka S, Suzuki S, Nagasako K (1971) The diagnosis of early gastric cancer through fibergastroscopic biopsy. Gann Monogr Cancer Res 11: 232–242
43. Tatsuta M, Okuda S, Taniguchi H (1983) Diagnosis of minute cancers by the endoscopic congo red-methylene blue test. Endoscopy 15: 252–256
44. Tomenius J (1950) An instrument for gastrobiopsies. Gastroenterology 15: 489–504
45. Tsuneoka K (1966) Early diagnosis of gastric cancer with fibergastroscope. Gann Monogr 3: 177–179
46. Vyberg M, Hougen HP, Tonnesen N (1983) Diagnostic accuracy of endoscopic gastrobiopsy in carcinoma of the stomach. A histopathological review of 101 cases. Acta Pathol Microbiol Immunol Scand [A] 91: 483–487
47. Whitehead R (1973) Mucosal biopsy of the gastrointestinal tract. Saunders, Philadelphia
48. Whitehead R (1968) Interpretation of mucosal biopsies from the gastrointestinal tract. In: Dyke SC (ed) Recent advances in clinical pathology, ser 5. Churchill, London, pp 375–400
49. Williams DG, Truelove SC, Gear NWL, Massarelia GR, Fitzgerald NW (1968) Gastroscopy with biopsy and cytological sampling under direct vision. Br Med J 1: 535–539
50. Wood IJ (1949) Gastric biopsy. Report in 55 biopsies using a new flexible gastric biopsy tube. Lancet 1: 18–21
51. Yamakawa T, Panish J, Berei G et al. (1971) The correlation of target biopsy and contact smear cytology under direct visual control in malignant gastric lesions. Gastrointest Endosc 17: 164–168

9. Theories on the Histogenesis and Pathogenesis of Gastric Cancer

As described in Chap. 5, there is a close correlation between the histological nature of minute gastric cancers (MGC) and that of the mucosa surrounding the cancer, and a similar general histological picture is also observed in cases of EGC and AGC. Therefore, for a basic understanding of the histogenesis of gastric cancer it is necessary to know what the biological nature of the gastric mucosa is at the cellular level.

Histological Correlation Between MGC and the Surrounding Mucosa from the Viewpoint of Generative Cells

Studies on the cell kinetics of gastric mucosa by flash labeling autoradiography with tritiated thymidine revealed that the labeled cells capable of synthesizing DNA are always seen regularly in a narrow transitional zone between foveolar tubules and gastric glands, which is called the generative cell layer. In a general view of the histological specimen, this zone is seen in the lower one-third of the mucosa in the region of the antrum and angulus, while it is distributed in the layer of the mucosa below the surface in the region of the corpus and fundus (Fig. 184).

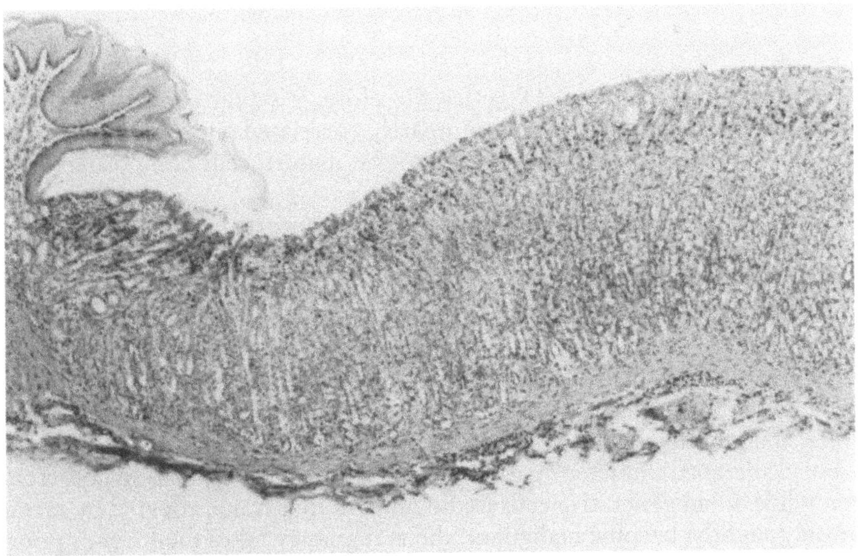

Fig. 184. Flash labeling of the fundic mucosa of rat by IP injection of tritiated thymidine. Labeled cells capable of DNA synthesis are seen only in the generative cells zone between gastric foveolae and fundic glands. (× 15)

The distribution pattern of mitotic epithelial cells, which can also be recognized with a standard optical microscope, corresponds closely to this layer. It is known from these and other findings that the generative cells are the only cells responsible for renewal of the epithelium of the gastric mucosa, which they accomplish by their activities of mitosis, migration, differentiation, maturation, and loss from the surface. In the normal stomach, the balance of cell production and loss is well maintained, and as a result of this dynamic equilibrium of epithelial cells the mucosa assumes a constant histological appearance.

It is also known from autoradiographic studies that when intestinal metaplasia occurs in the mucosa of the antrum, the generative cell layer identified by flash labeling shifts toward the deepest layer of the mucosa, owing to gradual regression of the ability of the generative cells to form pyloric glands (Fig. 185).

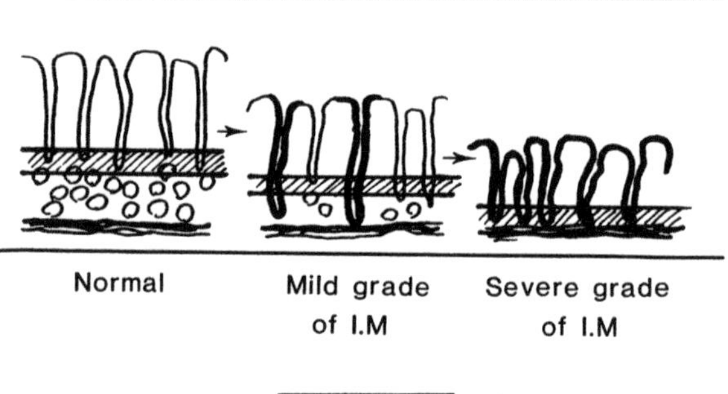

Fig. 185. Development and progression of intestinal metaplasia *(I. M)* in gastric mucosa

From the viewpoint of cell kinetics, therefore, it is quite certain that the appearance of metaplastic epithelium is intimately correlated with a decreased ability of the generative cells to differentiate into the mature cells composing the gastric glands proper.

Thus, it is reasonable to suppose that the generative cells of nonmetaplastic mucosa and of metaplastic mucosa have different biological potentials in the sense of cellular differentiation and maturation.

The reason for the intimate histological correlation between the grade of intestinal metaplasia of gastric mucosa and the histological type of cancer developing from the mucosa seems to be based on this principle. As shown in the schema, when generative cells in the mucosa affected by severe intestinal metaplasia become malignant, they are destined to take on the histology of well-differentiated tubular adenocarcinoma or gastric cancer of intestinal type, as in colorectal cancer, while when generative cells in the mucosa that is not affected by metaplasia, or only slightly, become malignant, the malignancy takes the form of poorly differentiated adenocarcinoma, often containing signet-ring cells or gastric cancer of diffuse type (Fig. 186); thereafter intestinal metaplasia of the affected mucosa may well occur, owing to the atrophic nature of the mucosa, and extend its area gradually during the latent period of the cancerous growth. This may be one reason why infiltration of signet-ring cancer cells is not infrequently seen in the mucosa of several grades of intestinal metaplasia (Fig. 187). In other words, these histological correlations between cancer and the cancer-bearing mucosa are part of the mimicry of parent tissue that is common phenomena to all cancerous tissues.

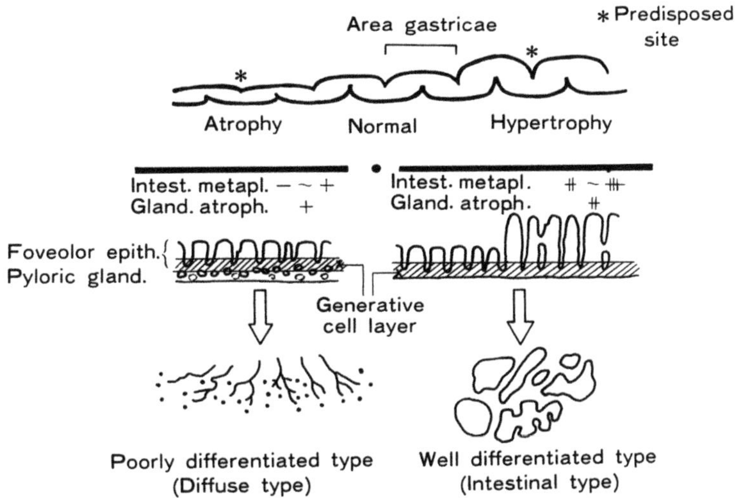

Fig. 186. Schematic showing histogenesis of gastric cancer

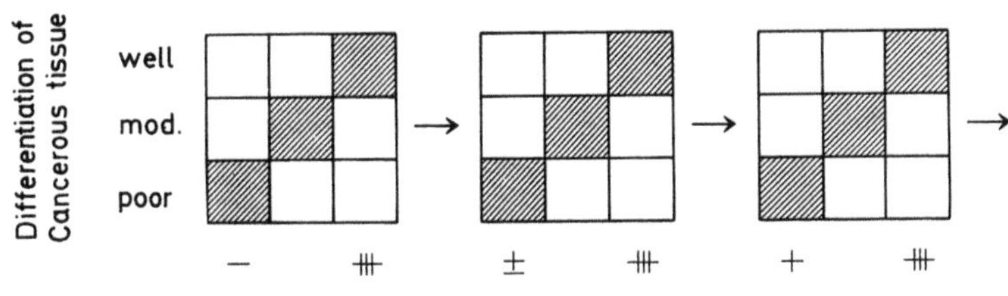

Fig. 187. Possible chronological correlation between histological types of gastric cancer and grades of intestinal metaplasia in the stomach affected by cancer

Morphogenesis of the Depressed Lesion of MGC and EGC

As described in previous chapter, MGC developing in a flat mucosa generally takes the form of tiny focal depressions or tiny and shallow erosions. From the viewpoint of histology and cell kinetics, the following phenomena seem to be intimately correlated with these macroscopical characteristics. In minute cancerous lesions with intestinal-type histology, generative cells responsible for maintaining

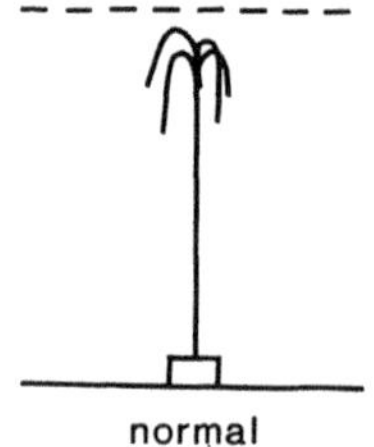

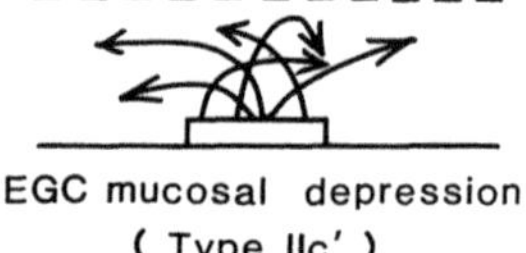

Fig. 188. Schematic showing height of normal gastric mucosa and of that affected by EGC with mucosal depression

a constant height of the mucosa have disappeared, and thus the part of the mucosa undergone malignant transformation has lost its renewal system and mitosis occurs at random. Moreover, the rate of mitosis in the cancerous tubules is lower than that of the generative cell layer in nonmalignant mucosa. For these reasons, the cancerous lesions become thinner than the surrounding metaplastic but nonmalignant mucosa. This situation is analogous to the principle of a fountain (Fig. 188). Owing to their extending and expanding nature, depressed lesions of MGC and EGC with intestinal-type histology always have a clear boundary from the surrounding mucosa, and the elevated mucosa around the focal mucosal depression is resulted from reactive hyperplasia of the metaplastic mucosa. In contrast, in MGC or EGC with diffuse-type histology the surface of the affected mucosa is liable to erosion owing to the peptic and digestive action of gastric juice, and the lowered resistance of the affected mucosa is due to diffuse infiltration of cancer cells in the upper half of the mucosa.

The morphogenesis of the two types of MGC is therefore entirely different even though they are similar in appearance, and the difference has been made more evident by recent studies on labeling indices and ploidy patterns of gastric cancer of the intestinal and the diffuse types [14].

Autoradiographic studies on the cell kinetics of gastrointestinal mucosa commenced around 1960. In the early stages, tritiated thymidine or other radioactive DNA precursors were injected into experimental animals and the distribution, movement pattern, and frequency of the labeled cells in several organs and tissues were examined at predetermined intervals after the injection. These methods allowed some insight into cell renewal systems in the gastric mucosa, life-span and generation time of each epithelial component, doubling time of the tumor, etc. [4, 11–13, 15, 16, 20].

Now the method has been applied to biopsies taken from human tissues with in vitro cultures or ex vivo methods and by these the cell kinetics of human gastric mucosa in both normal and diseased conditions is largely understood, even though some disadvantages of the method compared with in vivo labeling have still not been completely overcome [1–3, 6, 14, 17–19, 22–27].

The theories on histogenesis of human gastric cancer described above are derived mostly from the results obtained in recent studies on cell kinetics.

Histological Conditions in Gastric Mucosa Before Development of Cancer

Even if malignant transformation occurs in a cell or cells of the generative cell layer, as suggested by several investigators [5, 10, 21], the transformed cell will not have enough time to stay and divide there, but will move upward in the course of cell flow and be lost from the surface like other benign epithelial cells, unless it is out of the cell renewal flow.

On the basis of intensive studies on the cell kinetics of gastric mucosa by means of tritiated thymidine autoradiography, and of scanning electron micrography of the cut surface of the mucosa, FUJITA [7–9] stressed the possibility that such transformed cells might be separated or escaped from the cell renewal flow to grow up to recognizable neoplasm. If his hypothesis is correct, our basic ideas on the mechanism of the pathogenesis of gastric cancer will need to be rethought.

Development of Gastric Cancer from the Viewpoint of Animal Experiment and Basic Study

The etiology of human gastric cancer and the mechanism of its development have not yet been fully elucidated, but from experimental and epidemiologic studies it seems almost certain that the disease is caused mainly by environmental factors, especially food and drink.

After more than 50 years of animal experiments on chemical carcinogenesis it is now possible to induce gastric cancer in test animals – mostly rats and dogs – with a high degree of consistency, and the major progress in the field of stomach cancer is summarized in Table 2. Various animal experiments in the induction of gastric cancer have revealed that the two-step theory generally accepted for chemical carcinogenesis is also applicable to the stomach. For the development of gastric carcinoma, a first step of initiating malignancy of the generative cells – target cells in the stomach – by causing a chemical carcinogen or its metabolite to interact with DNA of the target cells and a second step of promoting these initiated cells to become a visible tumor by noncarcinogenic but growth-stimulating substances are both necessary.

It seems probable from several in vitro and in vivo studies that nitroso compounds formed in the stomach from several noncarcinogenic precursors by the action of acidic gastric juice may initiate malignant transformation of generative cells in the gastric mucosa. For promotion of the development of gastric cancer, the intake of high concentrations of sodium chloride, bile reflux, etc. are reported to bring about secondary changes in the environment of the stomach. Hypoacidity and intestinal metaplasia due to exogenous and endogenous factors and an increase in the number of immature regenerative epithelial cells formed by repeated erosion or ulceration, which are proven to be quite susceptible to the carcinogenic substances, can be included amongst the promoting factors. Genetic factors also cannot be completely ruled out in the etiology of human gastric cancer, as shown in the results of statistical investigation of family histories of gastric cancer patients (Fig. 7).

When data obtained in human series and in animal experiments are considered, human gastric cancer is presumed to arise as illustrated in Fig. 8; that is to say cancer can develope when two or three factors overlap (crosshatched are in Fig. 8) in the stomach.

Resistance of the host tissue not allowing rapid proliferation of newly born cancer cells in gastric mucosa may be a reason for long latent period before manifestation of cancer, and such resistance seems to be due chiefly to the immune response of cells in the lymphatic cell series.

Finally it should be added here that theories relating to prevention of gastric cancer have gained their scientific basis from recent experimental studies. When vitamin C or ascorbic acid was added to the culture medium of the Ames' test system the mutagenicity of the cultured bacteria resulting from the formation of nitrosoamine from secondary amine and nitrite was greatly reduced [20a]. The result of this in vitro study has been applied to humans and confirmed [21a].

References

1. Denekamp J, Kallmann RF (1973) In vitro and in vivo labelling of animal tissues with tritiated thymidine. Cell Tissue Kinet 6: 217–227
2. Deshner E, Tamura K, Bralow SP (1979) Sequential histopathology and cell kinetic changes in rat pyloric mucosa induced by MNNG. J Natl Cancer Inst 63: 171–179
3. Deshner E, Lipkin M (1978) Proliferation and differentiation of gastrointestinal cells in health and disease. In: Lipkin K, Good RA (eds) Gastrointestinal tract cancer. Plenum, New York, pp 3–24
4. Deshner E, Winawer SH, Lipkin M (1972) Patterns of nucleic acid and protein synthesis in normal human gastric mucosa and atrophic gastritis. J Natl Cancer Inst 48: 1567–1574
5. Eder M (1974) Problem of formal genesis of carcinoma of the stomach. Grundmann E, et al. (eds) Early gastric cancer. Current status of diagnosis. Springer, Berlin Heidelberg New York, pp 27–33
6. Fabrikant JI, Wisseman CL, Vitak MJ (1969) The kinetics of cellular proliferation in normal and malignant tissue. Radiology 92: 1309–1320
7. Fujita S (1983) Natural history of human gastric carcinoma in terms of their genesis and progression. Asian Med J 26: 787–805
8. Fujita S, Hattori T, Fukuda M (1979) Sogenannte präcanceröse Veränderungen in der Magenschleimhaut und ihre Bedeutung bei der Carcinogenese. Verh Dtsch Ges Pathol 63: 261–263
9. Fujita S, Hattori T (1977) Cell proliferation, differentiation and maturation in the gastric mucosa. A study of the background of carcinogenesis. In: Farber E, et al. (eds) Pathophysiology of carcinogenesis in digestive organs. University of Tokyo Press, Tokyo, pp 21–36
10. Grundmann E (1975) Histologic types and possible initial stages in early gastric carcinoma. Beitr Pathol 154: 256–280
11. Hattori T, Hosokawa Y, Fukuda M et al. (1984) Analysis of DNA ploidy patterns of gastric carcinomas of Japanese. Cancer 54: 1591–1597
12. Hattori T, Fujita S (1979) Tritiated thymidine autoradiographic study on histogenesis and spreading of intestinal metaplasia in human stomach. Pathol Res Pract 164: 224–237
13. Hattori T, Fujita S (1976) Tritiated thymidine autoradiographic study of cellular migration in the gastric glands of the golden hamster. Cell Tissue Res 175: 171–184

14. Hattori T (1974) On cell proliferation and differentiation of the fundic mucosa of the golden hamster. Fractographic study combined with microscopy and 3H-thymidine autoradiography. Cell Tissue Res 148: 213–226

15. Hughes WL, Bond VP, Brecher G et al. (1958) Cellular proliferation in the mouse as revealed by autoradiography with tritiated thymidine. Proc Natl Acad Sci USA 5: 476–483

16. Hunt TE, Hunt EA (1961) Thymidine 3H radioautographs of the gastric mucosa of rat after stimulation with compound 48/80. Anat Rec 139: 240–241

17. Johnson HA, Bond VP (1961) A method of labeling tissue with tritiated thymidine in vitro and its use in comparing rates of cell proliferation in duct epithelium, fibroadenoma and carcinoma of human breast. Cancer 14: 639–643

18. Lipkin M (1977) Neoplastic transformation of cells in the gastrointestinal tract of man and rodent. In: Farber E, et al. (eds) Pathophysiology of carcinogenesis in digestive Organs. University of Tokyo Press, Tokyo, pp 413–428

19. Lipkin M, Sherlock P, Bell B (1963) Cell proliferation kinetics in the gastrointestinal tract of man. II. Cell renewal in stomach, ileum, colon and rectum. Gastroenterology 45: 721–729

20. Messier B, Lebrond CF (1960) Cell proliferation and migration as revealed by radioautography after injection of thymidine into rats and mice. Am J Anat 106: 247–284

20a. Mirvish SS, Wallcave L, Eagen M, Shubik P (1972) Ascorbate-nitrite reaction: possible means of blocking the formation of carcinogenic N-nitroso compounds. Science (Wash D.C.) 177: 65–68

21. Murakami T (1952) Studies on the histogenesis of early gastric cancer. Acta Pathol Jpn 2: 10–22

21a. Ohshima H, Bartsch H (1981) Quantitative estimation of endogenous nitrosation in humans by monitoring N-nitrosoproline excreted in the urine. Cancer Res 41: 3658–3662

22. Ravetto C, Santamaria L (1981) Dysplasia and morphogenesis of gastric cancer. Cancer Detect Prev 4: 369–376

23. Sasaki M (1977) Measurement of tritiated thymidine labelling index by incubation in vitro of surgically removed cervical cancer. Gann 68: 307–313

24. Sasaki K, Takahashi M, Ogino T, Okuda S (1984) An autoradiographic study on the labeling index of biopsy specimens from gastric mucosa. Cancer 54: 1307–1309

25. Steel GG, Bensted JPM (1965) In vitro studies of cell proliferation in tumours. I. Critical appraisal of method and theoretical considerations. Eur J Cancer 1: 275–297

26. Steenbeck LF, Wolff G (1971) Histoautoradiographische Untersuchung der menschlichen Magenschleimhaut bei chronischer Gastritis und Magenkarzinom. Arch Geschwulstforsch 38: 132–138

27. Winawer SJ, Lipkin M (1969) Cell proliferation kinetics in the gastrointestinal tract of man. IV. Cell renewal in the intestinalized gastric mucosa. J Natl Cancer Inst 42: 9–17

10. Subject Index